Critical Race Theory in Education

Critical Race Theory (CRT) is an international movement of scholars working across multiple disciplines; some of the most dynamic and challenging CRT takes place in education. This collection brings together some of the most exciting and influential CRT in education.

CRT scholars examine the race-specific patterns of privilege and exclusion that go largely unremarked in mainstream debates. The contributions in this book cover the roots of the movement, the early battles that shaped CRT, and key ideas and controversies, such as the problem of color-blindness, racial microaggressions, the necessity for activism, how particular cultures are rejected in the mainstream, and how racism shapes the day-to-day routines of schooling and politics.

Of interest to academics, students, and policy-makers, this collection shows how racism operates in numerous hidden ways and demonstrates how CRT challenges the taken-for-granted assumptions that shape educational policy and practice.

Laurence Parker is Professor of Educational Leadership and Policy and Associate Dean of the Honors College, University of Utah, USA.

David Gillborn is Professor of Critical Race Studies and Founding Director of the Centre for Research in Race and Education, University of Birmingham, UK.

Education and Social Theory
Series Editor: Stephen J. Ball, Institute of Education, University College London, UK

Social theory can help us to make sense of many aspects of contemporary education by providing analytic concepts and insights. Social theories are tools of analysis and interpretation for educational researchers that enable us to make sense of the processes, effects, and outcomes of educational experiences and institutions.

Drawing together selections from the best work previously published in Taylor and Francis journals to create powerful and effective collections, this series highlights and explores the social theories critical to educational writers, researchers and scholars. Each book focuses a different key writer or field of theory, with the overarching aim of providing an overview of the social theories important to education research, but also of showing how these theories can be applied in a practical manner in the current education landscape.

Books in the Series:

Critical Race Theory in Education
Edited by Laurence Parker and David Gillborn

Foucault and Education
Edited by Stephen J. Ball

Marxisms and Education
Edited by Noah De Lissovoy

Revisiting Actor-Network Theory in Education
Edited by Tara Fenwick and Richard Edwards

Feminist Posthumanisms, New Materialisms and Education
Edited by Jessica Ringrose, Katie Warfield and Shiva Zarabadi

Freud, Lacan, Zizek and Education
Edited by Claudia Lapping

The Education Assemblage
Edited by Greg Thompson

Bourdieu and Education
Edited by Diane Reay

Judith Butler and Education
Edited by Judith Butler

Nancy Fraser, Social Justice and Education
Edited by Carol Vincent

Basil Bernstein, Code Theory and Education
Edited by Parlo Singh

Critical Race Theory in Education

Edited by
Laurence Parker and David Gillborn

Routledge
Taylor & Francis Group
LONDON AND NEW YORK

First published 2020
by Routledge
2 Park Square, Milton Park, Abingdon, Oxon, OX14 4RN

and by Routledge
52 Vanderbilt Avenue, New York, NY 10017

Routledge is an imprint of the Taylor & Francis Group, an informa business

British Library Cataloguing in Publication Data
A catalogue record for this book is available from the British Library

ISBN13: 978-0-367-43607-0

Typeset in Plantin
by Newgen Publishing UK

Publisher's Note
The publisher accepts responsibility for any inconsistencies that may have arisen during the conversion of this book from journal articles to book chapters, namely the inclusion of journal terminology.

Disclaimer
Every effort has been made to contact copyright holders for their permission to reprint material in this book. The publishers would be grateful to hear from any copyright holder who is not here acknowledged and will undertake to rectify any errors or omissions in future editions of this book.

Contents

Citation Information vii
Notes on Contributors ix

Introduction 1
David Gillborn and Laurence Parker

1 Just what is critical race theory and what's it doing in a *nice* field like education? 9
Gloria Ladson-Billings

2 "Race is… race ain't": an exploration of the utility of critical race theory in qualitative research in education 27
Laurence Parker

3 Forging community in race and class: critical race theory and the quest for social justice in education 40
David Stovall

4 Towards an interest-convergence in the education of African-American football student athletes in major college sports 57
Jamel K. Donnor

5 Interest-divergence and the colour of cutbacks: race, recession and the undeclared war on black children 80
David Gillborn

6 "I don't think I'm a racist": critical race theory, teacher attitudes, and structural racism 95
Sabina E. Vaught and Angelina E. Castagno

7 Whose culture has capital? A critical race theory discussion of community cultural wealth 114
Tara J. Yosso

8 Racial microaggressions as a tool for critical race research 137
Lindsay Pérez Huber and Daniel G. Solorzano

9 Against the politics of desperation: educational justice, critical race theory, and Chicago school reform 161
David Stovall

10 You can't erase race! Using CRT to explain the presence of race and racism in majority white suburban schools 172
Thandeka K. Chapman

11 Pedagogy of fear: toward a Fanonian theory of 'safety' in race dialogue 189
Zeus Leonardo and Ronald K. Porter

Index 208

Citation Information

The chapters in this book were previously published in a selection of different journals. When citing this material, please use the original journal name and page numbering for each article, as follows:

Chapter 1

Just what is critical race theory and what's it doing in a nice *field like education?*
Gloria Ladson-Billings
International Journal of Qualitative Studies in Education, volume 11, issue 1 (1998), pp. 7–24

Chapter 2

"Race is... race ain't": an exploration of the utility of critical race theory in qualitative research in education
Laurence Parker
International Journal of Qualitative Studies in Education, volume 11, issue 1 (1998), pp. 43–55

Chapter 3

Forging community in race and class: critical race theory and the quest for social justice in education
David Stovall
Race Ethnicity and Education, volume 9, issue 3 (2006), pp. 243–259

Chapter 4

Towards an interest-convergence in the education of African-American football student athletes in major college sports
Jamel K. Donnor
Race Ethnicity and Education, volume 8, issue 1 (2005), pp. 45–67

Chapter 5

Interest-divergence and the colour of cutbacks: race, recession and the undeclared war on Black children
David Gillborn
Discourse: Studies in the Cultural Politics of Education, volume 34, issue 4 (2013), pp. 477–491

Chapter 6

"I don't think I'm a racist": Critical Race Theory, teacher attitudes, and structural racism
Sabina E. Vaught and Angelina E. Castagno
Race Ethnicity and Education, volume 11, issue 2 (2008), pp. 95–113

Chapter 7

Whose culture has capital? A critical race theory discussion of community cultural wealth
Tara J. Yosso
Race Ethnicity and Education, volume 8, issue 1 (2005), pp. 69–91

Chapter 8

Racial microaggressions as a tool for critical race research
Lindsay Pérez Huber and Daniel G. Solorzano
Race Ethnicity and Education, volume 18, issue 3 (2015), pp. 297–320

Chapter 9

Against the politics of desperation: educational justice, critical race theory, and Chicago school reform
David Stovall
Critical Studies in Education, volume 54, issue 1 (2013), pp. 33–43

Chapter 10

You can't erase race! Using CRT to explain the presence of race and racism in majority white suburban schools
Thandeka K. Chapman
Discourse: Studies in the Cultural Politics of Education, volume 34, issue 4 (2013), pp. 611–627

Chapter 11

Pedagogy of fear: toward a Fanonian theory of 'safety' in race dialogue
Zeus Leonardo and Ronald K. Porter
Race Ethnicity and Education, volume 13, issue 2 (2010), pp. 139–157

Notes on Contributors

Angelina E. Castagno, Northern Arizona University, USA.

Thandeka K. Chapman, University of California, San Diego, USA.

Jamel K. Donnor, College of William and Mary, USA.

David Gillborn, University of Birmingham, UK.

Gloria Ladson-Billings, University of Wisconsin, Madison, USA.

Zeus Leonardo, University of California, Berkeley, USA.

Laurence Parker, University of Utah, USA.

Lindsay Pérez Huber, California State University, Long Beach, USA.

Ronald K. Porter, University of California, Berkeley, USA.

Daniel G. Solorzano, University of California, Los Angeles, USA.

David Stovall, University of Illinois, Chicago, USA.

Sabina E. Vaught, Columbia University, USA.

Tara J. Yosso, University of California, Santa Barbara, USA.

Introduction

David Gillborn and Laurence Parker

What's all the fuss about?

'Theory' is a word that has many connotations. Sometimes 'theory' is seen as detached, removed from the everyday, as in '*That might work in theory but not in practice*'. In academe, 'theory' is usually assumed to relate to weighty, conceptual matters that are complicated and even frightening. Graduate students have to demonstrate their competent use of an appropriate theory; in universities 'theory' is often used as a weapon to alienate, isolate, or demonstrate the imagined superiority of a speaker (Becker, 2008, 135–136). Critical Race Theory (CRT) is not like that. CRT is dedicated to understanding and changing the world as it is experienced by minoritized people subject to racist oppression and exclusion. CRT is serious, applied, and constantly developing.

CRT challenges mainstream conventions and assumptions in numerous ways. The approach puts race and racism at the heart of its analysis, and rejects conventional assumptions about what counts as knowledge and how research should be conducted – because traditional approaches have been shaped by, and serve to reinforce, existing racial biases. For example, CRT puts a premium on the experiential knowledge and voice of marginalized groups, who are usually absent from official accounts. Some of the most famous and influential CRT scholarship takes the form of counterstories, which use fictionalized characters and situations as a vehicle to explore real-world examples of race inequality and the processes that sustain and normalize a racist status quo.

Contrary to the deliberate and/or lazy misrepresentations that are peddled by its many detractors, CRT does not ignore other forms of oppression (such as class, gender, sexuality, disability); in fact, it was a critical race scholar, Kimberlé Crenshaw, who coined the notion of *intersectionality* (an approach that focuses on the cross-cutting operation of multiple forms of discrimination). Many critical race scholars are keen to apply an intersectional approach; some have even led the development of 'off-shoot' movements that focus explicitly on the intersection of racism and other factors, such as *Disability Critical Race Theory* (DisCrit) (Annamma et al., 2013; Connor et al., 2016). However, the starting point for all CRT is a focus on racism as a deeply ingrained, hugely destructive but often taken-for-granted aspect of everyday life:

> Although Critical Race scholarship differs in object, argument, accent, and emphasis, it is nevertheless unified by two common interests. The first is to understand how a regime of white supremacy and its subordination of people of color have been created and maintained... The second is a desire not merely to understand the vexed bond between law and racial power but to change it. (Crenshaw et al., 1995, p. xiii)

CRT does not restrict its understanding of 'White supremacy' to the obvious, fascistic hate groups who are usually associated with the term; instead, CRT focuses on a much more widespread, insidious, and far-reaching version of White supremacy – one so ubiquitous that it is often seen as unremarkable, 'normal', 'business as usual' (see Delgado & Stefancic, 2000, p. xvi):

> [By] 'white supremacy' I do not mean to allude only to the self-conscious racism of white supremacist hate groups. I refer instead to a political, economic, and cultural system in which whites overwhelmingly control power and material resources, conscious and unconscious ideas of white superiority and entitlement are widespread, and relations of white dominance and non-white subordination are daily reenacted across a broad array of institutions and social settings. (Ansley, 1997, p. 592)

This focus alone is enough to generate fierce hostility inside and outside the academy, where CRT is frequently portrayed as anti-White and even racist:

> For all its supposed academic credentials, critical race theory boils down to one simple claim: "If you are white you are racist!" ... what is being created is a permanent hostility between racialised groups. Critical race theory is recreating racism. (Hayes, 2013)

This, of course, is nonsense; but the quotation sums up one of several recurring lines of attack. Conservative commentators typically argue that any attention to race risks incitement to hopelessness – even violence – and threatens the meritocratic ideals that they believe are already enshrined in practice. Their outrage reaches new heights when they realize that CRT views the very notion of meritocracy itself (and equally sacrosanct ideals such as objectivity and neutrality) as mechanisms that act to defend and camouflage the vested interests of White elites. In addition, as Ladson-Billings (2013) has noted, from the very first public outing for CRT in education, 'friendly fire' has been a constant presence as the approach draws the ire of self-proclaimed 'progressives' who publicly avow their commitment to advancing equity but object to CRT's bold decision to put race and racism at the forefront of the analysis. In the UK, for example, the most persistent and one-sided attacks on CRT in education have originated from a small group of mostly White Marxist academics whose 'wilful misreading of CRT has become something of an academic mini-industry' (Warmington, 2019, p. 11). The attacks frequently claim a comradely, constructive motivation but descend into patronizing dismissals that chastise critical race theorists for their failure to understand the proper place of class at the heart of all meaningful critiques. As Warmington notes, such criticisms echo earlier 'discourses of derision' that similarly caricatured and rejected Black scholarship in the 1960s and 1970s.

The ferocity of the attacks on CRT is a measure of its distinctiveness and its ability to cut through the fog of traditional approaches to race inequity, where racism seems to be viewed as a kind of residual issue that can only legitimately be considered *after* all other possible issues (from class and gender to diet and air pollution) have been exhausted (Preston & Bhopal, 2012). Its radical approach has helped to make CRT a compelling and vitally important voice in academic and activist work:

> CRT has become a rare space for resistance. For race-conscious, anti-racist scholars, it has promoted international dialogue and offered conceptual tools with which to bring to the fore issues of race and racism at a time of rising populism and white nationalism. (Warmington, 2019, p. 15)

By unapologetically putting racism at the heart of its analyses, CRT stands apart from numerous other approaches that focus on inequality in society but are often ambiguous about the status of race and racism. CRT views 'race' as a *social construct* – it is not a fixed biological 'fact' but a malleable social category that has been defined differently in different societies and has changed its meaning over time. Nevertheless, the socially constructed nature of 'race' does nothing to diminish the very real, material impact of racism on the lives of millions of people. CRT's preparedness to name racism and deal with the day-to-day reality of inequity, no matter how difficult the conversations may be for some, is an aspect of *racial realism* – one of the characteristic elements of a CRT approach (see Parker in this volume).

A living theory

Several of the chapters in this volume include a description of the distinctive ideas and approaches that characterize CRT in education. There is no single unchanging statement of rules and regulations that defines CRT; rather, it is an ongoing project, a developing set of ideas, tools, and concepts that add up to one of the most important and fastest-growing approaches in contemporary social science. Although CRT has grown into an international approach that is applied in numerous different disciplines, the field of education has become one of the most important areas.

As Ladson-Billings (this volume) describes, CRT emerged from the struggles of people of color, working and studying in U.S. law schools, who found their concerns with anti-racism sidelined and shouted down. Crenshaw has described how the name came into being:

> I began to scribble down words associated with our objectives, identities, and perspectives, drawing arrows and boxes around them to capture various aspects of who "we" were and what we were doing... Mixing them up and throwing them together in various combinations, one proposed combination came together in a

> way that seemed to capture the possibility we were aiming to create... We would signify the specific political and intellectual location of the project through "critical," the substantive focus through "race," and the desire to develop a coherent account of race and law through the term "theory." (Crenshaw, 2002, pp. 1360–1361)

This is a hugely significant insight into the nature of CRT. The name itself was coined with a deliberate sense of purpose and self-confidence; as Crenshaw continues, mixing a declaration of intent and a challenge to the established hierarchies: 'the name Critical Race Theory... was basically made up, fused together to mark a possibility' (p. 1361). The inclusion of 'theory' is especially important because it signals a conscious rejection of the patronizing dismissal that frequently meets any attempt to put race/racism at the center of analysis:

> ...criticisms that were beginning to emerge from Stanford quarters in the form of a counter-critique to our early work, characterizing it as essentialist. Whether intended or not, in that critique some of us heard a crude characterization of our work as theoretically unsophisticated and politically backward. (Crenshaw, 2002, p. 1357)

As Warmington (2019) notes, CRT continues to be challenged about the use of the term 'theory' and yet CRT is no less a theory than any of the more widely acceptable/higher-status versions usually associated with dead White (European) men: Bourdieu, Foucault, Marx etc. CRT has a distinctive set of conceptual tools and understands the world in relation to the operation of racialized power. As we have noted (above), critical race theorists tend to be more open to new ideas and collaborations than adherents to some other approaches but CRT has proven remarkably perceptive about the constant ebb and flow of policy and practice. Apparent race equality gains are proven to be short-lived or even illusory, with race inequity soon remade and retrenched (Thompson Dorsey & Venzant Chambers, 2014). CRT has even proven adept at predicting the future, where its reading of the deeper currents of race oppression are a better indicator of future trends than the superficial rhetoric of policy-makers. For example, Ladson-Billings (2009) accurately identified many of the key obstacles that limited genuine progress under the Obama presidency, while readers of Gillborn's analysis of the racialized impact of recessions and cutbacks (this volume) will not have been surprised by the United Nations' subsequent verdict that the UK's 'austerity' program had 'been disproportionately detrimental to members of racial and ethnic minority communities' (United Nations, 2019).

Critical Race Theory: Then, now, the future...

The chapters in this volume are part of the conceptual foundation of CRT in education. These writings aim to point out the importance of the social construction of race and racism, how CRT emerged from a critique of the law; and its subsequent movement into a critical analysis of education at the primary, secondary and post-secondary levels. Carbado (2002, p. 181) noted that a collection such as this stresses the importance of racecentricity – an explicitly race-conscious approach to education. When one reads, for example, the chapter by Gloria Ladson-Billings, 'Just what is critical race theory doing in a *nice* field like education?', Tara J. Yosso's 'Whose culture has capital? A critical race theory discussion of community cultural wealth' or the chapter by Leonardo and Porter, CRT is utilized as a lens through which to examine the ways that White supremacy and structural racism within education policy impacts student/teacher relations, what gets taught in terms of curriculum, how schools are financed; and how community cultural wealth refers to forms of knowledge that are shared as part of surviving and resisting racism and other forms of oppression. Yosso's genealogy of CRT is particularly useful in that she carefully documented Derrick Bell's use of counterstories and counternarratives as theoretical and pedagogical tools to disrupt the formalistic legal concepts of reasoning; as well as how the CRT foundations were grounded in diverse specific emerging disciplines and activisms of Black Studies, Chicana/o studies, Asian American Studies, Tribal Nation/Indigenous Studies, and Women's/Gender studies.

Another point to consider when reading this volume is the emphasis on applying CRT to an analysis of teaching in the primary and secondary levels, as well as athletics and sports and the presence of racism in White suburban schools. Vaught and Castagno show how CRT can be used to dismantle teacher assumptions of not being racist by critiquing teacher discourse and actions that show the opposite effects of racism's impact on students of color. Donnor's chapter applies Bell's concept of interest-convergence to examine the ways that Black and Pacific Islander students, particularly in US college football, are viewed as part of the racial capitalist agenda for universities to make noble claims on diversity; but for marketing and branding purposes primarily, with very little concern for these student athletes or racial conditions on campus (see Leong, 2013 for racial capitalism in higher education). The Chapman and Gillborn chapters show how and why White supremacy operates in suburban schools, and how state and national governments will use the rhetoric of fiscal responsibility to justify drastic cuts in spending that disproportionately affect Black children. One of the main points here is how CRT can be used to document the forces of state-sanctioned racism, in the form of fiscal policy that has a direct discriminatory impact on students of color and on their material conditions in schools.

CRT in relation to research methodology in education, both qualitative and quantitative, has made headway recently as more education research scholars, social scientists, and social justice lawyers have used it to analyze the impact of the law and race to study structural racism, racial capitalism, and the social psychology of racism (Carbado & Roithmayr, 2014; Parks et al., 2008). Here the works of Parker, and Pérez Huber and Solórzano call for using CRT as an interpretive methodological framework: qualitative methods with an emphasis on critical race methodology. In this way, CRT methodology provides an interpretive lens through which to view the subjective everyday experiences of students and persons of color in schools. CRT methodology is important to examine specific moments, incidents, practices, and situations that contribute to an overarching pattern of a denial of racial equity in education. Centering and documenting race and racial contexts (with intersections of class, race, and, gender), these readings cover the overarching patterns of inequity in education through the powerful medium of counternarratives and counterstories.

Critical race methodology serves as a bridge to the chapters by Stovall, whose CRT writings and activism are rooted in viewing CRT as a 'call to work'. These chapters illustrate the importance of the centering of race and culture in student advocacy and community engagement. Stovall's chapters evoke the notion of CRT as a means to change academic achievement, and making racial spaces truly beneficial for students of color. Through this scholarship we can see how CRT serves as a useful analytical methodological framework and call for actions to address daily racial microaggressions and use racial cultural capital to situate community empowerment for change. A key point here is Stovall's argument that we should view CRT in education as a verb to act:

> The present is the future for Black and Brown students. They are asking, 'what are we doing now to build for tomorrow? The now is what is taking us to the future but it is informed by the past…' what does it mean to make a way where there is no way available? Black youth are saying to us now that whatever we need we will get it because we need it. (Personal communication, Stovall presentation at UCLA CRT/RAC led by Daniel Solórzano, January 23, 2018)

Stovall's point, about CRT as a verb to engage in action, was evident in the 2019 Critical Studies in Education Association (CRSEA) annual meeting at the University of Southern California in Los Angeles. At this conference, sessions were devoted to exploring critical reflections and implications of CRT frameworks from the perspective of scholars, practitioners, and youth on what it means to do critical race work that is impactful, praxis-driven, and collaborative with communities of interest in respectful ways. The conference sessions also featured presentations and research that pushed the boundaries of what intersectionality means through lived experiences. For example, a panel of scholars of color had a session on Deaf CRiT in which they shared how they used critical race theories in their scholarship to address and illuminate injustices in the greater aural-based society and among Deaf and signing communities (Fernandez-Garcia et al., 2019). These and other sessions used intersectional lenses to expand thinking and usages of CRT as it relates to education and powerfully demonstrate the continued vibrancy of CRT as a perspective that continues to grow and challenge the boundaries of accepted scholarship.

The chapters in this volume represent some of the most important foundational elements of the field. CRT in education's content is a blended synthesis of the anthropological, sociological, and historical scholarship on the idea of race, and how this socially constructed idea became connected to the scientific method to justify racial hierarchies, and its connection to power and authority and the building of capitalist and colonial empires through law. As Carbado (2019) has pointed out, critical race theorists in the law have long demonstrated the ways in which the US Supreme Court in particular, and laws, statutes, and policies in general, have effectively 'constitutionalized racial inequality' and that this has been accelerated under the 45th President's administration (2016–2020), such that the 'body of law all but ensures the continued marginalization of people of color from everything; from employment discrimination, to voting rights, to policing, to the war on terrorism, to affirmative action, to mass incarceration and the death penalty' (p. 3). The Courts have limited the scope of constitutional rights for persons of color, and as a result Carbado posits that we are in a critical race 'state of continuity'. By this he means that systems and technologies of power-ideologies and discourses are continuous through different historical periods, geographic boundaries, public and private spaces, and social categories (Carbado, 2019, pp. 4–5). This does not mean that the systems of oppression are set in stone (they morph to new historic conditions and opportunities) but the line of continuity, and the central role of White supremacy, is clear.

References

Annamma, S.A., Connor, D. & Ferri, B. (2013). Dis/ability critical race studies (DisCrit): Theorizing at the intersections of race and dis/ability. *Race Ethnicity and Education*, 16(1): 1–31, doi:10.1080/13613324.2012.730511

Ansley, F.L. (1997). White supremacy (and what we should do about it), in R. Delgado & J. Stefancic (eds). *Critical White Studies: Looking Behind the Mirror*. Philadelphia: Temple University Press, pp. 592–595.

Becker, H.S. (2008). *Writing for Social Scientists: How to Start and Finish Your Thesis, Book, or Article*. 2nd edn. Chicago: University of Chicago Press.

Carbado, D.W. (2002). Afterword: (E)Racing education. *Equity & Excellence in Education*, 36(2): 181–194.

Carbado, D.W. (2019). States of continuity or state of exception: Race, law and politics in the age of Trump. *Constitutional Commentary*, 34(1): 1–15.

Carbado, D.W. & Roithmayr, D. (2014). Critical race theory meets social science. *Annual Review of Law & Social Science*, 10(1): 146–167.

Connor, D.J., Ferri, B.A. & Annamma, S.A. (eds) (2016). *DisCrit: Disability Studies and Critical Race Theory in Education*. New York: Teachers College Press.

Crenshaw, K. (2002). The first decade: Critical reflections, or foot in the closing door. *UCLA Law Review*, 49(5): 1343–1373.

Crenshaw, K., Gotanda, N., Peller, G. & Thomas, K. (eds) (1995). *Critical Race Theory: The Key Writings That Formed the Movement*. New York: New Press.

Delgado, R. & Stefancic, J. (eds) (2000). *Critical Race Theory: The Cutting Edge*. 2nd edn. Philadelphia: Temple University Press.

Fernandez-Garcia, C., Riedel-Moges, R., Guerreo-Cantor, J. & Ramirez-Stapleton, L. (2019, May 29–June 1). *Deaf CRiT Panel*. Plenary session presented at the Critical Race Studies in Education Association annual meeting. Los Angeles, CA: University of Southern California.

Hayes, D. (2013). Teaching students to think racially. *Spiked*. www.spiked-online.com/2013/03/19/teaching-students-to-think-racially (accessed August 10, 2019).

Ladson-Billings, G. (2009). Education for everyday people: Obstacles and opportunities facing the Obama administration. *Harvard Educational Review*, 79(2): 345–359.

Ladson-Billings, G. (2013). Critical Race Theory—What it is not! in M. Lynn & A.D. Dixson (eds). *Handbook of Critical Race Theory in Education*. New York: Routledge, pp. 34–47.

Leong, N. (2013). Racial capitalism. *Harvard Law Review*, 126(8): 2153–2226.

Parks, Gregory S., Jones, S. & Cardi, J.W. (eds) (2008). *Critical Race Realism: Intersections of Psychology, Race and Law*. New York: The New Press.

Preston, J. & Bhopal, K. (2012). Conclusion: Intersectional theories and 'race': From toolkit to 'mash-up', in K. Bhopal & J. Preston (eds). *Intersectionality and 'Race' in Education*. London: Routledge, pp. 213–220.

Thompson Dorsey, D.N. &Venzant Chambers, T.T. (2014). Growing C-D-R (Cedar): Working the intersections of interest convergence and whiteness as property in the affirmative action legal debate. *Race Ethnicity and Education*, 17(1): 56–87.

United Nations (2019). United Kingdom: UN expert condemns entrenched racial discrimination and inequality, *Press release*. www.ohchr.org/EN/NewsEvents/Pages/DisplayNews.aspx?NewsID=24698&LangID=E (accessed August 10, 2019).

Warmington, P. (2019). Critical race theory in England: Impact and opposition. *Identities*, doi:10.1080/1070289X.2019.1587907

Just what is critical race theory and what's it doing in a *nice* field like education?

GLORIA LADSON-BILLINGS

Critical race theory (CRT) first emerged as a counterlegal scholarship to the positivist and liberal legal discourse of civil rights. This scholarly tradition argues against the slow pace of racial reform in the United States. Critical race theory begins with the notion that racism is normal in American society. It departs from mainstream legal scholarship by sometimes employing storytelling. It critiques liberalism and argues that Whites have been the primary beneficiaries of civil rights legislation. Since schooling in the USA purports to prepare citizens, CRT looks at how citizenship and race might interact. Critical race theory's usefulness in understanding education inequity is in its infancy. It requires a critique of some of the civil rights era's most cherished legal victories and educational reform movements, such as multiculturalism. The paper concludes with words of caution about the use of CRT in education without a more thorough analysis of the legal literature upon which it is based.

Introduction

Almost five years ago a colleague and I began a collaboration in which we grappled with the legal scholarship known as "critical race theory" (Delgado, cited in Monaghan, 1993). So tentative were we about this line of inquiry that we proceeded with extreme caution. We were both untenured and relatively new to our institution. We were unsure of how this new line of inquiry would be received both within our university and throughout the educational research/scholarly community. Our initial step was to hold a colloquium in our department. We were pleasantly surprised to meet with a room filled with colleagues and graduate students who seemed eager to hear our ideas and help us in these new theoretical and conceptual formulations.

That initial meeting led to many revisions and iterations. We presented versions of the paper and the ideas surrounding it at conferences and professional meetings. Outside the supportive confines of our own institution, we were met with not only the expected intellectual challenges, but also outright hostility. Why were we focusing only on race? What about gender? Why not class? Are you abandoning multicultural perspectives? By the fall of 1995 our much discussed paper was published (Ladson-Billings & Tate, 1995). We have, however, held our collective intellectual breaths for almost a year because, despite the proliferation of critical race legal scholarship, we have seen scant evidence that this work has made any impact on the educational research/scholarly community. Thus, seeing critical race theory (CRT) as a theme in an educational journal represents our first opportunity to "exhale."

> It had been a good day. My talk as a part of the "Distinguished Lecture" Series at a major research university had gone well. The audience was receptive; the questions were challenging, yet respectful. My colleagues were exceptional hosts.

> I spent the day sharing ideas and exchanging views on various phases of their work and my own. There had even been the not so subtle hint of a job offer. The warm, almost tropical climate of this university stood in stark contrast to the overly long, brutal winters of my own institution. But it also had been a tiring day – all that smiling, listening with rapt interest to everyone's research, recalling minute details of my own, trying to be witty and simultaneously serious had taken its toll. I could not wait to get back to the hotel to relax for a few hours before dinner.
>
> One of the nice perks that comes with these lecture "gigs" is a decent hotel. This one was no exception. My accommodation were on the hotel's VIP floor – equipped with special elevator access key and private lounge on the top floor overlooking the city. As I stepped off the elevator, I decided to go into the VIP lounge, read the newspaper, and have a drink. I arrived early, just before the happy hour, and no one else was in the lounge. I took a seat on one of the couches and began catching up on the day's news. Shortly after I sat down comfortably with my newspaper, a White man peeked his head into the lounge, looked at me sitting there in my best (and conservative) "dress for success" outfit – high heels and all – and said with a pronounced Southern accent, "What time are y'all gonna be servin'?"

I tell this story both because storytelling is a part of critical race theory and because this particular story underscores an important point within the critical race theoretical paradigm, i.e. race [still] matters (West, 1992). Despite the scientific refutation of race as a legitimate biological concept and attempts to marginalize race in much of the public (political) discourse, race continues to be a powerful *social* construct and signifier (Morrison, 1992):

> Race has become metaphorical – a way of referring to and disguising forces, events, classes, and expressions of social decay and economic division far more threatening to the body politic than biological "race" ever was.
>
> Expensively kept, economically unsound, a spurious and useless political asset in election campaigns, racism is as healthy today as it was during the Enlightenment. It seems that it has a utility far beyond economy, beyond the sequestering of classes from one another, and has assumed a metaphorical life so completely embedded in daily discourse that it is perhaps more necessary and more on display than ever before. (p. 63)

I am intrigued by the many faces and permutations race has assumed in contemporary society. Our understanding of race has moved beyond the bio-genetic categories and notions of phenotype. Our "advanced ideas" about race include the racialization of multiple cultural forms. Sociologist Sharon Lee (1993) suggests that "questions of race have been included in all U.S. population censuses since the first one in 1790" (p. 86). Although racial categories in the U.S. census have fluctuated over time, two categories have remained stable – Black and White. And, while the creation of the category does not reveal what constitutes within it, it does create for us a sense of polar opposites that posits a cultural ranking designed to tell us who is White or, perhaps more pointedly, who is *not* White!

But determining who is and is not White is not merely a project of individual construction and/or biological designation. For example, in early census data, citizens of Mexican descent were considered White, though over time, political, economic, social, and cultural shifts have forced Mexican Americans out of the White category. Conversely, Haney López (1995) pointed out that some groups came to the USA and brought suit in the courts to be declared White. Omi and Winant (1993) argue, however, that the polar notions of race as either an ideological construct or as an objective condition both have shortcomings. That is, thinking of race strictly as an ideological concept denies the reality of a racialized society and its impact on people in their everyday lives. On the other hand, thinking of race solely as an objective condition denies the problematic aspects of race – how to decide who fits into which racial classifications.

Our notions of race (and its use) are so complex that even when it fails to "make sense" we continue to employ and deploy it. I want to argue, then, that our conceptions of race, even in a postmodern and/or postcolonial world, are more embedded and fixed than in a previous age. However, this embeddedness or "fixed-ness" has required new language and constructions of race so that denotations are submerged and hidden in ways that are offensive though without identification. Thus, we develop notions of "conceptual whiteness" and "conceptual blackness" (King, 1995) that both do and do not map neatly on to bio-genetic or cultural allegiances. Conceptual categories like "school achievement," "middle classness," "maleness," "beauty," "intelligence," and "science" become normative categories of whiteness, while categories like "gangs," "welfare recipients," "basketball players," and "the underclass" become the marginalized and de-legitimated categories of blackness.

The creation of these conceptual categories is not designed to reify a binary but rather to suggest how, in a racialized society where whiteness is positioned as normative, *everyone* is ranked and categorized in relation to these points of opposition. These categories fundamentally sculpt the extant terrain of possibilities even when other possibilities exist. And, although there is a fixedness to the notion of these categories, the ways in which they actually operate are fluid and shifting. For example, as an African American female academic, I can be and am sometimes positioned as conceptually White in relation to, perhaps, a Latino, Spanish-speaking gardener. In that instance, my class and social position override my racial identification and for that moment I become "White."

The significance of race need not be overly debated in this paper. But, as Toni Morrison argues, race is always already present in every social configuring or our lives. Roediger (1991) asserts, "Even in an all-white town, race was never absent" (p. 3). However, more significant/problematic than the omnipresence of race is the notion that "whites reach the conclusion that their whiteness is meaningful" (Roediger, p. 6). It is because of the meaning and value imputed to whiteness that CRT becomes an important intellectual and social tool for deconstruction, reconstruction, and construction: deconstruction of oppressive structures and discourses, reconstruction of human agency, and construction of equitable and socially just relations of power. In this paper, then, I am attempting to speak to innovative theoretical ways for framing discussions about social justice and democracy and the role of education in reproducing or interrupting current practices.

I hope to provide a brief synopsis of Critical Race Theory[1] and discuss some of its prominent themes. Then I will discuss its importance to our understanding of the citizen in a democracy, its relationship to education and finally some cautionary implications for further research and study. As is true of all texts, this one is incomplete (O'Neill, 1992). It is incomplete on the part of both the writer and the reader. However, given its incompleteness, I implore readers to grapple with how it might advance the debate on race and education.

What is Critical Race Theory?

Most people in the USA first learned of critical race theory (CRT) when Lani Guinier, a University of Pennsylvania Law Professor, became a political casualty of the Clinton administration. Her legal writings were the focus of much scrutiny in the media. Unschooled and unsophisticated about the nature of legal academic writing, the media vilified Guinier and accused her of advocating "un-American" ideas. The primary focus of the scorn shown Guinier was her argument for proportional representation.

Guinier (1991) asserted that in electoral situations where particular racial groups were a clear (and persistent) minority, the only possibility for an equitable chance at social benefits and fair political representation might be for minority votes to count for more than their actual numbers. Guinier first proposed such a strategy as a solution for a postapartheid South Africa. Because Whites are in the obvious minority, the only way for them to participate in the governing of a new South Africa would be to insure them some seats in the newly formed government.

Guinier made a similar argument in favor of African Americans in the USA. She saw this as a legal response to the ongoing lack of representation. Unfortunately, her political opponents attacked her scholarship as an affront to the American tradition of "one person, one vote." The furor over Guinier's work obscured the fact that as an academic, Guinier was expected to write "cutting-edge" scholarship that pushed theoretical boundaries (Guinier, 1994). Her work was not to be literally applied to legal practice. However, in the broad scope of critical race legal studies, Guinier may be seen as relatively moderate and nowhere near the radical the press made her out to be. But, her "exposure" placed critical race theory and its proponents in the midst of the public discourse.

According to Delgado (1995, p. xiii), "Critical Race Theory sprang up in the mid-1970s with the early work of Derrick Bell (an African American) and Alan Freeman (a white), both of whom were deeply distressed over the slow pace of racial reform in the United States. They argued that the traditional approaches of filing *amicus* briefs, conducting protests and marches, and appealing to the moral sensibilities of decent citizens produced smaller and fewer gains than in previous times. Before long they were being joined by other legal scholars who shared their frustration with traditional civil rights strategies.

Critical race theory is, thus, both an outgrowth of and a separate entity from an earlier legal movement called critical legal studies (CLS). Critical legal studies is a leftist legal movement that challenged the traditional legal scholarship that focused on doctrinal and policy analysis (Gordon, 1990) in favor of a form of law that spoke to the specificity of individuals and groups in social and cultural contexts. Critical legal studies scholars also challenged the notion that "the civil rights struggle represents a long, steady, march toward social transformation" (Crenshaw, 1988, p. 1334).

According to Crenshaw (1988), "Critical [legal] scholars have attempted to analyze legal ideology and discourse as a social artifact which operates to recreate and legitimate American society" (p. 1350). Scholars in the CLS movement decipher legal doctrine to expose both its internal and external inconsistencies and reveal the ways that "legal ideology has helped create, support, and legitimate America's present class structure" (Crenshaw, p. 1350). The contribution of CLS to legal discourse is in its analysis of legitimating structures in the society. Much of the CLS ideology emanates from the work of Gramsci (1971) and depends on the Gramscian notion of "hegemony" to describe the continued legitimacy of oppressive structures in American society.

However, CLS fails to provide pragmatic strategies for material social transformation. Cornel West (1993) asserts that:

> ... critical legal theorists fundamentally question the dominant liberal paradigms prevalent and pervasive in American culture and society. This thorough questioning is not primarily a constructive attempt to put forward a conception of a new legal and social order. Rather, it is a pronounced disclosure of inconsistencies, incoherences, silences, and blindness of legal formalists, legal positivists, and legal realists in the liberal tradition. Critical legal studies is more a concerted attack and assault on the legitimacy and authority of pedagogical strategies in law school than a comprehensive announcement of what a credible and realizable new society and legal system would look like. (p. 196)

CLS scholars critique mainstream legal ideology for its portrayal of U.S. society as a meritocracy but failed to include racism in its critique. Thus, CRT became a logical outgrowth of the discontent of legal scholars of color.

CRT begins with the notion that racism is "normal, not aberrant, in American society" (Delgado, 1995, p. xiv), and, because it is so enmeshed in the fabric of our social order, it appears both normal and natural to people in this culture. Indeed, Bell's major premise in *Faces at the bottom of the well* (1992) is that racism is a permanent fixture of American life. Thus, the strategy becomes one of unmasking and exposing racism in its various permutations.

Second, CRT departs from mainstream legal scholarship by sometimes employing storytelling to "analyze the myths, presuppositions, and received wisdoms that make up the common culture about race and that invariably render blacks and other minorities one-down" (Delgado, 1995, p. xiv). According to Barnes (1990) "Critical race theorists... integrate their *experiential knowledge* (emphasis added), drawn from a shared history as 'other' with their ongoing struggles to transform a world deteriorating under the albatross of racial hegemony" (pp. 1864–1865). Thus, the experience of oppressions such as racism or sexism has important aspects for developing a CRT analytical standpoint. To the extent that Whites (or in the case of sexism, men) experience forms of racial oppression, they may develop such a standpoint. For example, the historical figure John Brown suffered aspects of racism by aligning himself closely with the cause of African American liberation.[2] Contemporary examples of such identification may occur when White parents adopt transracially. No longer a White family, by virtue of their child(ren), they become racialized others. A final example was played out in the infamous O. J. Simpson trials. The criminal trial jury was repeatedly identified as the "Black" jury despite the presence of one White and one Latino juror. However, the majority White civil case jury was not given a racial designation. When Whites are exempted from racial designations and become "families," "jurors," "students," "teachers," etc. their ability to apply a CRT analytical rubric is limited. One of the most dramatic examples of the shift from non-raced to CRT perspective occurred when Gregory Williams (1995) moved from Virginia where he was a White boy to Muncie, Indiana, where his family was known to be Black. The changes in his economic and social status were remarkable, and the story he tells underscores the salience of race in life's possibilities. The primary reason, then, that stories, or narratives, are deemed important among CRT scholars is that they add necessary contextual contours to the seeming "objectivity" of positivist perspectives.

Third, CRT insists on a critique of liberalism. Crenshaw (1988) argues that the liberal perspective of the "civil rights crusade as a long, slow, but always upward pull"

(p. 1334) is flawed because it fails to understand the limits of current legal paradigms to serve as catalysts for social change and its emphasis on incrementalism. CRT argues that racism requires sweeping changes, but liberalism has no mechanism for such change. Rather, liberal legal practices support the painstakingly slow process of arguing legal precedence to gain citizen rights for people of color.

Fourth, and related to the liberal perspective, is the argument posed by CRT that Whites have been the primary beneficiaries of civil rights legislation. For example, although under attack throughout the nation, the policy of affirmative action has benefited Whites, a contention that is validated by the fact that the actual numbers reveal that the major recipients of affirmative action hiring policies have been White women (Guy-Sheftall, 1993). One might argue, then, that many of these White women have incomes that support households in which other Whites live – men, women, and children. Thus, these women's ability to find work ultimately benefits Whites, in general.

In contrast, let us look at some of the social benefits African Americans have received due to affirmative action policies. Even after 20 years of affirmative action, African Americans constitute only 4·5% of the professorate (Hacker, 1992). In 1991 there were 24 721 doctoral degrees awarded to U.S. citizens and noncitizens who intended to remain in the USA, and only 933 or 3·8% of these doctorates went to African American men and women. If every one of those newly minted doctorates went into the academy, it would have a negligible effect on the proportion of African Americans in the professorate. In addition, the majority of the African Americans who earn PhDs earn them in the field of education, and of that group, most of the degrees are in educational administration where the recipients continue as school practitioners (Hacker, 1992).

Thus, CRT theorists cite this kind of empirical evidence to support their contention that civil rights laws continue to serve the interests of Whites. A more fruitful tack, some CRT scholars argue, is to find the place where the interests of Whites and people of color intersect. This notion of "interest-convergence" (Bell, 1980, p. 94) can be seen in what transpired in Arizona over the Martin Luther King, Jr. Holiday commemoration.

Originally, the state of Arizona insisted that the King Holiday was too costly and therefore failed to recognize it for state workers and agencies. Subsequently, a variety of African American groups and their supporters began to boycott business, professional, and social functions in the state of Arizona. When members of the National Basketball Association and the National Football League suggested that neither the NBA All-Star Game nor the Super Bowl would be held in Arizona because of its failure to recognize the King Holiday, the decision was reversed. Hardly anyone is naive enough to believe that the governor of Arizona had a change of heart about the significance of the King Holiday. Rather, when his position on the holiday had the effect of hurting state tourist and sports entertainment revenues, the state's interests (to enhance revenue) converged with that of the African American community (to recognize Dr. King). Thus, converging interests, not support of civil rights, led to the reversal of the state's position.

In a recent compilation of CRT key writings (Crenshaw et al., 1995) it is pointed out that there is no "canonical set of doctrines or methodologies to which [CRT scholars] all subscribe" (p. xiii). But, these scholars are unified by two common interests – to understand how a "regime of white supremacy and its subordination of people of color have been created and maintained in America" (p. xiii) and to change the bond that exists between law and racial power.

In the pursuit of these interests, legal scholars, such as Patricia Williams (1991) and Derrick Bell (1987; 1992), were among the early critical race theorists whose ideas reached the general public. Some might argue that their wide appeal was the result of their abilities to tell compelling stories into which they embedded legal issues.[3] This use of story is of particular interest to educators because of the growing popularity of narrative inquiry in the study of teaching (Carter, 1993; Connelly & Clandinin, 1990). But, just because more people are recognizing and using story as a part of scholarly inquiry does not mean that all stories are judged as legitimate in knowledge construction and the advancement of a discipline.

Lawrence (1995) asserts that there is a tradition of storytelling in law and that litigation is highly formalized storytelling, though the stories of ordinary people, in general, have not been told or recorded in the literature of law (or any other discipline). But this failure to make it into the canons of literature or research does not make the stories of ordinary people less important.

Stories provide the necessary context for understanding, feeling, and interpreting. The ahistorical and acontextual nature of much law and other "science" renders the voices of dispossessed and marginalized group members mute. In response, much of the scholarship of CRT focuses on the role of "voice" in bringing additional power to the legal discourses of racial justice. Indeed, Delgado (1990) argues that people of color speak with experiential knowledge about the fact that our society is deeply structured by racism. That structure gives their stories a common framework warranting the term "voice." Consequently, critical race theorists are attempting to interject minority cultural viewpoints, derived from a common history of oppression, into their efforts to reconstruct a society crumbling under the burden of racial hegemony (Barnes, 1990).

The use of voice or "naming your reality" is a way that CRT links form and substance in scholarship. CRT scholars use parables, chronicles, stories, counterstories, poetry, fiction, and revisionist histories to illustrate the false necessity and irony of much of current civil rights doctrine. Delgado (1989) suggests that there are at least three reasons for "naming one's own reality" in legal discourse:

1. much of "reality" is socially constructed;
2. stories provide members of outgroups a vehicle for psychic self-preservation; and
3. the exchange of stories from teller to listener can help overcome ethnocentrism and the dysconscious (King, 1992) drive or need to view the world in one way.

The first reason for naming one's own reality involves how political and moral analysis is conducted in legal scholarship. Many mainstream legal scholars embrace universalism over particularity. According to Williams (1991), "theoretical legal understanding" is characterized, in Anglo-American jurisprudence, by the acceptance of transcendent, acontextual, universal legal truths or procedures. For instance, some legal scholars might contend that the tort of fraud has always existed and that it is a component belonging to the universal system of right and wrong. This world-view tends to discount anything that is nontranscendent (historical), or contextual (socially constructed), or nonuniversal (specific) with the unscholarly labels of "emotional," "literary," "personal," or false (Williams, 1991).

In contrast, critical race theorists argue that political and moral analysis is situational – "truths only exist for this person in this predicament at this time in history" (Delgado, 1991, p. 11). For the critical race theorist, social reality is constructed by the formulation and the exchange of stories about individual situations (see, for example, Matsuda, 1989). These stories serve as interpretive structures by which we impose order on experience and it on us (Delgado, 1989).

A second reason for the naming one's own reality theme of CRT is the psychic preservation of marginalized groups. A factor contributing to the demoralization of marginalized groups is self-condemnation (Delgado, 1989). Members of minority groups internalize the stereotypic images that certain elements of society have constructed in order to maintain their power. Historically, storytelling has been a kind of medicine to heal the wounds of pain caused by racial oppression. The story of one's condition leads to the realization of how one came to be oppressed and subjugated, thus allowing one to stop inflicting mental violence on oneself.

Finally, naming one's own reality with stories can affect the oppressor. Most oppression, as was discussed earlier, does not seem like oppression to the perpetrator (Lawrence, 1987). Delgado (1989) argues that the dominant group justifies its power with stories, stock explanations, that construct reality in ways that maintain their privilege. Thus, oppression is rationalized, causing little self-examination by the oppressor. Stories by people of color can catalyze the necessary cognitive conflict to jar dysconscious racism.

The "voice" component of CRT provides a way to communicate the experience and realities of the oppressed, a first step in understanding the complexities of racism and beginning a process of judicial redress. For example, the voice of people of color is required for a deep understanding of the educational system. Delpit (1988) argues one of the tragedies of the field of education is how the dialogue of people of color has been silenced. Delpit begins her analysis of the process-oriented versus the skills-oriented writing debate with a statement (or story) from an African American male graduate student at a predominantly white university who is also a special education teacher in an African American community:

> There comes a moment in every class where we have to discuss "The Black Issue" and what's appropriate education for Black children. I tell you, I'm tired of arguing with those White people, because they won't listen. Well, I don't know if they really don't listen or if they just don't believe you. It seems like if you can't quote Vygotsky or something, then you don't have any validity to speak about your own kids. Anyway, I'm not bothering with it anymore, now I'm just in it for a grade. (p. 280)

The above comment and numerous other statements found in Delpit's analysis illustrate the frustration of teachers of color that is caused by being left out of the dialogue about how best to educate children of color. Further, Delpit raises several very important questions:

> How can such complete communication blocks exist when both parties [Black and Whites] truly believe they have the same aims? How can the bitterness and resentment expressed by educators of color be drained so that all sores can heal? What can be done? (p. 282)

Critical race theory and citizenship

One of the places to begin understanding CRT is to examine how conceptions of citizenship and race interact. Although connections of CRT and citizenship are numerous and complex, in this paper I will attempt to detail only one of the central connections that is important in understanding the relationship of this scholarship to educational issues. That central connection is the "property issue" (Ladson-Billings & Tate, 1995). CRT scholars assert that the USA is a nation conceived and built on property rights (Bell, 1987; Harris, 1993). In the early history of the nation only propertied White males enjoyed the franchise. The significance of property ownership as a prerequisite to citizenship was tied to the British notion that only people who *owned* the country, not merely those who *lived* in it, were eligible to make decisions about it.[4]

The salience of property often is missed in our understanding of the USA as a nation. Conflated with democracy, capitalism slides into the background of our understanding of the way in which U.S. political and economic ideology are entangled and read as synonymous. But it is this foundation of property rights that make civil rights legislation so painfully slow and sometimes ineffective. Civil rights are wedded to the construction of the rights of the individual. Bell (1987) argues that "the concept of individual rights, unconnected to property rights, was totally foreign to these men of property," (p. 239) in his explanation of how men who expressed a commitment to liberty and justice could uphold the repression of African Americans, the indigenous peoples who inhabited the land, and women.

African Americans represented a particular conundrum because not only were they not accorded individual civil rights because they were not White and owned no property, but they were constructed *as* property! However, that construction was only in the sense that they could be owned by others. They possessed no rights of property ownership. Whites, on the other hand, according to Harris (1993), benefited from the construction of whiteness as the ultimate property. "Possession – the act necessary to lay basis for rights in property – was defined to include only the cultural practices of Whites. This definition laid the foundation for the idea that whiteness – that which Whites alone possess – is valuable and is property" (p. 1721).

This thematic strand of whiteness as property in the USA is not confined to the nation's early history. Indeed, Andrew Hacker's (1992) exercise with his college students illustrates the material and social value the students place on their possession of whiteness. Hacker uses a parable to illustrate that although the students insist that "in this day and age, things are better for Blacks" (p. 31), none of them would want to change places with African Americans. When asked what amount of compensation they would seek if they were forced to "become Black," the students "seemed to feel that it would not be out of place to ask for $50 million, or $1 million for each coming Black year" (p. 32). According to Hacker:

> And this calculation conveys, as well as anything, the value that white people place on their own skins. Indeed, to be white is to possess a gift whose value can be appreciated only after it has been taken away. And why ask so large a sum? .... The money would be used, as best it could, to buy protection from the discriminations and dangers white people know they would face once they were perceived to be black. (p. 32)

Thus, even without the use of a sophisticated legal rhetorical argument, Whites know they possess a property that people of color do not and that to possess it confers, aspects of citizenship not available to others. Harris's (1993) argument is that the "property functions of whiteness" (p. 1731) – rights of disposition, rights to use and enjoyment, reputation and status property, and the absolute right to exclude – make the American dream of "life, liberty, and the pursuit of happiness" a more likely and attainable reality for Whites as citizens. This reality also is more likely to engender feelings of loyalty and commitment to a nation that works in the interests of Whites. Conversely, Blacks, aware that they will never possess this ultimate property, are less sanguine about U.S. citizenship.

Patricia Williams (1995) explains these differential notions of citizenship as being grounded in differential experiences of rights because "one's sense of empowerment defines one's relation to law, in terms of trust–distrust, formality–informality, or right–no rights (or 'needs')" (pp. 87–88). An example of this differing relation (in this case to commerce) was shared in one of my classes. We were discussing McIntosh's (1990) article on "White privilege." One White woman shared a personal experience of going into a neighborhood supermarket, having her items rung up by the cashier, and discovering that she did not have her checkbook. The cashier told her she could take her groceries and bring the check back later. When she related this story to an African American male friend, he told her that was an example of the privilege she enjoyed because she was White. Her White property was collateral against the cart full of groceries. She insisted that this was the store's good neighbor policy, and the same thing would have happened to him. Determined to show his friend that their life experiences were qualitativedifferent, the young man went shopping a few days later and pretended to have left his checkbook. The young woman was standing off to the side observing the interaction. The same cashier, who had been pointed out by the woman as the "neighborly one," told the young African American man that he could push the grocery items to the side while he went home to get his checkbook. The White woman was shocked as the African American male gave her a knowing look.

These daily indignities take their toll on people of color. When these indignities are skimmed over in the classrooms that purport to develop students into citizens, it is no wonder students "blow off" classroom discourse. How can students be expected to deconstruct rights, "in a world of no rights" (Williams, 1995, p. 98) and construct statements of need "in a world of abundantly apparent need?" (p. 89)

African Americans, thus, represent a unique form of citizen in the USA – property transformed into citizen. This process has not been a smooth one. When Chief Justice Taney concluded in the *Dred Scott* decision that African Americans had no rights that Whites were required to respect, he reinscribed the person-as-property status of African Americans. Later in *Plessy v. Ferguson* the high court once again denied full citizenship rights to African Americans as a way to assert White property rights – rights to use and enjoy and the absolute right to exclude.

Even the laudable decision of *Brown v. Board of Education* comes under scrutiny in the CRT paradigm. Lest we misread *Brown v. Board of Education* as merely a pang of conscience and the triumph of right over wrong, it is important to set *Brown in* context. First, historically the *Brown* decision helped the USA in its struggle to minimize the spread of communism to so-called Third World nations. In many countries, the credibility of the USA had been damaged by the widely broadcast inequitable social conditions that existed in the USA in the 1950s. Both the government and the NAACP lawyers argued the *Brown* decision would help legitimize the political and economic philosophies of the USA with these developing nations (Bell, 1980).

Second, *Brown* provided reassurance to African Americans that the struggle for freedom and equality fought for during World War II might become a reality at home. Black veterans faced not only racial inequality, but also physical harm in many parts of the South. And, the treatment of African Americans after the war in concert with the voice of African American leaders such as Paul Robeson may have greatly influenced the *Brown* decision. Robeson argued:

> It is unthinkable... that American Negroes [*sic*] would go to war on behalf of those who have oppressed us for generations... against a country [the Soviet Union] which in one generation has raised our people to the full human dignity of mankind. (in Foner, 1978, pp. 17–18)

According to Bell (1980), it is not unreasonable to assume that those in positions of power would recognize the importance of neutralizing Robeson and others who held similar views. Robeson's comments were an affront to the "national interests." Thus, racial decisions by the courts were pivotal in softening the criticism about the contradiction of a free and just nation that maintained a segment of its citizenry in second-class status based on race. Finally, there were White capitalists who understood that the South could be transformed from an Agrarian society to an industrialized sunbelt only when it ended the divisive battle over state-supported segregation. Here, segregation was read as a barrier obstructing the economic self-interest of U.S. profit makers.

At this writing, the electorate of California have passed Proposition 209, calling for an end to "preferential treatment" in state employment and state university admission policies based on race or gender. The trope of preferential treatment has help create a perception that ending affirmative action will lead to a more fair and equitable society, while, in reality, the proposition will be used to instantiate the hierarchical relations of power that once again privilege whiteness as the most valued property. Citizenship for people of color remains elusive.

Critical race theoretical approaches to education

Thus far in this paper I have attempted to explain the meaning and historical background of critical race theory in legal scholarship and the role of property rights in understanding citizenship. However, educators and researchers in the field of education will want to know what relevance CRT has to education. The connections between law and education are relatively simple to establish. Since education in the USA is not outlined explicitly in the nation's constitution, it is one of the social functions relegated to individual states. Consequently, states generate legislation and enact laws designed to proscribe the contours of education.

One of the earliest legislative attempts was Massachusetts' "old deluder Satan" act that required citizens of the state to provide education for its children to insure they received moral and religious instruction. In the modern era the intersection of school and law provided fertile ground for testing and enacting civil rights legislation. Thus, the landmark *Brown* decision generated a spate of school desegregation of Central High School in Little Rock, Arkansas, the New Orleans Public Schools, the University of Mississippi, the University of Alabama, and the University of Georgia. By the 1970s, school desegregation/civil rights battles were being fought in northern cities. The fight for school desegregation in Boston schools was among the most vicious in civil rights annals.

One recurring theme that characterized the school/civil rights legal battles was "equal opportunity." This notion of equal opportunity was associated with the idea that students of color should have access to the same school opportunities, i.e. curriculum, instruction, funding, facilities. as White students. This emphasis on "sameness" was important because it helped boost the arguments for "equal treatment under the law" that were important for moving African Americans from their second-class status.

But what was necessary to help African Americans to "catch up" with their White counterparts? Beyond equal treatment was the need to redress pass inequities. Thus, there was a move toward affirmative action and the creation of African Americans and other marginalized groups as "protected classes" to insure that they were not systematically screened out of opportunities in employment, college admission, and housing. If we look at the way that public education is currently configured, it is possible to see the ways that CRT can be a powerful explanatory tool for the sustained inequity that people of color experience. I will use the areas of curriculum, instruction, assessment, school funding, and desegregation as exemplars of the relationship that can exist between CRT and education.

Curriculum

Critical race theory sees the official school curriculum as a culturally specific artifact designed to maintain a White supremacist master script. As Swartz (1992) contends:

> Master scripting silences multiple voices and perspectives, primarily legitimizing dominant, white, upper-class, male voicings as the "standard" knowledge students need to know. All other accounts and perspectives are omitted from the master script unless they can be disempowered through misrepresentation. Thus, content that does not reflect the dominant voice must be brought under control, *mastered*, and then reshaped before it can become a part of the master script. (p. 341)

This master scripting means stories of African Americans are muted and erased when they challenge dominant culture authority and power. Thus, Rosa Parks is reduced to a tired seamstress instead of a long-time participant in social justice endeavors as evidenced by her work at the Highlander Folk School to prepare for a confrontation with segregationist ideology. Or, Martin Luther King, Jr. becomes a sanitized folk hero who enjoyed the full support of "good Americans" rather than a disdained scholar and activist whose vision extended to social justice causes throughout the world and challenged the USA on issues of economic injustice and aggression in Southeast Asia.

The race-neutral or colorblind perspective, evident in the way the curriculum presents people of color, presumes a homogenized "we" in a celebration of diversity. This perspective embraces a so-called multicultural perspective by "misequating the middle passage with Ellis Island" (King, 1992, p. 327). Thus, students are taught erroneously that "we are all immigrants," and, as a result, African American, Indigenous, and Chicano students are left with the guilt of failing to rise above their immigrant status like "every other group."

But it is not just the distortions, omissions, and stereotypes of school curriculum content that must be considered, it also is the rigor of the curriculum and access to what is deemed "enriched" curriculum via gifted and talented courses and classes. As Jonathan Kozol (1991) describes:

> The curriculum [the white school] follows "emphasizes critical thinking, reasoning and logic." The planetarium, for instance, is employed not simply for the study of the universe as it exists. "Children also are designing their own galaxies," the teacher says. (p. 96)

> In my [Kozol's] notes: "Six girls, four boys. Nine White, one Chinese. I am glad they have this class. But what about the others? Aren't there ten Black children in the school who could *enjoy* this also?"

This restricted access to the curriculum is a good illustration of Harris's (1993) explanation of the function of property in terms of use and enjoyment.

Instruction

CRT suggests that current instructional strategies presume that African American students are deficient. As a consequence, classroom teachers are engaged in a never-ending quest for "*the* right strategy or technique" to deal with (read: control) "at-risk" (read: African American) students. Cast in a language of failure, instructional approaches for African American students typically involve some aspect of remediation.

This race-neutral perspective purports to see deficiency as an individual phenomenon. Thus, instruction is conceived as a generic set of teaching skills that should work for all students. When these strategies or skills fail to achieve desired results, the students, not the techniques, are found to be lacking.

Fortunately, new research efforts are rejecting deficit models and investigating and affirming the integrity of effective teachers of African American students.[5] This scholarship underscores the teachers' understanding of the saliency of race in education and the society, and it underscores the need to make racism explicit so that students can recognize and struggle against this particular form of oppression.

Examples of counterpedagogical moves are found in the work of both Chicago elementary teacher Marva Collins and Los Angeles high school mathematics teacher Jaime Escalante. While neither Collins nor Escalante is acclaimed as a "progressive" teacher, both are recognized for their persistence in believing in the educability of all students. Both remind students that mainstream society expects them to be failures and prod the students to succeed as a form of counterinsurgency. Their insistence on helping students achieve in the "traditional" curriculum represents a twist on Audre Lorde's notion that one cannot dismantle the master's house with the master's tools. Instead, they believe one can only dismantle the master's house with the master's tools.

Assessment

For the critical race theorist, intelligence testing has been a movement to legitimize African American student deficiency under the guise of scientific rationalism (Alienikoff, 1991; Gould, 1981). According to Marable (1983), one purpose of the African American in the racial/capitalist state is to serve as a symbolic index for poor Whites. If the working-class White is "achieving" at a higher level than Blacks, then they feel relatively superior. This allows Whites with real power to exploit both poor Whites and Blacks. Throughout U.S. history, the subordination of Blacks has been built on "scientific" theories (e.g., intelligence testing) that depend on racial stereotypes about Blacks that make their condition appear appropriate. Crenshaw (1988) contends that the point of controversy is no longer that these stereotypes were developed to rationalize the oppression of Blacks, but rather, "[T]he extent to which these stereotypes serve a hegemonic function by perpetuating a mythology about both Blacks and Whites even today, reinforcing an illusion of a White community that cuts across ethnic, gender, and class lines" (p. 1371).

In the classroom, a dysfunctional curriculum coupled with a lack of instructional innovation (or persistence) adds up to poor performance on traditional assessment measures. These assessment measures – crude by most analyses – may tell us that students do not know what it on the test, but fail to tell us what students actually know and are able to do. A telling example of this mismatch between what schools measure and what students know and can do is that of a 10-year-old African American girl who was repeatedly told by the teacher that she was a poor math student. However, the teacher was unaware that the girl was living under incredible stresses where she was assuming responsibilities her drug-addicted mother could not. To ward off child welfare agents the child handled all household responsibilities, including budgeting and paying all the household bills. Her ability to keep the household going made it appear that everything was fine in the household. According to the teacher, she could not do fourth-grade math, but the evidence of her life suggests she was doing just fine at "adult" math!

School funding

Perhaps no area of schooling underscores inequity and racism better than school funding. CRT argues that inequality in school funding is a function of institutional and structural racism. The inability of African Americans to qualify for educational advancements, jobs, and mortgages creates a cycle of low educational achievement, underemployment and unemployment, and standard housing. Without suffering a single act of personal racism, most African Americans suffer the consequence of systemic and structural racism.[6]

Jonathan Kozol's *Savage inequalities* (1991) created an emotional and ethical stir within and beyond the education community. White colleagues talked of how moved both they and their students were as they read Kozol's descriptions of inequity in school settings. Some talked of being "moved to tears" and "unable to read more than a few pages at a time." Others talked of how difficult it was for their students to read the book. Interestingly, many African American colleagues indicated that although Kozol had been precise and passionate in his documentation, he had not revealed anything new about the differences that exist between African American and White schools. But, Kozol's research did give voice to people of color. His analysis of funding inequities provides insight into the impact of racism and White self-interest on school funding policies.

CRT argues that the import of property provides another way to consider the funding disparity. Schooling, as a function of individual states, is differentially administered by the various state legislatures. But, one of the most common aspects of these 50 different schooling agencies is the way they are funded. Almost every state funds schools based on property taxes. Those areas with property of greater wealth typically have better funded schools. In the appendix of Kozol's book are comparisons showing the disparities within three different areas. In the Chicago area, for the 1988–89 school year, the funding disparity was an almost a $4,000 per pupil difference. Chicago schools were spending $5,265 per pupil, while the suburban Niles Township High School District was spending $9,371. In the New Jersey area the differences between Camden Schools and Princeton Schools was about $4,200 in per pupil spending. In the New York City area the difference was almost $6,000 in per pupil spending.

Talking about the disparity between per pupil spending often invites the critique that money doesn't matter. Studies as far back as Coleman et al. (1966) and Jencks et al. (1972) have argued that family and individual effects are far more powerful than schools in determining poor school performance. Whether or not school spending is a determining factor in school achievement, no one from the family and individual effects camp can mount an ethical case for allowing poor children to languish in unheated, overcrowded schools with bathrooms that spew raw sewage while middle-income White students attend school in spacious, technology rich, inviting buildings. If money doesn't matter, then why spend it on the rich?

CRT takes to task school reformers who fail to recognize that property is a powerful determinant of academic advantage. Without a commitment to redesign funding formulas, one of the basic inequities of schooling will remain in place and virtually guarantee the reproduction of the status quo.

Desegregation

Although desegregation is not occurring in every school district, its impact on the national level is important enough to be included with the more common school experiences of curriculum, instruction, assessment, and funding. Despite the recorded history of the fight for school desegregation, CRT scholars argue that rather than serving as a solution to social inequity, school desegregation has been promoted only in ways that advantage Whites (Bell, 1990)

Lomotey and Staley's (1990) examination of Buffalo's "model desegregation" program revealed that African American students continued to be poorly served by the school system. African American student achievement failed to improve, while suspension, expulsion, and dropout rates continued to rise. What, then, made Buffalo a model desegregation program? In short, the answer is the benefits that Whites derived from the program and their seeming support of desegregation. As a result of the school desegregation program, Whites were able to take advantage of special magnet school programs and free extended child care. Thus, the dominant logic is that a model desegregation program is one that insures that Whites are happy (and do not leave the system altogether).

The report of school desegregation in Buffalo is not unlike the allegorical story presented by CRT dean, Derrick Bell (1987). The story, entitled "The sacrificed Black children," illustrates how the failure to accept African American children into their community schools causes a White school district to ultimately end up begging the students to come because their presence was intimately tied to the economic prosperity of the community. It is this realization that civil rights legislation in the USA always has benefited Whites (even if it has not always benefited African Americans) that forms the crux of the CRT argument against traditional liberal civil rights legislation. The CRT argument provides an important segue into the final section of this paper – the need for caution in proceeding with the integration of CRT into educational research.

Words of caution

It is the pattern in educational research for a new idea or innovation to take hold and proliferate. Sometimes an idea takes a while to take root, but once it does, most likely its creators lose control of the idea. Consider what happened with the notion of cooperative learning. When Cohen and Roper (1972) proposed cooperative classroom structures to equalize the status of White and African American students, their work held great promise for helping teacher to develop curricular and instructional strategies for improving the academic performance of all children in desegregated classrooms. However, somehow their findings got distilled into day-long workshops and five-step lesson plans. School systems throughout the USA were adopting cooperative learning without any thought to improving the performance of children of color.

A similar transmutation of theory is occurring in the area of multicultural education. Although scholars such as James Banks, Carl Grant, and Geneva Gay[7] began on a scholarly path designed to change schools as institutions so that students might be prepared to reconstruct the society, in its current practice iteration, multicultural education is but a shadow of its conceptual self. Rather than engage students in provocative thinking about the contradictions of U.S. ideals and lived realities, teachers often find themselves encouraging students to sing "ethnic" songs, eat ethnic foods, and do ethnic dances. Consistently, manifestations of multicultural education in the classroom are superficial and trivial "celebrations of diversity."

What, then, might happen to CRT in the hands of educational researchers and school personnel? Well, to be honest, like Lani Guinier, I doubt if it will go very far into the mainstream. Rather, CRT in education is likely to become the "darling" of the radical left, continue to generate scholarly papers and debate, and never penetrate the classrooms and daily experiences of students of color. But, students of color, their families, and communities cannot afford the luxury of CRT scholars' ruminations any more than they could afford those of critical and postmodern theorists, where the ideas are laudable but the practice leaves much to be desired.

As excited as I may be about the potential of CRT for illuminating our thinking about school inequity, I believe educational researchers need much more time to study and understand the legal literature in which it is situated. It is very tempting to appropriate CRT as a more powerful explanatory narrative for the persistent problems of race, racism, and social injustice. If we are serious about solving these problems in schools and classrooms, we have to be serious about intense study and careful rethinking of race and education. Adopting and adapting CRT as a framework for educational equity means that we will have to expose racism in education *and* propose radical solutions for addressing it. We will have to take bold and sometimes unpopular positions. We may be pilloried figuratively or, at least, vilified for these stands. Ultimately, we may have to stand, symbolically, before the nation as Lani Guinier and hear our ideas distorted and misrepresented. We may have to defend a radical approach to democracy that seriously undermines the privilege of those who have so skillfully carved that privilege into the foundation of the nation. We will have to adopt a position of consistently swimming against the current. We run the risk of being permanent outsiders, but, as Wynter (1992) suggests, we must operate from a position of *alerity* or *liminality* where we may "call into question the rules of functioning on whose basis the United States conceptualizes itself as a generically 'White' nation, and elaborate its present system of societal self-knowledge" (p. 19). But, I fear we (educational researchers) may never assume the liminal position because of its dangers, its discomfort, and because we insist on thinking of ourselves as permanent residents in a *nice* field like education.

Notes

1. For a richer description of critical race theory, see Tate (1997).

2. Scholars such as Peggy McIntosh (1990) and Ruth Frankenberg (1993) have begun to deconstruct whiteness through their position of otherness as women. Their work suggests possibilities for Whites to deploy a CRT analysis.

3. Williams is known for her Benetton story where she was locked out of the trendy clothing store in New York because of her race. Some doubted the "generalizability" of Williams story until television personality Oprah Winfrey reported a similar incident. Bell's "Space Traders'" story is an allegorical tale that suggests that White America would gladly "give away" African Americans to space aliens if the aliens made a good enough trade.

4. Of course in America the concept of "ownership" of the land has to be contested by the indigenous people's rights to that land. However, that discussion is beyond the scope of this one.

5. See for example, Foster and Newman (1989), Henry (1992), and Ladson-Billings (1995).

6. The impact of racism generally is tied to the everyday lives of poor and underclass people of color. Recently, revelations of major U.S. corporations (e.g., Texaco and Avis) indicate that they systematically perpetuate racism in hiring, promotion, and customer service.

7. Banks, Grant, and Gay are but a few of the notables who were in the forefront of the intellectual genesis of multicultural education. Gwendolyn Baker, Carlos Cortez, and Margaret Gibson are others. Any attempt to name them all would fall short.

References

Alienikoff, T. A. (1991). A case for race-consciousness. *Columbia Law Review, 91*, 1060–1125.

Barnes, R. (1990). Race consciousness: The thematic content of racial distinctiveness in critical race scholarship. *Harvard Law Review, 103*, 1864–1871.

Bell, D. (1980). *Brown* and the interest-convergence dilemma. In D. Bell (Ed.), *Shades of Brown: New perspectives on school desegregation* (pp. 90–106). New York: Teachers College Press.

Bell, D. (1987). *And we are not saved: The elusive quest for racial justice*. New York: Basic Books.

Bell, D. (1990). *Brown* and the interest-convergence dilemma. In D. Bell (Ed.), *Shades of Brown: New perspectives on school desegregation* (pp. 90–106). New York: Teachers College Press.

Bell, D. (1992). *Faces at the bottom of the well*. New York: Basic Books.

Carter, K. (1993). The place of story in the study of teaching and teacher education. *Educational Researcher, 22* (1), 5–12.

Cohen, E. G., & Roper, S. S. (1972). Modification on interracial interaction disability: An application of status characteristics theory. *American Sociological Review, 37*, 643–657.

Coleman, J. S., Campbell, E. G., Hobson, C. J., McPartland, J., Mood, A. M., Weinfeld, F. D. & York, R. L. (1966). *Equality of educational opportunity*. Washington, DC: U.S. Government Printing Office.

Connelly, F. M., & Clandinin, D. J. (1990). Stories of experience and narrative inquiry. *Educational Researcher, 19* (5), 2–14.

Crenshaw, K. (1988). Race, reform, and retrenchment: Transformation and legitimation in anti-discrimination law. *Harvard Law Review, 101* (7), 1331–1387.

Crenshaw, K., Gotanda, N., Peller, G., & Thomas, K. (Eds.) (1995). *Critical race theory: The key writings that formed the movement*. New York: Free Press.

Delgado, R. (1989). Symposium: Legal storytelling. *Michigan Law Review, 87*, 2073.

Delgado, R. (1990). When a story is just a story: Does voice really matter? *Virginia Law Review, 76*, 95–111.

Delgado, R. (1991). Brewer's plea: Critical thoughts on common cause. *Vanderbilt Law Review, 44*, 1–14.

Delgado, R. (Ed.). (1995). *Critical race theory: The cutting edge*. Philadelphia: Temple University Press.

Delpit, L. (1988). The silenced dialogue: Power and pedagogy in educating other people's children. *Harvard Educational Review, 58*, 280–298.

Foner, P. (Ed.). (1978). *Paul Robeson speaks*. New York: Citadel Press.

Foster, M., & Newman, J. (1989). "I don't know nothin' about it:" Black teachers' code-switching strategies in interviews. *Working papers in educational linguistics* (WPEL).

Philadelphia: Graduate School of Education, University of Pennsylvania.

Frankeberg, R. (1993). *White women, race matters: The social construction of whiteness*. Minneapolis: University of Minnesota Press.

Gordon, R. (1990). New developments in legal theory. In D. Kairys (Ed.), *The politics of law: A progressive critique* (pp. 413–425). New York: Pantheon Books.

Gould, S. J. (1981). *The mismeasure of man*. New York: W. W. Norton.

Gramsci, A. (1971). Selections from the prison notebooks. Q. Hoare & G. N. Smith (Eds. and Trans.) New York: International Publishers.

Guinier, L. (1991). No two seats: The elusive quest for political equality. *Virginia Law Review, 77*, 1413–1514.

Guinier, L. (1994). *The tyranny of the majority: Fundamental fairness is representative democracy*. New York: Free Press.

Guy-Sheftall, B. (1993 April). *Black feminist perspective on the academy*. Paper presented at the annual meeting of the American Educational Research Association, Atlanta.

Hacker, A. (1992). *Two nations: Black and White, separate, hostile, unequal*. New York: Ballantine Books.

Haney López, I. (1995). White by law. In Delgado, R. (Ed.), *Critical race theory: The cutting edge* (pp. 542–550). Philadelphia: Temple University Press.

Harris, C. (1993). Whiteness as property. *Harvard Law Review, 106*, 1707–1791.

Henry, A. (1992). African Canadian women teachers' activism: Recreating communities of caring and resistance. *Journal of Negro Education, 61*, 392–404.

Jencks, C., Smith, M., Acland, H., Bane, M. J., Cohen, D., Gintis, H., Heyns, B., & Michelson, S. (1972). *Inequality: A reassessment of the effect of family and schooling in America*. New York: Basic Books.

King, J. (1991). Dysconscious racism: Ideology, identity and the miseducation of teachers, *Journal of Negro Education, 60*, 133–146.

King, J. (1992). Diaspora literacy and consciousness in the struggle against miseducation in the Black community. *Journal of Negro Education, 61*, 317–340.

King, J. (1995). Culture-centered knowledge: Black studies, curriculum transformation, and social action. In J. Banks & C. M. Banks (Eds.), *Handbook of research on multicultural education* (pp. 265–290). New York: Macmillan.

Kozol, J. (1991). *Savage inequalities*. New York: Basic Books.

Ladson-Billings, G. (1995). "But that's just good teaching!" The case for culturally relevant teaching. *Theory Into Practice, 34*, 159–165.

Ladson-Billings, G., & Tate, W. F. (1995). Toward a critical race theory of education. *Teachers College Record, 97*, 47–68.

Lawrence, C. (1987). The id, the ego, and equal protection: Reckoning with unconscious racism. *Stanford Law Review, 39*, 317–388.

Lawrence, C. (1995). The word and the river: Pedagogy as scholarship and struggle. In Crenshaw, K., Gotanda, N., Peller, G., & Thomas, K. *Critical race theory: The key writings that formed the movement*. (pp. 336–351). New York: Free Press.

Lee, S. M. (1993). Racial classifications in the U.S. census: 1890–1990. *Ethnic and Racial Studies, 16*, 75–94.

Lomotey, K., & Staley, J. (1990, April). *The education of African Americans in Buffalo Public Schools*. Paper presented at the annual meeting of the American Research Association, Boston.

Marable, M. (1983). *How capitalism underdeveloped Black America*. Boston: South End Press.

Matsuda, M. (1989). Public response to racist speech: Considering the victim's story. *Michigan Law Review, 87*, 2320–2381.

McIntosh, P. (1990). White privilege: Unpacking the invisible knapsack. *Independent School*, Winter, 31–36.

Monaghan, P. (1993, June 23). 'Critical race theory' questions the role of legal doctrine in racial inequity. *Chronicle of Higher Education*, A7, A9.

Morrison, T. (1992). *Playing in the dark: Whiteness and the literary imagination*. Cambridge, MA: Harvard University Press.

Omi, M., & Winant, H. (1993). *Racial formation in the United States from the 1960s to the 1990s* (2nd ed.). New York: Routledge.

O'Neill, M. (1992). Teaching literature as cultural criticism. *English Quarterly, 25* (1), 19–24.

Roediger, D. (1991). *The wages of whiteness: Race and the making of the American working class*. London: Verso.

Swartz, E. (1992). Emancipatory narratives: Rewriting the master script in the school curriculum. *Journal of Negro Education, 61*, 341–355.

Tate, W. (1997). Critical Race Theory and education: History, theory, and implications. In M. Apple (Ed.), *Review of Research in Education, 2* (pp. 191–243) Washington, DC: American Educational Research Association.

West, C. (1992, Aug. 2). Learning to talk of race. *New York Times Magazine, 24*, 26.

West, C. (1993). *Keeping faith*. New York: Routledge.

Williams, G. H. (1995). *Life on the color line*. New York: Plume.

Williams, P. (1991). *The alchemy of race and rights: Diary of a law professor*. Cambridge, MA: Harvard University Press.

Williams, P. (1995). Alchemical notes: Reconstructing ideals from deconstructed rights. In R. Delgado (Ed.), *Critical race theory: The cutting edge* (pp. 84–94). Philadelphia: Temple University Press.

Wynter, S. (1992). "*Do not call us Negros*": *How multicultural textbooks perpetuate racism*. San Francisco: Aspire.

"Race is... race ain't": an exploration of the utility of critical race theory in qualitative research in education

LAURENCE PARKER

Critical race theory (CRT) has garnered increasing attention from various circles and disciplines as an emerging perspective in jurisprudence scholarship addressing race. CRT scholarship encompasses and borrows from a myriad set of sociopolitical and philosophical critiques that challenge the objective reality of the law and of legal doctrine and interpretation. CRT scholars have argued that racism is an endemic part of U.S. social relations and this racism has shaped the laws and policies of U.S. institutions. Recently, scholars in education have started to explore the utility of CRT and the ways theories about race can explain the social construction and operation of racism in educational institutions. This paper continues this inquiry by briefly illustrating how CRT can be used in the higher education affirmative action debate surrounding the *Hopwood v. Texas* decision (1996). Specifically, the presentation of definitive race-neutral legal interpretations of narratives vs. counterstories of race is discussed with summary attention paid to the implications for qualitative research on race and education.

The picture and the purpose[1]

Email message, received by Larry Parker at the University of Utah-Salt Lake City, UT (February 3, 1997): "Larry can you please send a short narrative and a picture of yourself because I think they are going to do some publicity for your talk here in April on Critical Race Theory and Education. Thanks."

In my mind I know that I should send a picture to my friend and colleague along with a brief description of my Critical Race Theory and Education talk on April 28 at a university on the west coast of the USA. But it is the middle of the quarter here, and I am heavily involved in the usual academic stuff like teaching, serving on committees, working with doctoral students on proposals, starting to get organized for the Research Focus on Black Education SIG activities at the upcoming annual meeting of AERA (American Educational Research Association), and fielding requests for campus and local speaking engagements during Black History Month. So juggling everything has been mind boggling. I have known my colleague for over 10 years, through her research and at professional meetings, and she has invited me out to her university to give this talk in April. I want to send her the picture, but I just do not have the time. Besides, I never like the way those instamatic small headshot pictures of me come out. I end up looking like another "black male suspect" featured in the FBI wanted shots of the most sought after criminals that one sees in the post office from time to time.

So I respond to her email with, "I am sorry, but I just do not think I will have time to get a picture to you. I can send a brief description of the talk so you can use it for publicity purposes soon OK? Thanks, Larry."

April 26, 1997 – I am flying to the largest town nearby my colleague's campus a few days before I am scheduled to give the talk on critical race theory and education. My colleague and her partner meet me at the airport. After we exchange greetings and get into the truck to head over to my hotel, my friend says, "Larry I wished you had sent a picture in for the publicity for the talk, because you should see what they did instead." "They drew a picture of you, and you look like this tall white guy." "Really," I said, and she responded, "Yes, for some reason that is who they imagined would be giving the talk, and by the time I saw the flyers with the illustration they already had them printed up." We laughed about it and discussed racial assumptions through images as we made our way to my hotel and then off to dinner.

April 28, 1997 (around 9 a.m.) – I get to the campus, and my friend shows me the publicity flyer for my talk, and the illustration of me, and, sure enough, it is a drawing that looks similar to a tall white male, but one with hair.

April 28, 1997 (around 4:20 p.m.) – After a late start, I explain the purpose of today's discussion on critical race theory to the small audience of students, faculty, and staff. I introduce the talk as an overview on how critical race theory has emerged from the legal arena and the race-based critique of the law and legal policy. I also want to highlight how it connects to race and education through the previous works of Gloria Ladson Billings, William Tate, and the recent paper submissions to the special issue of the *International of Qualitative Studies in Education*. I conclude the introduction with a comment about the publicity flyer for the talk by saying that a purpose of critical race theory is to question social constructions and assumptions of race, particularly concerning whiteness, and as I pulled out the flyer to show the audience, I said "see, this is an illustration supposed to represent the speaker for today, but do I match these white male features in this drawing?" "Besides, this drawing has me with hair and no earrings," and while I was saying this for added emphasis and a bit of humor, I took my left hand and rubbed it over my shaved bald head and touched my two hoop earrings that I happened to be wearing that day.

April 28, 1997 (around 5:10 p.m.) – After the overview of critical race theory and a summary of one of the featured papers, my friend, acting as moderator, opens it up for questions and comments. In my mind, I am expecting that the audience will ask questions about the research issues related to critical race theory, such as how is it different in epistemology and methodology from critical theory and how does CRT borrow from feminism or postmodernism? I am also anticipating that they will ask how is it grounded in the law and education? Is it just another form of racial identity politics that critiques the ideology of whiteness and privilege? How does it intersect with gender, race, social class, and other areas of difference regarding research? These are the types of questions asked about critical race theory when I presented on this before.[2] So I was not prepared for the first set of questions from a Chinese-American female student who pointedly asked me, "Well, that theory you discussed is fine, but what does it have to do with dealing with what students of color have to deal with here on this campus, like single mothers who need child care here and many other issues that are of concern to students of color?" Immediately an African-American female student followed up with a second concern. "She is right; we need to talk about the racism and homophobia on this very campus that is of concern to students of color and gay and lesbian students and how this ideal of diversity sometimes gets ignored." To be sure, the other questions related to research methods, methodology, epistemology and the law did come up. However, the initial questions of the students – related to their concerns about race, single mothers, and homophobia on this campus – undergirded the conversation that eventually took all of us well into the evening potluck dinner and discussion.

The intent of this story is to illustrate the major tenets of critical theory (CRT) as it relates to qualitative studies in education. A major point of CRT is to place race at the center of analysis with respect to how many White European Americans and institutions in U.S. society assume normative standards of whiteness, which in turn ignores or subjugates African-Americans, American Indians, Chicanos–Chicanas, Chinese-Americans, and other marginalized racial groups.[3] In the personal narrative, I did not send a photograph in which I felt I would look like a racialized black criminal. However, the illustration used in its place was drawn with assumed white male characteristics of a guest speaker at a college campus. Critical race theory serves to illustrate how, despite the progress of civil rights laws and good intentions to eradicate racism, it is still an endemic part of life in the USA. CRT maintains that racism has been ingrained through historical consciousness and events and that racist ideologies have directly shaped the law, racial categories, and racial privilege (Crenshaw, Gotanda, Peller, & Thomas, 1995; Delgado, 1995; Harris, 1994; Symposium, 1994).

However, the second part of the story directly questions the utility of critical race theory in institutional sites of struggle. The students raised the issues of "what will this new theory do for us marginalized groups on this campus?" To be sure, CRT scholars have expanded their use of the theory to analyze or purpose race-based solutions regarding important public policy issues, such tax law and its impact on African-Americans (Moran & Whitford, 1996) or the effects of minimum wage laws on low-income Latino and African-Americans (Hutchinson, 1997). Furthermore, critical race feminists have voiced their informed perspectives on historical and present-day intersections and conflicts related to racism, sexism, and the law (Cleaver, 1997; Harris, 1997). The critical race feminists have used personal/political racial narratives intertwined with legal analysis to address key areas of concern, such as race and sexual harassment (Cho, 1997); jobs, welfare, and mothering (Augustin, 1997); domestic violence (Rivera, 1997); and international issues related to work, patriarchy, and immigration (Calvo, 1997; Carbado, 1997). Still, the question of the utility of a "new theory on race" for empowerment is a legitimate issue of contention (Nebeker, 1997).[4] In addition, Ladson-Billings expressed caution at the beginning of this special issue about rushing too quickly to embrace CRT in that it may result in the dilution of this critique by the mainstream educational establishment.

There are two points that I hope to cover in the remainder of this article. First, the *Hopwood v. Texas* (1996) ruling, which concerned race-based admissions and reverse discrimination claims by White European Americans, has important CRT implications for affirmative action in higher education. This judicial decision by the 5th Circuit Federal Appeals Court held that U.S. statutes and civil rights legislation are color-blind and race neutral. With that ideological reasoning, the Court banned the use of race as a consideration for admission to the University of Texas-Austin law school (and subsequently all public graduate and undergraduate programs in Texas).[5] However, a critical race theory position on *Hopwood* and the recent passage of Proposition 209 in California, which ended affirmative action in public higher education in that state, would argue for a continuation of affirmative action to remedy past discrimination that still affects present-day normative perceptions and policy actions against racially marginalized groups on university campuses. Critical race theory seeks to uncover the legal history of racial subordination and trace how ideology (Omi & Winant, 1994) and the "language as racism and the experience of racism" (Bartolome & Macedo, 1997, p. 225) are linked to political decisions and legal rulings. These policies have a disparate impact on shaping racial conflicts between those who hold the "color-blind" perspective in the academy and the racial concerns of African-Americans, Chicano–Chicanas, or Asian-Americans as expressed by the two students in the opening narrative.

Second, I will offer suggestions concerning the utility of CRT in education and qualitative research. Critical race theory can be viewed with skepticism in that it may not add anything different to the qualitative research debate in terms of epistemology, methodology, and methods that some researchers (e.g., feminists, critical ethnographers) have been undertaking in terms of participatory studies related to social justice issues (Donmoyer, 1997). Getting into the pros and cons of the race-based epistemological debate and CRT is beyond the scope of this paper.[6] However, the critical centering of race (together with social class, gender, sexual orientation, and other areas of difference) at the locations where the research is conducted and discussions are held can serve as a major link between fully understanding the historical vestiges of past discrimination and the present-day racial manifestations of that discrimination. This in turn can lead to discussions and analyses of "data" through a critical race-centered interpretive framework. Furthermore, rather than ask what can this theory do for qualitative studies in education, an alternate inquiry I would propose is what can qualitative research in education do to illuminate and address the salient features of CRT with respect to race and racism in educational institutions and the larger society?

Racial neutrality versus racial reality

The most recent controversy surrounding affirmative action emerged in *Hopwood v. Texas*. This case centred on whether the University of Texas-Austin had compelling state justification for using dual racial categories for affirmative action purposes for law school admissions. In 1992, four White European American applicants were denied admission to the University of Texas-Austin school. At the time, the law school used admissions procedures that considered the applications of nonminority students, but a separate committee reviewed the applications of African-American and Chicano/Chicana students. The four rejected White European American applicants sued in Federal district court (*Hopwood v. Texas*, 1994), alleging that this system violated their Equal Protection rights under the 14th Amendment and civil rights statutes. The Federal district court held in favor of the plaintiffs but refused to bar the law school from using race in the admissions review process. The appeal went to the Federal Fifth Circuit Court of Appeals, which reversed the district court and ruled that the University of Texas Law School should not use race to achieve diversity, because the 14th Amendment required state actions in governmental affairs to be color-blind and race-neutral.

The Federal 5th Circuit Court of Appeals ruled that the law school had failed to show any notable present effects of past discrimination. Furthermore, even though African-American and Chicano/Chicana students perceived that the University of Texas-Austin was a hostile environment for minorities, this stemmed from their own perceptions of present prejudice and were not the result of direct policies created by the law school (*Hopwood v. Texas*, p. 953). The Court of Appeals reasoned that since the 1960s and the entrance of the first African-Americans into the law school, the University of Texas had attempted various affirmative action efforts to increase racial diversity. Therefore, the university was not really guilty of institutional discrimination after that time. The Appeals Court also posited that traditional thinking about affirmative action and race-based admissions treated campus racial diversity as a solidified group category, and this perpetuated biases and ignored a person's individuality in terms of how someone should be viewed:

> Diversity fosters, rather than minimizes, the use of race. It treats minorities as a group, rather than as individuals. It may further remedial purposes but, just as likely, it may promote improper racial stereotypes, thus fueling racial hostility. The use of race, in and of itself, to choose students simply achieves a student body that looks different. Such a criterion is no more rational on its own terms than would be choices based upon the physical size or blood type of applicants. (*Hopwood v. Texas*, 1996, p. 945)

In the court's view, it would be even worse to keep distinctive race-based admissions that odiously repeated the "separate but equal" status of the Jim Crow era. The Appeals Court relied on the claims of the rejected white student applicants who were victims of reverse discrimination and denied their Equal Protection rights. The judges' opinion in *Hopwood* also cited plaintiff Cheryl Hopwood as an example of fostering diversity through her status of individual achievement as a member of the Armed Forces, a wife, and the mother of a severely disabled child, as opposed to her race. In essence, the Fifth Circuit Federal Appeals Court did not view the use of race in the admissions process as fulfilling a compelling government objective to remedy past discrimination.

From a CRT perspective, the *Hopwood* opinion reinforces affirmative action being viewed as allowing lower qualified applicants into the academy or as taking jobs and admissions slots away from White European Americans. This is opposed to seeing affirmative action as a means by which the law could enable institutions to "Do the Right Thing" and be held accountable on diversity in admissions and faculty hiring (Nelson & Pellet, 1997). Ware (1996) has commented on how *Hopwood* represents the current thinking among many supporters of race-neutrality. Namely, that racial discrimination is a historical event associated with slavery and Jim Crow legal segregation. To the extent that it exists today, it is isolated and sporadic, and "the current generation should not have to bear the cost associated with creating opportunities for minorities. From here we should just play fair" (p. 45). Ware argues that this view of race-neutrality would serve to ossify the advantages of racial privilege and grant amnesty to white European Americans responsible for an unequal system. Ware also points out that the supporters of the color-blind approach have always cited merit in higher education admissions as standards to uphold for all individuals. Yet, in reality, the rule of law operates to preserve existing race, gender, and social class relations of power and privilege. This, in turn, undergirds what Ware (1996) refers to as "anecdotes of opportunities lost to less qualified minorities and women that abound in every faculty lounge" (p. 90). In addition, he challenges the position that minorities are first and foremost individuals:

> One of the latest arguments made against affirmative action is that it is divisive and encourages people to think of themselves in terms of their ethnicity and group identity rather than as individuals. Racism, not affirmative action, is the culprit for these circumstances. African Americans have always had to confront society as members of a disfavored minority, since they are often judged on the basis of that status rather than as individuals. This began long before the development of any affirmative action program. (Ware, 1996, p. 90)

Critical race theory seeks to de-cloak the institutional and ideological racial purpose behind the "color-blind" myth of merit and individualism embedded in the anti-affirmative action arguments. The CRT perspective in *Hopwood* also links and traces the historical connection of discrimination at the university to the current realities of racism as seen and felt by racial minority groups on predominantly white campuses. For example, during the Jim Crow segregation period the University of Texas law school barred African-Americans from attending the campus. The *Sweatt v. Painter* (1950) U.S. Supreme Court ruling addressed discrimination against African-Americans by the University of Texas law school. This ruling was part of the initial set of higher education cases preceding *Brown v. Board of Education* (1954), the ruling that led to the eventual dismantling of legal segregation in educational institutions such as the University of Texas law school. Yet, even with the removal of the legal barriers, a climate of "sponsored discrimination" continued through the 1960s and 1970s against the Chicanas/Chicanos and African-American law school students as they were assigned to segregated housing and excluded from law school organizations (Lauer, 1996, p. 123–124).

Additionally, there were other publicized incidents of historical racial discrimination at predominantly white universities, ranging from former Gov. George Wallace's attempt to block the first black students admitted to the University of Alabama to the shooting of Medgar Evers when he tried to enroll in the University of Mississippi during the civil rights era. More recently, Feagin's (1992) interviews with African-American students have illustrated the continuing presence of racism on predominantly white campuses. Some, for example, have reporting having "confederate flags slapped in their faces and called niggers by white fraternities during parades while authorities did nothing" (p. 550). These racial incidents were treated with indifference or even hostile reactions by campus police and administrators.

In fact, as the *Hopwood* decision calls for African-American and Chicano/Chicana students to be viewed as individuals, Feagin's interviews revealed that white faculty still view minority students in stereotypical group terms. An African-American graduate student reflected on her observations and encounters with a prominent department chairperson on a predominantly white campus. The chair made assumptions about race and a black undergraduate in the department who was doing research on black–white achievement:

> Apparently, she assumed that this one undergraduate somehow spoke for all Black people. And this professor would ask her things like, "Well, I don't know what you people want. First you want to be called Negro, then you want to be called Black. Now you want to be called African American. What do you people want anyway? And why don't Black people show up in class more? Why is that I can't get enough Blacks to sit on my classes?" So every now and then that sort of racist mentality comes out. (Feagin, 1992, p. 556)

These interviews revealed patterns of the barriers in the white campus world that African-American students face from students, faculty, and staff. The hostile or discriminatory actions ranged from aggression to exclusion, dismissal, or typecasting. Feagin (1992) posited that when all of the patterns from the interviews and reflections were analyzed, they revealed a process and culture of "cumulative discrimination" (p. 575). This type of racism manifests itself as blatant or subtle actions and has a severely oppressive and cumulative effect on these students. From a critical race theory perspective, this 'cumulative discrimination" can be traced back to the history of institutional racism in the academy and the ways it has a significant impact on present-day racism and its manifestations.

Therefore, the initial decreases in minority interest and attendance at the University of Texas law school and other public universities in California after Prop. 209 should not be surprising.[7] For example, the number of Latino students accepted to all graduate programs at the University of California-Berkeley fell from 246 in 1996 to 180 in 1997 (Burdman, 1997, p. A1). Also, only one of the 17 Black students admitted actually planned to attend the UC-Berkeley law school (Appelbome, 1997b). A critical race theory analysis thus points out the problems (and their effects, such as decreased enrollment) with the legality of the "color-blind" admissions process, particularly as race now looms even larger on predominantly white colleges and universities since Chicano/Chicana and African-American students do not see these campuses as a welcoming environment for them. Furthermore, to obtain an education at the more elite universities, racial minority students must overcome the vestiges of discrimination that appear in the current campus environment of color-blindness.

Borrowing from Delgado (1989), CRT serves an important role through its use of the storytelling and narratives of racially marginalized students on predominantly white campuses. These narratives comprise an integral part of historical and current testimonies and findings of fact in legal and political policy battles surrounding race in higher education. The Federal Courts and the White European American majority should be interested in these "stories" because, as Delgado asserts, it is only through listening that "one can acquire the ability to see the world through others eyes" (Delgado, 1989, p. 2439). Critical race theory exposes the color-blind position to the light. Through narratives and other historical evidence, it documents minority student exclusion and the ways some have had to compromise their race to survive at predominantly white colleges and universities. Furthermore, CRT offers avenues for a different thinking about affirmative action, a thinking that challenges the "one-size that fits all" notion of merit in admissions and faculty hires (Sturm & Guinier, 1996, p. 957). Instead, more complex and innovative approaches that emphasize assessments through educational experiences are necessary to enhance affirmative action and expand the diversity mission of most educational institutions.[8]

"Race is ... race ain't": can CRT answer this question?

The nexus of critical race theory from the legal arena, and qualitative research methods and methodologies in education, provides a framework to understand the centrality of racism in school and university settings. The narratives generated from qualitative research serve as a powerful link between historical vestiges of past racism and the effects of what the color-blind perspective omits with its present-day orientation. To be sure, legal criticisms have dismissed the use of narrative and storytelling in CRT, positing that stories about racism are unreliable, unverifiable. This has been a particularly poignant criticism of legal scholars (Farber & Sherry, 1993, 1994) who have had problems with the lack of objective measures of evidence. They have also questioned the factual objectivity of the personal accounts of racism and fictional stories about racial dilemmas in the USA presented by CRT scholars such as Patricia Williams (1991, 1995) or Derrick Bell (1987, 1992).

However, Di Toro commented (in her review of Williams, 1995) that the subjective narrative authority and personal voice of an African-American professional woman who has experienced racism forces readers to question their own subject positions as opposed to the authority of empirical evidence:

> As readers, we are asked to grant Williams absolute authority over her personal experience, and to acknowledge our own participation in making that experience sometimes excruciatingly difficult for her ... engaging with Williams in this way can raise a potentially disabilitating personal dilemma: If we are white, we want neither to disbelieve her nor presume to sanction her story from a position of white privilege. The former leaves the reader in a position of racist skepticism towards a black narrator; the latter may have equally oppressing effects: When the white reader believes, she may be positioning herself as a 'legitimator' of the black narrator. (Di Toro, 1996, p. 1469)

The use of narrative in critical race theory adds to the racial dimension and purpose of qualitative inquiry and ethnographic research in education. Previously, Stanfield (1993, 1994) and Foster (1994) noted the controversy surrounding how qualitative research has presented various aspects of black life and the African-American community. The processes used to engage in this description has been fraught with problems. They have ranged from subject exploitation and misuse of power by researchers to a general failure of critical self-questioning and the problematic nature of university status and privilege. However, CRT and qualitative research in education both utilize personal narratives (of the self and others) that can also use fiction or performance-based texts (Denzin, 1997), to illustrate, from a critical position, the historical and current connections and effects of racial issues and concerns. Since the analysis of race is at the center of CRT, then qualitative researchers can provide myriad ways to reconceptualize and challenge racial policies and their images and patterns of representation. Not only can this be done through more conventional means of qualitative research, but also through the use of various forms of political artistic expressions and literary presentations of "racial data" that challenge the social constructions of racial experiences and the way they are presented in the larger society (White & Bonner, 1997).[9]

The legal narratives of racism and racial discrimination can serve to challenge the prevailing notion of race neutrality in educational institutions. The thick descriptions of sites (e.g., conducting and analyzing interviews and long-term participant-observations) that are characteristic of educational anthropology (Wolcott, 1994) not only serve an illuminative purpose, but can also be used to document overt and institutional racism. Deyhle's (1995) ten-year ongoing relationships and work with the Navajos in southern Utah and northern Arizona has resulted in research that fully describes how racism plays out in the larger community between Anglos and Navajos. This racism was central to analyzing relations between Anglos and Navajos. Racism was reflected in the conflicts over power regarding Navajo self-determination in education versus Anglo teachers' and administrators' control of school policies. Her work also documents the Navajo community's legal attempts to maintain cultural integrity and fight for equitable remedies in the Federal courts to address racial discrimination pertaining to tracking, high suspension–expulsion rates, and inequitable funding of schools.

The importance that critical race theory places on historical links to contemporary social constructions of race also has implications for qualitative studies in schools and colleges. This can be pursued through an examination of the vestiges and representations of the ideology of color-blindness in educational institutions. For example, *Hopwood*'s reliance on individual merit and the irrelevance of race is similar to the rhetoric of individual success and color-blindness among white teachers that Lipman (1977) found in her study of school restructuring. An area for future research linking qualitative studies to critical race theory may, thus, involve tracing how the racial ideology of color-blindness plays a role in shaping the experiences of African-American or Latino–Latina students from the high schools to the postsecondary education level. Since the current political climate and legal positions dictate that schools and colleges should be race-neutral in a meritocratic society, then critical race theory and qualitative research in education can provide racial counter-insights as a critique of this meritocracy. Furthermore, CRT and qualitative research can show how the ideology of race neutrality and "ethno-culturalism" (Diamond, 1996, p. 163) can take on various shapes and forms (e.g., Prop. 187 in California banning public services for illegal immigrants, English-only mandates, xenophobic attitudes, etc.). This in turn reinforces structural racism and fuels overt bigotry in schools and colleges over issues such as language, national origin, and immigration as shown in the documentary film "Fear and Learning at Hoover Elementary School" by Laura Sĭmon (1977).

Finally, the theorizing about race from critical perspectives can attempt to connect to already ongoing daily realities and struggles about race and other areas of discrimination.[10] For example, the talk I gave at the university in the opening narrative served, in hindsight, as an opportunity for students, faculty, and administrators to express their concerns about student diversity and single mothers, racism, sexism, homophobia, and the ways they played out on their institution. Previously at this campus, there had been a series of racial incidents between white European American and African-American students. These incidents also led to verbal and email attacks on lesbian and gay students as well. Although the racial harassment arose out of a black–white conflict, the subsequent discussion led to various groups voicing concerns about how the racial conflict triggered more open hostilities by some students toward other marginalized groups and how this resulted in a campus-wide climate of harassment and tension. The discussion which took place after the talk on CTR also centred on different ways to look at discrimination on campus. For example, some focussed on the historical establishment of the university as a source of the problem, while others discussed how these issues can lead to future teaching and action in areas related to diversity and social justice. The centering of student, faculty, and administrator narratives on race and other areas of difference can give rise to future connections between CRT and education, particularly if it stimulates or adds to ongoing efforts addressing educational diversity and social change.

Conclusion: CRT and connections and dilemmas for the future

The future of critical race theory and its place in education will partially depend on the efforts made by researchers and scholars to explore its possible connections to the racism in U.S. schools and communities of color (Tate, 1997). Qualitative research can also inform critical race theory as to how the ideology and resulting legal mandate of color-blindness in schools and universities further serve as racist barriers for students of color. Critical race theory can be a useful framework for studying whiteness, especially by students and scholars of color who study whites and issues related to white racism. The critiques of whiteness, power, and privilege (Fine, Weis, Powell, and Wang Mun Wong, 1997), also serves as a useful point of dialogue with some white European American students and multiracial student groups who are trying to comb racism as well (Garza, 1997; Kelley, Schuwerk, Krishnamurthy, and Kao, 1997).

Still, my main dilemma is one posed in the opening narrative by the two students. Namely, how does critical race theory address their interest related to campus racism, homophobia, sexism, etc.? The talk and follow-up discussion at the pot-luck dinner serendipitously created a safe space that led to honest open-ended conversations on the broad implications of the campus's racial and homophobic incidents. Yet, I would have to agree with Jervis (1996) that, overall, schools and universities tend to ignore the most prominent matters related to race, culture, and ethnicity. Until now, for the most part, it has been the legal scholars in CRT who have placed racism at the center of the ideological discussion related to law, policy, and the social construction of race. Their borrowing of various methods from the social sciences and liberal arts demonstrate the effects of the vestiges of racism and present-day perspectives on race in the USA. I believe that qualitative researchers in education have added and will continue to add even more to the development of critical race theory and other initiatives that address racism in educational institutions, its disparate impact on students of color, and the ways they are striving for self-determination to obtain the equitable education they deserve.

Notes

1. The author would like to sincerely thank Frank Margonis and the QSE editorial group on this special issue for their helpful comments on this paper. Special acknowledgments are also given to my colleagues and associates at the university in the western USA where the opening narrative took place.
2. Questions and issues raised about epistemology, methodology, and ideology in race-based scholarship and education were initially raised by Marjorie Davis, Melanie Carter, and Cynthia Tyson at a seminar conducted by Patti Lather at Ohio State University, November 15, 1996.
3. In this paper, I will use African-Americans and blacks, whites and white European Americans, Chicano/Chicana, and Latino/Latina interchangeably, even though there are differences among these groups as well as distinctions among Asian-Americans and American Indians.
4. Nebeker (1997) made a similar claim to that of Ellsworth (1989) in her critique of critical pedagogy and empowerment in education. Nebeker argued that CRT may indeed provide a solid theoretical understanding of the complexity of race in the USA. However, that did not translate into how the theory could help empower the vast majority of students of color in the schools. Furthermore, she argued that CRT scholarship left little room for sympathetic whites who shared the ideals of CRT regarding emphasis on racial justice. However, I would propose that CRT is an emerging theoretical framework subject to change as it moves into education. Furthermore, CRT does have a place for white European Americans because it was partially built on the legal critique of whiteness and white privilege (Haney López, 1996) and the sudden emergence of white studies from a critical perspective.
5. Despite the fact that *Hopwood* only covers the states of the 5th Circuit (Texas, Mississippi, and Louisiana), some politicians and news commentators have argued for "need-based" or social-class-based affirmative action to replace race and gender. However, Feinberg (1996) has put forth strong social and philosophical arguments against such policies as replacements for gender and race.
6. Critical race theory comes more out of the legal and sociopolitical criticism, and it may not add to the discussions related to race and research epistemologies. However, CRT can be used as a vehicle to open the conversation about race-based research epistemologies, such as black feminist thought (Collins, 1991) and Africana studies (Asante, 1997; Kershaw, 1992). Some of the calls for race-based epistemological work (Stanfield, 1994) will also be useful to illustrate how racial minorities act as individuals and/or act as collective communities to resist the notion of color-blindness and attempt to foster success for their students. These issues for African-American education have been discussed in important works edited by Lomotey (1992) and Shujaa (1994; 1996).
7. One student, Bruce Rideaux, who is a senior at the University of Texas now, said he would not consider going to the Austin campus if he were applying to college now, "there are 50000 students here and so few of them are black, with all this going on, I probably would have gone to a black or smaller university" (Applebome, 1997a, p. C24). Malcolm Lavergne, who was the first African-American to send in a tuition deposit to attend the University of Texas law school, later changed his mind because after *Hopwood*, "it would be like going to a country club there" (Applebome, 1997c, p. A10). There is some speculation that the drop

in interest and enrollment is due to higher admissions standards after Hopwood and Prop. 209. However, this just highlights racism and the apparent return to the Jim Crow era except that now merit through grades test scores, and "other forms of diversity" form the basis of how one gets into the elite universities. As Sturm and Guinier (1996) have pointed out, this type of meritocracy merely exacerbates racial, social class, and gender discrimination in higher education admissions.

8. Sturm and Guinier (1996) argue that the current emphasis on standardized testing to determine entrance into law schools, graduate schools, etc., constricts opportunities for women and minorities to participate fully in U.S. society since political, social, and economic status and influence are directly determined by the gatekeeping function of the test and the institutional acceptance of the questionable validity of these tests. Sturm and Guinier also assert that the battle should really be over how affirmative action can truly lead to a more equitable and just society as opposed to a narrow battle over numbers of minorities and reverse discrimination in an institution.

9. In this presentation, White and Bonner used poetry, video, rap music and other creative forms of expression to draw from their own epistemologies of color as African-Americans, and they in turn also explored how different methodologies and methods can be used to address race, gender, and other aspects of diversity in the urban education context.

10. CRT can provide a theory about race with respect to the seemingly intractable nature of the black–white conflict as well as the emergence of race, culture, and language regarding other groups. A CRT perspective can provide insights as to how Asian-Americans are sometimes viewed as "honorary whites" for political purposes in the affirmative action debate, yet have been discriminated against in higher education admissions (Tagaki, 1992). However, more work is needed to explore how critical race theory can or cannot be used in the international education context when one considers the central questions of transnationalism, diaspora, postcolonialism (Chow, 1993; Fanon, 1967; Gilroy, 1993).

References

Applebome, P. (1997a, March 19). Universities report less minority interest after action to ban preferences. *New York Times*, p. C24.

Applebome, P. (1997b, June 28). In 2 law schools, black enrollment scarcely exists. *New York Times*, pp. 1, 7.

Applebome, P. (1997c, July 2, 1997). Affirmative action bar transforms law school. *New York Times*, p. A10.

Asante, M. K. (1997). Afrocentricity and the quest for method. In J. L. Conyers, Jr. (Ed.), *Africana studies: A disciplinary quest for both theory and method* (pp. 69–90). Jefferson, MC: McFarland.

Augstin, N. A. (1997). Learnfare and black motherhood: The social construction of deviance. In A. K. Wing (Ed.), *Critical race feminism: A reader* (pp. 144–150). New York: New York University.

Bartolome, L. I., & Macedo, D. P. (1997). Dancing with bigotry: The poising of racial and ethnic identities. *Harvard Educational Review*, *67*, 222–246.

Bell, D. A. (1987). *And we are not saved: The elusive quest for racial justice.* New York: Basic Books.

Bell, D. A. (1992). *Faces at the bottom of the well: The permanence of racism*. New York: Basic Books.

Brown v. *Board of Education*, 347 U.S. 483 (1954).

Burdman, P. (1997, June 26). UC Berkeley minority admissions dropping. *San Francisco Chronicle*, pp. A1, A19.

Calvo, J. M. (1997). Spouse-based immigration laws: The legacy of coverture. In A. K. Wing (Ed.) *Critical race feminism: A reader* (pp. 380–386). New York: New York University.

Carbado, D. W. (1997). Motherhood and work in cultural context: One woman's patriarchal bargain. In A. K. Wing (Ed.), *Critical race feminism: A reader* (pp. 339–350). New York: New York University.

Cho, S. K. (1997). Converging stereotypes in racialized sexual harassment: Where the model minority meets Suzie Wong. In A. K. Wing (Ed.), *Critical race feminism: A reader* (pp. 203–220). New York: New York University.

Chow, R. (1993). *Writing diaspora: Tactics of intervention in contemporary cultural studies.* Bloomington, IN: Indiana University Press.

Cleaver, K. N. (1997). Racism, civil rights, and feminism. In A. K. Wing (Ed.), *Critical race feminism: A reader* (pp. 35–43). New York: New York University.

Collins, P. H. (1991). *Black feminist thought: Knowledge, consciousness, and the politics of empowerment.* New York: Routledge.

Crenshaw, K., Gotanda, N, Peller, G., & Thomas, K. (Eds). (1995). *Critical Race Theory: Key writings that formed the movement.* New York: New Press.

Denzin, N. K. (1997). *Interpretive ethnography: Ethnographic practices for the 21st century.* Newbury Park, CA: Sage.

Delgado, R. (1989). Storytelling for oppositionist and others: A plea for narrative. *Michigan Law Review*, *87*, 2411–2441.

Delgado, R. (Ed.). (1995). *Critical race theory: The cutting edge*. Philadelphia, PA: Temple University Press.

Deyhle, D. (1995). Navajo youth and Anglo racism: Cultural integrity and resistance. *Harvard Educational Review*, *65*, 403–444.

Diamond, S. (1996). Right-wing politics and the anti-immigration cause. *Social Forces*, *23*, 154–168.

Di Toro, J. A. (1996). Casting the outsider [Review of the book *The rooster's egg*]. *Stanford Law Review*, *48*, 1469–1486.

Donmoyer, R. (1997). This issue: Visions of educational research's past and future. *Educational Researcher, 26*, 2.

Ellsworth, E. (1989). Why doesn't this feel empowering? Working through the repressive myths of critical pedagogy. *Harvard Educational Review, 59*, 297–324.

Fanon, F. (1967). *Black skin: White masks*. New York: Grove.

Farber, D. A., & Sherry, S. (1993). Telling stories out of school: An essay on legal narratives. *Stanford Law Review, 45*, 807–856.

Farber, D. A., & Sherry, S. (1994). The 2000,000 cards of Dimitri Yurasov: Further reflections on scholarship and truth. *Stanford Law Review, 46*, 647–662.

Feagin, J. R. (1992). The continuing significance of racism: Discrimination against black students in white colleges. *Journal of Black Studies, 6*, 546–578.

Feinberg, W. (1996). Affirmative action and beyond: A case for a backward-looking gender and race-based policy. *Teachers College Record, 97*, 362–399.

Fine, M., Weis, L., Powell, L. C., & Wang Mun Wong, L. (Eds.). (1997). *Off-white: Readings on race, power and society*. New York: Routledge.

Foster, M. (1994). The power to know one thing is never the power to know all things: Methodological notes on two studies of Black American teachers. In A. Gitlin (Ed.), *Power and method: Political activism and educational research* (pp. 129–146). New York: Routledge.

Garza, A. (1997). New abolitionist students: Austin, Texas. *Race Traitor, 7*, 6–8.

Gilroy, P. (1993). *The black atlantic: Modernity and double consciousness*. Cambridge: Harvard University Press.

Haney López, I. F. (1996). *White by law: The legal construction of race*. New York: New York University Press.

Harris, A. P. (1994). Forward: The jurisprudence of reconstruction. *California Law Review, 82*, 741–785.

Harris, A. P. (1997). Race and essentialism in feminist legal theory. In A. K. Wing (Ed.), *Critical race feminism: A reader* (pp. 11–18). New York: New York University.

Hopwood v. Texas, 861 F. Supp. 551 (W.D. Tex. 1994).

Hopwood v. Texas, 78 F.3d 932 (5th Cir. 1996).

Hutchinson, H. (1997). Toward a critical race reformist conception of minimum wage regimes: Exploding the power of myth, fantasy, and hierarchy. *Harvard Journal of Legislation, 34*, 93–134.

Jervis, K. (1996). "How come there are no brothers on that list?" Hearing the hard questions all children ask. *Harvard Educational Review, 66*, 546–576.

Kelley, S., Schuwerk, R., Krishnamurthy, P., & Kao, J. (1997). Abolitionism on the campus: Students for the abolition of whiteness: Chicago. *Race Traitor, 7*, 1–6.

Kershaw, T. (1992). Afrocentrism and the Afrocentric method. *The Western Journal of Black Studies, 16*, 160–168.

Ladson-Billings, G. (1998). Just what is critical race theory and what's it doing in a *nice* field like education? *International Journal of Qualitative Studies in Education, 11*, 7–24.

Lauer, R. A. (1996). *Hopwood* v. *Texas*: A victory for equality that denies reality. *St. Mary's Law Journal, 28*, 110–145.

Lipman, P. (1997). Restructuring in context: A case study of teacher participation and the dynamics of ideology, race, and power. *American Educational Research Journal, 34*, 3–38.

Lomotey, K. (Ed.). (1990). *Going to school: The African-American experience*. Albany, NY: SUNY.

Moran, B. I., & Whitford, W. (1996). A black critique of the internal revenue code. *Wisconsin Law Review, 1996*, 752–803.

Nebeker, K. C. (1997). *Critical race theory: A white masters student takes on this growing genre*. Unpublished manuscript, University of Utah.

Nelson, S., & Pellett, G. (Producers and Directors). (1997, March 5). PBS Special: *Shattering the silences: Minority faculty on white campuses*. New York: Public Broadcasting Service.

Omi, M., & Winant, H. (1994). *Racial formation in the United States: From the 1960s to the 1990s* (2nd ed.). New York: Routledge.

Rivera, J. (1997). Domestic violence against Latinas by Latino males: An analysis of race, national origin, and gender differentials. In A. K. Wing (Ed.), *Critical race feminism: A reader* (pp. 259–268). New York: NYU.

Shujaa, M. J. (Ed.). (1994). *Too much schooling, too little education: A paradox of black life in white societies*. Tenton, NJ: Africa World Press.

Shujaa, M. J. (Ed.). (1996). *Beyond desegregation: The politics of quality in African American schooling*. Thousand Oaks, CA: Corwin.

Símon, L. (Director–Producer). (1997, July 1). *Point of view: Fear and learning at Hoover Elementary*. New York: Public Broadcasting Service.

Stanfield, J. H. II (1993). Methodological reflections: An introduction. In J. H. Stanfield & R. M. Dennis (Eds.), *Race and ethnicity in research methods*. (pp. 175–188). Newbury Park, CA: Sage.

Stanfield, J. H. (1994). Ethnic modeling in qualitative research. In N. K. Denzin & Y. S. Lincoln (Eds.), *Handbook of qualitative research* (pp. 175–188). Thousand Oaks, CA: Sage.

Sturm, S., & Guinier, L. (1996). The future of affirmative action: Reclaiming the innovative ideal. *California Law Review, 84*, 953–1035.

Sweatt v. Painter, 339 U.S. 629 (1950).

Symposium. (1994). Critical race theory [Special Issue]. *California Law Review, 82,* (4).

Takagi, D. Y. (1992). *The retreat from race: Asian American admissions and racial politics.* New Brunswick: Rutgers University Press.

Tate, W. F. IV. (1997). Critical race theory and education: History, theory and implications. *Review of Research in Education, 22* (pp. 191–243). Washington, DC: American Educational Research Association.

Ware, L. (1996). Tales from the crypt: Does strict scrutiny sound the death knell for affirmative action in higher education? *Journal of College and University Law, 23,* 43–90.

White, C., & Bonner, W. J. (1997, June 20). *Re-claiming voice: At play in the fields of the Lord.* Paper and performance session presented at the Ethnographic Inquiry and Qualitative Research in a Postmodern Age Conference, University of Southern California, Los Angeles, CA.

Williams, P. J. (1991). *The alchemy of race and rights.* Cambridge: Harvard University Press.

Williams, P. J. (1995). *The rooster's egg.* Cambridge: Harvard University Press.

Wolcott, H. H. (1994). *Transforming qualitative data: Description, analysis, and interpretation.* Newbury Park, CA: Sage.

Forging community in race and class: critical race theory and the quest for social justice in education

David Stovall

Among the communities of critical race theorists and its detractors in education, there is an apparent rift as to what theoretical construct best contributes to the social justice project in education. Conferences and meetings have served as quasi-battle grounds for theorists, activists and scholars to go back and forth about what theoretical construct has the greatest bearing on educational praxis. Debate notwithstanding, the following document argues critical race theory (CRT hereafter) as a viable theoretical construct to address issues of social justice in education. In so doing, the following document couches the discussion in three tasks. The first is to identify the contributions of CRT in education. Second, the document argues for a closer read of the theoretical construct and its subsequent application. The concluding task will be an example of how the points of contention and compliance can be located through an example (in this case narrative) of a school with a social justice agenda at its center. As Yamamoto suggests, the occupation of the socially conscious scholar is to participate in the activities that challenge hegemony at both the grassroots and intellectual levels. From this we can engage CRT in education with a concerted effort to change our present realities.

Social justice, CRT, critical race praxis, and White supremacy: working definitions

For the purposes of this document, definitions in this section should be considered 'working' descriptions in that they are not exhaustive of the literature on social justice, CRT, racialization and White supremacy. Operating as a subset of the larger body of literature, the following section provides a base of understanding from which to operate.

Beginning with social justice, a definition is borrowed from Maxine Greene in that the project in education includes teaching:

> … for enhanced perception and imaginative explorations, for the recognition of social wrongs, of sufferings, of pestilences wherever and whenever they arise … it is to teach so that the young may be awakened to the joy of working for transformation in the smallest places, so that they may become healers and change their worlds. (Greene, cited in Ayers *et al.*, 1998, p. xiv)

In essence the process becomes to engage young people (in this case) to answer the question 'what is powerful, important and ours?' Throughout this process those who work with young people in the capacity of educator, community organizer, social service provider or academic come to embrace numerous theoretical concepts and constructs to explain the varied realities in which they operate. Where most theories in this concept would be considered 'grounded theory' in that they are informed by the situations in which we work, CRT contributes to such knowledge in the valuing of daily experiences with racism as necessary qualitative data.

In its most explicit definition of its operation in education, Gloria Ladson-Billings uses CRT to name and highlight the function of White supremacy through five tenets. Essentially, the CRT project in education becomes the attempt to:

1. Name and discuss the pervasive, daily reality of racism in US society which serves to disadvantage people of color.
2. Expose and deconstruct seemingly 'colorblind' or 'race neutral' policies and practices which entrench the disparate treatment of people of non-White persons.
3. Legitimize and promote the voices and narrative of people of color as sources of critique of the dominant social order which purposely devalues them.
4. Revisit civil rights law and liberalism to address their inability to dismantle and expunge discriminatory socio-political relationships.
5. Change and improve challenges to race neutral and multicultural movements in education which have made White student behavior the norm (Ladson-Billings, 1998).

Central to the following account, the third tenet operates as a means by which to challenge detractors of CRT and legitimize the importance of working towards social justice in communities of color. In response to the adversarial relationship that many communities of color have experienced with urban school systems, a counter story is needed to identify the desire for said communities for quality education despite mainstream accounts that depict communities of color as 'anti-school' or 'anti-intellectual'. Such counter stories become the foundation by which to pose alternatives to education systems that operate to further marginalize communities of color. Borrowing from the work of Solorzano and Yosso (2002), a counter story asks readers to 'suspend judgement, listen for the story's points, test them against (their) own version of reality (however conceived), and use the counter story as a theoretical conceptual, methodological, and pedagogical case study' (Solorzano & Yosso, 2002, p. 23).

Acknowledging similar experiences in the international scope of imperialism and domination, CRT positions itself on the continuum of scholars who have unambiguously named the nature of oppression in US education (see Anderson, 1988; Delpit, 1995; Ladson-Billings & Tate, 1995; Mills, 1997; Woodson, 2000; Watkins, 2001).

Instead of separating the authors due to method or discipline, CRT invokes a call to an interdisciplinary approach in naming the function of educational domination. Accounts in the humanities, social sciences (education included), and legal scholarship converge in CRT to identify the structures by which we understand the forces that work in opposition to the social justice project in education.

Again, CRT recognizes the complexity of racial dynamics. Such intricacy requires the ability to speak across numerous boundaries to highlight common points of interest that not only seek to eliminate White supremacy, but on the most practical level engage communities in building coalitions. Eric Yamamoto, by encouraging a critical race praxis, promotes increased attention to a critical rethinking of what race is, how civil rights claims may be both empowering and debilitating and whether legal process and its alternatives foster or impede racial healing (Yamamoto, 1998, p. 129)

The process of developing praxis (theory plus practice) becomes an inclusive strategy aimed at facilitating an understanding between groups of color of the systemic structures that impede development and justice. In education this can operate at numerous levels where students and parents may experience levels of discrimination based on language, socioeconomic status, or stereotype. Where a more specific example will be discussed in later sections, the understanding of White supremacy as a structural phenomenon informs our work in developing proactive stances in addressing needs and concerns of communities of color. The process is useful in education because it challenges scholars to 'spend less time on abstract theorizing and more time on actual community based anti-subordination practice' (Yamamoto, 1997, p. 873). Referenced by Dixson and Rousseau (2005), CRT 'mandates that social activism be a part of any CRT project' (Dixon & Rousseau, 2005, p. 12). In the following section we are introduced to the author's attempt at such an endeavor.

Although highly debated in academic circles on the viability of its function, a working definition of White supremacy provides a space from which to develop a concentrated understanding of CRT. In so doing, this account borrows a definition of White supremacy from Frances Lee Ansley (2003), in recognizing it as:

> A political, economic and cultural system in which Whites overwhelmingly control power and material resources, conscious and unconscious ideas of White superiority and entitlement are widespread, and relations of White dominance and non-White subordination are daily re-enacted across a broad array of institutions and social settings. (Ansley, cited in Mills, 2003, p.179)

Where many would argue this to be a de facto summation of public schooling in the US, others have critiqued it as too narrow a concept to encapsulate the complexities of social relationships. Despite such critique, CRT scholars would add that this concept is of critical importance as we investigate what shape the project of social justice will take, depending on the situation.

The following account will also refer to situations as 'racialized'. Borrowing from Bonilla-Silva's (1996) concept of racialized social systems, it refers to 'societies in which economic, political, social, and ideological levels are partially structured by the placement of actors in racial categories or races' (Bonilla-Silva, 1996, p. 469). A concrete example would be the more fluid concepts of race throughout Central America, the Carribean and South America. In opposition to overt racist acts, there is a subtle social hierarchy based on 'social estimations' (e.g., one group 'looking better' or 'being smarter' than another based on physical attributes or family lineage). Where many Latino/a households watch novellas, many of the main characters remain European in appearance. Darker-skinned characters are still given roles as troublemakers, scarlets, or evildoers. As the common denominator remains language, hierarchy is actualized in roles assigned to certain groups. Such subtleties become important in later sections of the text due to the interplay of race and class analysis.

Although rarely equated with CRT in education, parallels can be made with much of socialist critique in education in its analysis of power and domination. William Watkins, in his analysis of White rule of African-American education from 1865 to 1954, points to the earlier colonial period in discussion of how education was 'designed to control, pacify, and socialize subject people' (Watkins, 2001, p. 1). In connecting the education of African-Americans to state politics and the labor market, Watkins engages meticulous analysis of the structure and function of power. In calling for a 'critical theory of racism that can grapple with a radical remaking of democracy in the age of a globalized post-industrial economy', Darder and Torres place a call to engage social justice with an understanding of the totalizing system of capitalism (Darder & Torres, 2003, p. 260). In breaking the hegemonic hold of standards-based education and its devaluing of students of color, the remainder of the document seeks synergy between the two camps in regards to what it will take to 'critically' engage education for those concerned with social justice.

Ideological connections: CRT's response to its detractors

Offering a critique of CRT, Darder and Torres (2003) are correct in that CRT is a theory critical of the common assumptions placed within the context of race. To make the point more salient, CRT *should be* discussed as a critical theory of race and racism. The critique of Darder and Torres in this sense is more semantic in nature in that they make the point that CRT scholars do not make the necessary distinction between 'race' and 'racism.' However, they are correct in that

> … dramatic national and international changes, both economic and political, have created conditions which, on the one hand, racialized structures, processes and representations are more intricate and elusive, yet, on the other hand, the historically entrenched inequities persist. (Darder & Torres, 2003, p. 245).

Operating as a theory critical of race and racism, the push becomes for CRT scholars to highlight the dynamic, but consistently oppressive nature of racism over the last 500 years in the western hemisphere. Darder and Torres are correct in that race is not a monolithic concept that encapsulates every experience of people of color. It is instead a construct that has been historically utilized to justify political, economic, and social inequality. Because it is socially constructed, race can have multiple meanings based on site-specific experiences and relationships to structures of power (i.e., state sanctioned education). Race as a concept has no biological foundation. However, it would be a critical mistake to deny the lived realities of racism in daily life.

In reference to capitalism, Darder and Torres are also correct in defining capitalism as a 'totalizing system of social relations' (2003, p. 247). The concept of White supremacy in CRT should be understood in the same light. Moreover, the concept should 'play the same roll in CRT that "capitalism" does in class society and "patriarchy" respectively play in Marxist and feminist political theory' (Mills, 2003, p. 182). Again, in its totalizing method, we would be remiss to deny the impact race has on a macro-construct like capitalism. To concur, capitalism does act as a homogenizing force instead of a diversifying one. Right-wing think tanks in the US like the American Civil-Rights Institute, The Center for Equal Opportunity, The Center for Individual Rights and the Hoover Institute make this clear in their recent co-option of civil rights language to influence public policy in education (i.e., Proposition 209 in California, Initiative 200 in Washington state, Proposition 203 in Arizona, etc). The argument has shifted to one that downplays the significance of race for language supporting economic concerns that will supposedly supercede or solve the social concerns of the present day. In the eyes of the conservative right in the US, affirmative action policies have become plans of 'racial preference,' and violations of civil rights. The domestic and global influence of the Right shape their viewpoints by 'rearticulating the Civil Rights legacy's moderate agenda of "rights" and opportunities in an ideology of individualism and meritocracy' (Winant, 2001, p. 151). Where Ward Connerly's (chairman of the American Civil Rights Institute) quote 'race has no place in American life or law' (www.acri.org) is viewed as questionable in reference to CRT ideology, it has become the Right's new lingua franca.

Conceptualized as a response to the critical legal studies (CLS hereafter) movement of the 1970s, CRT made the explicit point that class was too narrow a concept to explain the detrimental effects of hegemony in the US. As one of the common interests of CRT as stated by Crenshaw *et al.* (1995), the theory in its legal inception sought to;

> … understand how a regime of White supremacy and its subordination of people of color have been created and maintained in America and … to examine the relationship between the social structure and professed ideals such as 'the rule of law' and equal protection (Crenshaw *et al.*, 1995, p. 1)

With legal theory at its center, CRT critiqued liberalism and its reliance on systemic structures to address ills of the society at large. Its response to CLS came in the form of a critique of class as the dominant factor in addressing issues of inequality. Where CRT highlights the centrality of race, it should not perform such a task without substantive class analysis. Discussed in future sections, there are a number of CRT scholars who have initiated the process in education (see Lopez, 2003; Yosso, 2002; Torres, 1998).

The need for a closer read of CRT

Where the shortcomings of CRT are important to note in regards to class, it becomes equally important to discuss common misinterpretations of CRT. Reducing the construct to identity politics is an improper reading of the theoretical construct. Some argue the theory has used the construct of race:

> … as central category of analysis for interpreting the social conditions of inequality and marginalization. In turn, this literature has reinforced a racialized politics of identity and representation with its problematic emphasis on 'racial' identity as the overwhelming impulse for political action. (Darder & Torres, 2003, p. 246)

This interpretation is shortsighted for several reasons. First, it would be thoughtless not to place the realities of class discrimination as critical to any discourse on hegemony. However, it would also be incorrect to devalue the relationship between race and class in education. In this instance, race and class become a 'chicken and egg' argument as to which one is deemed most significant in analyzing and addressing issues of inequality. Both race and class are can be central to analysis of hegemony. CRT recognizes that one should not go without the other. It continues to function as a critical theory of racism. The use of the term 'race' in the title CRT is misinterpreted. It is not steeped in the narrow concept of 'race' as a monolith encapsulating the entirety of experiences of people of color. Instead, CRT recognizes in situations where class is argued to be the central theme, it would be just as damaging to exclude race and vice versa. The purpose in this instance is not for CRT to bemoan the issue of being considered secondary to class analysis. Instead, CRT is making the point to name the structural function of racism as relevant and significant, in addition to class. For education, CRT is making the attempt to confront White supremacy in the form of the power of Whites in the school system and the resources that the majority wealthy White districts have and refuse to relinquish (e.g., school funding in the US based on property taxes).

Where CRT agrees capitalism to be a 'totalizing' system, we should also consider White supremacy in the same instance. A prominent example would be the current 108th Senate of the US. CRT would suggest that it is not coincidence that 98 of the current 100 members are White. Instead, it is reflective of a totalizing system that has people of color on the margins in the law making process. Where socialist critique would couple members of the Senate as members of the ruling class, a CRT critique would remind us that this ruling class continues to be White, reflecting the views and values of a ruling elite. Surely there are those individual persons of color with conservative viewpoints that live affluently in their support of the status quo. There are even those that are chosen to act in leadership capacities for the ruling class. Yet, these persons are required to perform duties conducive to the prescribed functions of the state. Despite their conservative viewpoints, they remain disposable employees of the ruling class. While those who invoke a class analysis in reference to the aforementioned as 'selling out,' one should understand such actions as supporting White supremacy. Their actions as people of color in serving the interests of the conservative right reifies current racialized power structures in that those who control the resources and social status to which they emulate remain White. Even in spaces where this may be debatable (Mexico, Brazil, Cuba, Puerto Rico, etc), one need must be reminded of Bonilla-Silva's (1996) point that racism, in addition to overt behaviors, can be 'subtle, indirect, or fluid' (Bonilla-Silva, 1996, p. 468).

Returning to a critique of capitalism, critics of CRT are incorrect in stating that CRT has not given the necessary credence to the severity of capitalism. Conversely, CRT in legal scholarship has performed this task in reference to Cheryl Harris's 'Whiteness as property'. Highlighting the synonymous development of racism and economics in creating the social, economic, and political systems in the US, Harris responds to critics of her interpretation of property interests.

> Because the law recognized and protected expectations grounded in White privilege (albeit not explicitly in all instances), these expectations became tantamount to property that could not permissibly be intruded upon without consent. As the law explicitly ratified those expectations in continued privilege or extended ongoing protection to those illegitimate expectations by failing to expose or to disturb them radically, the dominant and subordinate positions within the racial hierarchy were reified in law. (Harris, cited in Crenshaw *et al.*, 1995, p. 281)

Here the argument encapsulates the economic and social order as centered in racial ideology. 'Property' in Harris' sense operates on material and social levels, expressed in common assumptions on race. Contrary to Darder and Torres's point on CRT as divorcing itself from the 'realities of class struggle', it makes room for the realities of class while discussing them in the context of what race meant historically and what it has come to mean in contemporary analysis (Darder & Torres, 2003, p. 248). Because racial and ethnic groups can be approved and discarded over time by the ruling class, it remains critical to name those who make the decisions as to who are accepted and rejected. Again, it is not by happenstance that this group remains White. In order to engage the social justice project in education, it is of critical importance to name said 'realities' in the effort to change them.

CRT recognizes the problematic nature of the Black and White binary in discussions of race. Additionally, its interdisciplinary approach it welcomes discussions of class in naming and working to end oppression. In so doing, as a theoretical construct it has evolved into Lat crit, Asian-American crit and critical race feminism to recognize the fluid nature of oppression and what it can mean to particular groups. Hayman (1995) makes the point salient in that 'CRT is complex, nuanced and dynamic and is in constant dialogue with other contemporary movements' (Hayman, 1995, p. 62). In developing a series of tenets of CRT, Hayman's second point is critical in that critical race theorists 'reject the contention that texts and practices have objective, neutral meanings and insist instead on their relentless deconstruction and perhaps reconstruction' (p. 70). The subtleties at play in such a statement are critical. On a practical level, the application of CRT should not be a space where those employed in the academy continuously complain about the 'troubles of the world'.

Instead, it should be understood that a main component in developing praxis includes a recognition and understanding of the world in which you live. Experiential knowledge is critical in providing the necessary foundation upon which to build the necessary strategies to address the issues at hand. Calmore (1992), in recognizing the importance of research and activism, locates the necessity of synergy between the paradigms:

> While activist practice must be directed toward transforming the concrete situations that give rise to oppression, it is also valuable for intellectuals to intervene critically in confronting the culture of domination and the system and process of laws that support and maintain it. … CRT recognizes that revolutionizing a culture begins with the radical assessment of it. (Calmore, 1992, p. 4)

Where not as overt, one can visualize the subtle yet totalizing function of racism. The stereotype of the group of old White men convening in clandestine meetings plotting the demise of people of color is futile. Racism, like capitalism, is an accepted structural phenomenon centered in maintaining the status quo. It is not, and never has been, the result of individual bigotry it is often reduced to. Instead of race as a category, racism (i.e., White supremacy) should be understood as a set of systemic structures that maintain a racial ruling elite as demonstrated through enforcement of policies and laws that govern the land. One need only investigate public policy and the damaging affects it has on communities of color. Where language is less overt than edicts of the Jim Crow South, the de jure interpretations of policy remain racialized. Take for example a current loitering ordinance in an urban metropolis. The policy states any group of three or more people can be considered a gang if one of the persons is a 'known gang member'. If the previous is true, the entire party can be detained for questioning. CRT would require us to engage an empirical inquiry of the ordinance. A critical question to be considered would be to investigate the demographics (race, gender, ethnicity, place of residence, etc) of those detained in reference to the policy. Currently, conservatives in the state of California have suggested a 'racial privacy initiative' that would make access to such information illegal. If we are unable to access said data, how would we discern if law enforcement is enforcing the policy fairly? Would this green light the police force to make random stops on any group of three of more people? What constitutes a 'known gang member'?

Educational policy should be viewed in the same light. While many conservative groups are lauding the 2001 US federal initiative 'No Child Left Behind' (NCLB hereafter), it has been nightmarish for other school districts. A CRT analysis of the policy would require research on NCLB's impact on communities of color in urban areas (most of which are low income). Currently the greatest pressure is placed on the lowest performing schools to increase student outcomes (e.g., test performance). What is not discussed, is how the Federal Government plans to support the lowest performing schools to improve student outcomes. Improvement is disguised with the language of choice, in that parents whose children attend a local underperforming school can transfer their child to a school that is at or above grade level. The undercurrent removed from the conversation is that many of the parents who qualify for such transfers are unable to send their children to the higher performing school due to population concerns (most schools performing at or above grade level in urban districts are at or above capacity). While language continues to be neutral, the enforcement becomes racialized in urban areas when the schools that are placed on the 'watch list' for poor performance predominantly serve students of color. Again, it is correct that those with a socialist critique of NCLB are correct in that these students of color will also reside in predominantly 'low-income' areas. However, we would be negligent not to include the policy's racial impact.

Still, the politics of identity are viewed as 'grossly inept and unsuited for building and sustaining collective political movements for social justice and economic democracy' (Darder & Torres, 2003, p. 248). This statement requires a bit of unpacking. To critique CRT simply as 'identity politics' ignores the necessity of narrative in developing coalitions across racial and class boundaries. Education provides and excellent example in that many African-American and Latino/a communities in the US are plagued with under-resourced schools. Although the specifics of each school are nuanced, it still sheds light on the master narrative of White supremacy. Almaguer's (1998) point remains relevant in his discussion of racism in California in that race relations:

> Reverberated along a number of racial fault lines, they did not assume a simple binary form or erupt along on principal fault. The allocation of 'group position' along these social strata was the outcome of both cultural and material considerations. (Almaguer, cited in Delgado & Stefancic, 1998, p. 166)

Detractors of CRT state the socialist project in education calls for readers to address 'the material conditions under which students must achieve' (Darder & Torres, 2003, p. 251). Such material conditions contain the 'structure of society and the economic and political limitations' (p. 251). They remain correct in relation to education in that 'academic performance is determined by a interplay of complex social process' (p. 253). CRT scholarship would not disagree. Nevertheless, these material conditions are not the creation of capitalism alone. Charles Mills (2003), in his discussion of class and race, forges the significance of White Supremacy, stating that it:

> ... needs to be taken as a theoretical object in its own right—a global social system comparable in current significance ... to Marx's class society and feminist thinkers' patriarchy. If philosophy is about understanding the human condition, then it needs to understand the condition of humans as shaped and molded by these systems into capitalists and workers, men and women, whites and nonwhites. (Mills, 2003, p.178)

If we take such a stance on education, it becomes critical to recognize the potential systemic damage of educational policy. Colorblind policies may have no de jure mention of race (or class) but are interpreted to disparately affect communities of color. It is not to deny that issues of class are at play. However, the inclusion of racism continues to inform our work on the discrete, yet damaging effects of White supremacy. Instead of class analysis serving as the point of solidarity, a focus on White privilege is just as likely to create solidarity between workers (Whites included) across race. Where those who side with socialist critique would argue that the previous promotes an identity politic, I would argue the contrary. Whites should be included in the focus on White privilege in that the responsibility in educating other Whites rests heavily with them. Their experiential knowledge of the construct enables them to unpack the intricate and subtle functions of White privilege and its various rationales. They should not be excluded from the larger context of class struggle because such recognition is integral in any analysis of racialized social systems. Again, we are compelled to include Bonilla-Silva's assertion that:

> … the systemic salience of class in relation to race increases when the economic, political and social distance between races decreases substantially. Yet this broad argument generates at least one warning: The narrowing of within-class differences between racial actors usually causes more rather hat less racial conflict, at least in the short run, as the competition for resources increases … even when class-based conflict becomes more salient in a social order, the racial component survives until the races' life chances are equalized and the mechanisms and social practices that produce those differences are eliminated. (Bonilla-Silva, 1996, p. 471)

It is shortsighted of us not to recognize the history of racism in the worker's movement in the US. Countless communities of color continue to be 'spoken for' by well-meaning Whites claiming to 'understand' the struggles of communities of color. In response, CRT maintains that the communities of color in question remain and should be understood as the resident experts on their conditions. Any organizing effort that does not acknowledge and develop praxis on this level is doomed for failure.

Nevertheless, a 'critical theory of racism represents a bold and forthright challenge to common-sense notions of "race"' (Darder & Torres, 2003, p. 259). However, it is incorrect to state that CRT makes it 'nearly impossible to dismantle the external material structure of domination that sustain racialized inequalities in schools and the larger society' (p. 259). CRT would argue that while material structures are a concern, praxis (theory plus practice) provides tangible examples in addressing issues of White supremacy.

Critics of CRT seek a 'critical language and conceptual apparatus that makes racism the central category of analysis in our understanding of racialized inequality' (Darder & Torres, 2003, p. 261). It is the understanding by scholars in CRT that the theoretical construct has been nothing short of this summation. Vital to this misinterpretation is the semantics of referencing CRT as a critique solely of 'race'. In no CRT literature is there a claim to the unanimity of race. The critique has and continues to be one of the functions of White supremacy and the complexities of race. CRT recognizes the Black/White racial binary as useless in describing the conditions of people of color in the US. In fact, a parallel understanding can be located in the introduction of Crenshaw *et al.* CRT, from its inception:

> … understands that racial power is produced by and experienced within numerous vectors of social life. CRT recognizes too, that political interventions which overlook the multiple ways in which people of color are situated (and restricted) as communities, sub-communities, and individuals will do little to promote effective resistance to, and counter mobilization against, today's newly empowered right. (Crenshaw *et al.*, 1995, p. xxxii)

In these parallel constructs is the potential for synergy. As the conservative Right in the US continues to co-opt the language of the civil rights movement, it would behoove us in education to engage proactive strategies in securing the ability to instill change across educational, political, economic and social communities.

Possible unions: counter-story, praxis and the quest for social justice in education

Through counter story we are able to discover the relationships between nuanced experience, individual responses and macro-policy. Coupled with praxis, the social justice project in education becomes a tangible exercise as experiences are utilized to inform our theories. By placing CRT and socialist critique on the ground, educators, activists, academics, and organizers are challenged to engage the often messy, muddled and conflicting issues of race and racism.

Yamamoto (1998) argues for a critical race praxis that pays 'enhanced attention to theory translation and deeper engagement with frontline action' while providing 'increased attention to a critical rethinking of what race is' (p. 129). The challenge posed by Darder and Torres to make racism a central category in our understanding of inequality becomes integral to our process. Although Yamomoto's example is an account of combining the struggles of two communities of color from a legal standpoint, the following section attempts to apply his theoretical construct to an example in education.

As an educator who tries to forge tangible relationships between theory and practice, I have found myself engaging three specific fronts: community organizations, urban public secondary schools, and the academy. Throughout the process I have been supported and debated as to what will 'work' in the three spaces in addressing issues of race and racism. Each space presents unique challenges, but can be intimately connected in developing critical race praxis. Returning to the aforementioned tenets of Ladson-Billings, naming the 'pervasive, daily reality of racism in US society' calls for an approach that is immersed in the stories and processes by which communities confront the establishment. By developing a counter story through my current work, the hope is to contribute to the existing examples of the social justice project in education.

Currently I am a member of a design team for a high school scheduled to open in the Fall of 2005, in a major urban city in the midwest region of the US. This particular city is severely segregated due to various racial tensions and historical municipal policies that have prevented certain communities of color (African-American and Latino/a in this account) from living in integrated spaces. In terms of schooling, it has resulted in a separate and unequal system of public education. Many of the schools located in African-American and Latino/a neighborhoods are grossly under-resourced, resulting in a series of concerns (i.e., poor teacher–student relationships, poor school–community relationships, low student performance, low student engagement, high student mobility rates, increasing drop-out rates, etc). The coupling of class and race are explicit in that over 85% of students served in public schools in this city are African-American and Latino/a while 65% of this population would be categorized as 'low income'. CRT and class analysis are coupled in that one cannot be present without the other in recognizing the political, social, and economic factors that influence inequality.

In reference to the current plight of urban public education, the aforementioned account is typical of many urban areas in the US. This particular situation becomes unique in that the following narrative is of two communities' attempt to forge meaningful relationships through the development of a high school. Their struggle serves as counter story aimed at developing community across racial groups in the struggle for social justice in education.

It would be incorrect in stating that African-Americans and Latino/as in this city have been historically pitted against each other. Despite tensions between both groups, there are instances where both communities have worked in concert to address political, housing, and educational concerns. However, tensions do flare in the space between communities as lines of communication are frequently strained due to language barriers, residential segregation and general unfamiliarity with each other's culture. In developing critical race praxis, both communities (one Mexican/Mexican-American, the other African-American) have made the conscious attempt to develop a college preparatory community school, serving both neighborhoods.

The story is mired in issues of race and class. First, this major city was in a major reform effort to 'revitalize the city's ailing schools'. What was not mentioned, however, was that the majority of these funds (distributed in the years 1995–2000) for secondary schools went to selective-enrollment schools for high achieving students. As selective enrollment schools were established throughout the city, most of the students were from families that would be categorized as 'middle class'. As low-income students are not present in the selective enrollment schools, a socialist critique is appropriate in recognizing the prevalence of class.

In addition, selective enrollment schools require students have to have a high composite scores upon graduation from grade school to take the admissions test for admission to selective enrollment high schools. At this juncture CRT is valuable in the analysis of system-wide racial dynamics of selective enrollment schools in addition to previously discussed class components. Despite the system's 85% African-American and Latino/a population, the majority of White students remaining in public schools are found in the selective enrollment high schools. Currently the city in question has eight selective enrollment schools out of an existing 70 high schools. All selective enrollment schools boast high college acceptance rates, active parent support networks, and high rates of teacher efficacy. Few students come from families in the 'low-income' bracket and are provided the best teachers and academic programs the system has to offer. While other high schools may have problems purchasing books and managing payroll, many of the selective enrollment schools have early college enrollment courses and faculty members with doctorate degrees.

During the same reform effort, the previously mentioned Mexican-American neighborhood was promised a non-selective enrollment, community high school to serve its students. Students would not be required to take a test for admissions and the only qualifications for attending the high school was graduation from 8th grade and residence in the neighborhoods' residential borders. To provide a show of confidence to the community, land was purchased in 1998 on which to build the high school. The central education office, along with the city's mayor, boasted the successes of the city's reform efforts. Unmentioned in popular media outlets was the neighborhoods' chronic school overcrowding and lack of resources. Currently one public high school is in the neighborhood. Because there are over 7500 high school aged students in the area, it is impossible for many students to attend their neighborhood public school. In addition to the 7500 high school students in the Mexican-American neighborhood, another 3500 African-American high school aged students live in the neighboring community. Because the neighborhood high school is bursting at the seems with a population at nearly 2200 students to serve two communities, many young people in the neighborhood have to travel considerable distances to attend other high schools with admissions slots. Again the realities of CRT and socialist critique are present in that both communities, in addition to lack of resources, are racialized, thusly receiving inadequate attention to their educational needs. They are not excluded from educational resources solely on issues of class. Instead, they are excluded because they are poor and of color.

As the reform effort progressed, two selective enrollment high schools were built and another three were scheduled to open by the fall of 2002. When members from the Mexican-American community questioned central office on the building of their high school, they were told that the funds were spent despite the city's land purchase. Appalled and disappointed, members of the Mexican-American community began to organize among themselves. The conversations were centered in the community holding the city accountable for its inability to grant the community their high school. Community meetings, receiving input from, block clubs, community development organizations, church groups, and parent organizations within schools resulted in a drastic, yet-effective form of protest to draw attention to central office's impropriety.

The meeting of the minds resulted in a hunger strike. For 19 days beginning on 13 May 2001 a group of 14 students, parents, grandparents and concerned community members went without food, protesting the denial of their high school. The hunger strike drew national attention, forcing the city to answer to the concerns of the community. After weeks of negotiations with central office, the community was granted their high school. The school will be four small schools housed in one building. The themes of the four schools are (1) social justice; (2) math, science, and technology; (3) visual and performing arts; and (4) world languages. Each school will have a population not exceeding 400 students (with the building totaling 1600 students).

The school did not come without a consent decree from central office requiring at least 30% of the school's population be African-Americans from the adjacent community. This became a challenge to the Mexican-American contingency due to lack of communication between the two neighborhoods. Where some may view this as a point of contention, many of the hunger strikers engaged the mandate understanding that the school would be for all children, not just those who live in their particular neighborhood, due to the support they received from numerous communities throughout the city. The moment is evident of CRT praxis in that the Mexican-American community demonstrated a willingness to abide by the consent decree, by actively engaging the African-American community to participate in the school design process. It should be noted that preceding the consent decree, I was called in by some of the hunger strikers that I knew in other capacities to advise the group on curriculum development. Since that time I have been selected for membership on the design team to develop the social justice high school. CRT praxis continues to inform my work in that the design team has been given the charge to support work to tally the concerns of both African-American and Mexican-American communities to forge substantive curriculum and community inclusion to the school.

Currently the hunger strikers have developed an advisory board, responsible for the final negotiations with central office in developing the high school. The advisory board has oversight of the four design teams (for each of the high schools), along with supervision responsibilities for principal selection. Critical to the process has been buy-in from the African-American community. Where many of the Mexican families have supported the process since the hunger strike, many African-Americans are new to the process and remain skeptical due to their 'mandated' participation. However, many of the community members from the African-American contingency have been supportive of the process in developing education for both groups of children. However, the advisory board has a youth committee that has remained skeptical of the process. When members of the youth committee (at this time they were comprised of Mexican-American youth) were told the high school would also have African-American students, they responded the idea would never work due to existing tensions at the existing high school. The advisory board, in taking the issues and concerns of the young people seriously are currently involved in a massive effort to mobilize parents and youth from both communities in advising the design teams (along with the advisory board) on suggestions to ease possible tensions between both communities. Again, a critical race praxis is needed to unpack the realities of two low-income, communities of color that have hesitations of collaborative efforts with each other. Praxis is developed as both communities understand the dynamics of being poor and of color in the struggle for social justice. In this sense the third tenet of CRT in education is actualized by legitimizing and promoting 'the voices and narrative of people of color as sources of critique of the dominant social order which purposely devalues them' (Ladson-Billings, 1998). Central to building community between the two groups, the advisory board has organized community meetings in Mexican-American and African-American grade schools, community centers and churches to answer questions from both communities concerning the high school.

Coupled with considerable pressure from central office to comply with various regulations and liability policies, the advisory board and design teams are under considerable pressure to create a quality high school for African-American and Latino/a students. Where central office granted the high school to the community, they have not been helpful in the process of providing technical assistance for the development of the four schools. As the case with most central offices, their primary concern is with their liabilities in regards to state and federal standards. On numerous occasions members from central office have come into advisory board meetings and made attempts at hijacking the community process, with the claim that they still have the 'final say' as to what happens with the school. As a collective, they have remained reluctant in granting community requests for deadlines, neighborhood boundaries, and proposal requests. Dates are consistently reset, central office representatives remain rude and uncooperative while community members trudge through efforts to mobilize both communities, hire principals, and develop curriculum. The task may appear ominous, but community members from both neighborhoods have remained diligent in guaranteeing a version of community education for all.

In this specific instance, socialist critique and CRT can operate synergistically, while providing necessary analysis and practice. Both epistemologies address the racialized realities of both communities as they are continually under-resourced and neglected by elements of the ruling class. For being labeled 'low-income', to the structural inequalities they experience based on race, their struggle is critical in highlighting the necessity of forging both trains of thought.

Conclusion: a call to ceasefire

As stated in the introduction, the challenge is for those members of the scholarly community that engage communities through schools is to utilize CRT where applicable. Arguing across conference tables is useless. For those of us who are concerned with the social justice project in education, our work will be done on the frontline with communities committed to change. In order to make such synergy to work both groups should understand neither race nor class exists as static phenomena. Leornardo (2004) is correct in that 'marginalized people have created rich inventories of culture, whereas race is imposed by White domination' (Leonardo, 2004, p. 491). Understanding this as a constant, the social justice project in education will require the recognition of the interplay of race and class to assess political, social, racial and economic dynamic. Doing so will require those on the side of CRT to recognize that there may be intra-racial issues that need class analysis, while not separating them from the larger construct of White supremacy. Those who engage class analysis will have to recognize the dynamics of racialization in discussions of the ruling classes, in understanding that racism is not the sole byproduct of capitalism. Instead, as demonstrated in this account, the dynamics of race inextricably identify a system of shifting hierarchies that are not married to a stringent interpretation of class analysis.

Nevertheless, I maintain the belief that documentation for the historical record informs the future group of those employed in the academy that will take the risk of recording their community engagement in spite of individual recognition and compensation. Where many would argue this to be a sabotage of the academic process, I would offer the contrary. Because we exist in a society that is systemically racist, the challenge becomes to forge community with the purpose of producing agents of change. Again, it is noted that this is not the purpose of every person employed in the academy. However, for those who speak to the 'need for change' the call has been placed to make our words bond to our actions. If we do not, the mistakes are ours.

References

Apple, M. (2000) *Official knowledge: democratic education in a conservative age* (New York, Routledge).

American Civil Rights Institute (www.acri.org).

Anderson, J. (1988) *The education of blacks in the south: 1860–1935* (Chapel Hill, NC, University of North Carolina Press).

Arimitage, P. B. (2000) *Political relationship and narrative knowledge: a critical analysis of school authoritarianism* (Westport, CN, Bergin & Garvey).

Ayers, W. & Ford, P. (Eds) (1996) *City kids, city teachers: reports from the front row* (New York, The New Press).

Ayers, W., Hunt, J. A. & Quinn, T. (1998) *Teaching for social justice* (New York, The New Press).

Bannet, E. T. (1993) *Postcultural theory: critical theory after the Marxist paradigm* (New York, Paragon House).

Bonilla-Silva, E. (1996) Rethinking racism: toward a structural interpretation, *American Sociological Review,* 62(3), 465–480.

Carbado, D. & Gulati, M. (2003) The law and economics of critical race theory, *Yale Law Journal,* 112(7), 1752–1829.

Calmore, J. (1992) Critical race theory, Archie Shepp, and fire music. Securing an authentic intellectual life in a multicultural world, *Southern California Law Review,* 65, 1–60.

Carr, W. (1995) *For education: towards critical educational inquiry* (Philadelphia, Open University Press).

Crenshaw, K., Gotanda, N., Peller, G. & Thomas, K. (1996) *Critical race theory: the key writings that formed the movement* (New York, The New Press).

Darder, A. & Torres, R. D. (Eds) (2003) *The critical pedagogy reader* (New York, Routledge Farmer).

Dixson, A. & Rousseau, C. K. (2005) And we are still not saved: critical race theory in education ten years later, *race, ethnicity, and education,* 8(1), 7–27.

Delgado, R. & Stefancic, J. (Eds) (1998) *The Latino/a condition* (New York, New York University Press).

Delpit, L. (1995) *Other people's children: cultural conflict in the classroom* (New York, The New Press).

Feagin, J. & Vera, H. (2001) *Liberation sociology* (Boulder, CO, Westview Press).

Gutierrez-Jones, C. (2001) *Critical race narratives: a study of race, rhetoric and injury* (New York, New York University Press).

Haney Lopez, I. F. (1996) *White by law: the legal construction of race* (New York, New York University Press).

Harvard Law Review Association (1986) *Essays on critical legal studies: selected from the pages of the Harvard law review* (Cambridge, MA, Harvard University Press).

Hayman, R. (1995) The color of tradition: critical race theory and postmodern constitutional traditionalism, *Harvard Civil Rights-Civil Liberties Law Review,* 30, 57–108.

Ladson-Billings, G. (1998) Just what is critical race theory and what's it doing in a nice field like education?, *International Journal of Qualitative Studies in Education,* 11(1), 7–24.

Ladson-Billings, G. & Tate, W. (1995) Toward a critical race theory of education, *Teachers College Record,* 97(1), 47–68.

Leonardo, Z. (2004) The unhappy marriage between Marxism and race critique: political economy and the production of racialized knowledge, *Policy Futures in Education,* 2(3&4), 483–493.

Lopez, G. R. (2003) The (racially neutral) politics of education: a critical race theory perspective, *Education Administration Quarterly,* 39(1), 68–87.

Makler, A. & Shangory Hubbard, R. (2000) *Teaching for justice in the social studies classroom: millions of intricate moves* (Portsmouth, NH, Heinemann Press).

Marx, K. & Engels, F. (1985) *The communist manifesto* (New York, Penguin Books).

Marsh, J. L. (1995) *Critique, action and liberation* (Albany, NY, State University of New York Press).

McLellan, D. (1977) *Karl Marx: selected writings* (Oxford, Oxford University Press).

Mills, C. (1997) *The racial contract* (Ithaca, NY, Cornell University Press).

Mills, C. (2003) *From class to race: essays in white Marxism and black radicalism* (New York, Rowman and Littlefield Publishers).

Roediger, D. (1991) *The wages of whiteness: race and the making of the American working class* (New York, Verso Publishers).

Solorzano, D. & Yosso, T. (2002) Critical race methodology: counter-storytelling as an analytical framework fro education research, *Qualitative Inquiry,* 8(1), 23–44.

Torres, C. A. (1998) Democracy, education, and multiculturalism: dilemmas of citizenship in a global world, *Comparative Education Review,* 42(4), 421–448.

Ture, K. & Hamilton, C. (1992) Black power: the politics of liberation (New York, Vintage Press).

Watkins, W. (2001) *The white architects of black education: ideology and power in America, 1865–1954* (New York, Teachers College Press).

Winant, H. (2001) *The world is a ghetto: race and democracy since World War II* (New York, Basic Books).

Woodson, C. G. (2000) *The mis-education of the negro* (Trenton, NJ, Africa World Press).

Valdes, F., McCristal Culp, J. & Harris, A. P. (Eds) (2002) *Crossroads, directions and a new critical race theory* (Philadelphia, Temple University Press).

Yamamoto, E. (1999) *Interracial justice: conflict and reconciliation in post-civil rights America* (New York, New York University Press).

Yosso, T. (2002) Towards a critical race curriculum, *Equity and Excellence in Education,* 35(2), 93–108.

Towards an interest-convergence in the education of African-American football student athletes in major college sports

Jamel K. Donnor

The purpose of this article is to advance Derrick Bell's (1992b) interest-convergence principle as an analytical lens for understanding the complex role of race in the educational experiences of African-American football student athletes. Currently, there is a scarcity of educational research that employs a critical theoretical perspective on race to address the education of African-American students in general, and student athletes in particular. This article includes American law cases that attend to the educational experiences of student athletes participating in high profile intercollegiate football programs. The inclusion of the legal literature is meant to adhere to the intellectual and methodological origins of critical race theory and to demonstrate how educational differences are institutionalized through coercion and ideology. The article concludes with a discussion of the interest-convergence principle as a means of investigating and establishing alternative strategies on behalf of the student athlete in order to improve his educational experience and academic outcomes.

Introduction

> We cannot ignore and should learn from and try to recognize situations when there is a convergence of interests. (Derrick Bell, 2000, p. 9)

The profundity of Derrick Bell's statement resides in its analytical insight given its simplicity. The above quote represents a timely mechanism for understanding the current educational experiences of African-Americans as the US celebrates the fiftieth anniversary of its Supreme Court's decision to abolish sanctioned racial segregation of public schools. Some American legal and educational scholars have come to question the impetus for the decision. Moreover, they contend that *Brown vs Board of Education* 1954 has failed to improve the education of African-Americans (and Latino Americans) collectively (see Bell, 1972, 1983, 1987, 1992a, 1992b, 1995a, 1995b, 2000, 2004; Dudziak, 1988; Ladson-Billings, 1994; Siddle-Walker, 1996; Foster,

1997). Analysis of the causes and consequences of the *Brown* decision lends support to Bell's theory of the importance of interest convergence. This article applies Bell's (2000) convergence of interest construct to a contemporary example in an effort to understand the academic experiences of African-American male scholarship football student athletes in the US.[1]

The education of African-American male student athletes in major college sports (i.e., football and men's basketball) has received a significant amount of attention in recent years. Much of this attention has focused on the graduation rates of African-American male football student athletes at the Division IA level.[2] Black males constitute the majority of student–athletes participating in Division IA football, however less than half of them graduated from college between 1996 and 2002 (NCAA, 2003). According to the National Collegiate Athletic Association (NCAA) (2003) the graduation rate for African-American males in Division I football was 49%, compared to 61% for their white counterparts during the six-year period.[3] These figures include student athletes who have either transferred schools or withdrawn from college after their junior year to pursue a professional football career in the National Football League (NFL). In addition, the NCAA (2003) findings account for student athletes admitted into academic programs such as education and engineering that require additional coursework and pre-professional training, thus extending their enrolment beyond the traditional four years.[4]

The NCAA's (2003) findings are intriguing, for they counter earlier research that indicated a positive correlation between athletic participation and academic achievement in high school regardless of race (see Braddock, 1979, 1981, 1982; Trent, 1982; Harris, 1991, 1998).[5] Moreover, the NCAA's use of a six-year scale to measure the academic outcomes of student-athletes is troubling considering five years is the maximum a student athlete can receive financial assistance from an athletic scholarship.[6] This means that in addition to graduating at a lower rate than white male student athletes, African-American student athletes, if they earn a college degree, are more likely to do so once their athletic eligibility has expired. Social activist and sociologist Harry Edwards (1984) argued that race plays a role in the education of African-American male student-athletes in three ways:

> They must contend, of course, with the connotations and social reverberations of the traditional 'dumb jock' caricature. But [B]lack student athletes are burdened also with the insidiously racist implications of the myth of 'innate [B]lack athletic superiority', and the more blatantly racist stereotype of the 'dumb Negro' condemned by racial heritage to intellectual inferiority. Under circumstances where there exists a pervasive belief in the mutual exclusivity of physical and intellectual capability. (p. 8)

The aforementioned quote suggests that the low academic outcomes and the 'Black dumb jock' caricature are the result of a disparate educational experience (Edwards, 1984, p. 8).

The purpose of this article is to advance Derrick Bell's (1992b) interest-convergence principle as an analytical lens for understanding the role of race in the educational experiences of African-American football student athletes at elite intercollegiate athletic programs within the US. Rooted in American contemporary legal studies, the interest-convergence principle is an analytical construct of critical race theory (CRT) that explains how laws and policies established to promote equality maintain the status quo. Currently, there is a scarcity of educational research that employs a critical theoretical perspective on race to address the education of African-American students in general, and student athletes in particular. By examining the fundamental relationships among ideology, culture, status and action in the education of African-American male student athletes in college football, this article will illustrate through the legal literature how race continues to serve as a 'constitutive element and an organizing principle' in determining the life chances of African-Americans within the context of education (see Winant, 2001, p. 21). Lastly, the goal of this article is to contribute to the knowledge base on the education of African-American male student athletes by expanding the current discourse on the relationship between race and education conceptually and methodologically.

To achieve this goal, I will first articulate the popular perceptions of sport in America, African-American male participation in sports, and intercollegiate athletics in the US. Next, I will briefly discuss and critique the traditional theoretical frameworks (e.g., conflict and social psychological) used to explain the educational outcomes and experiences of Black males in major college football. This step is necessary in order to highlight the gaps in the literature and justify the call for a theoretical and analytical approach that is race-centred. Thirdly, I will explain critical race theory and its use in education. This article will also include cases from the American legal literature that attend to the educational experiences of African-American male student athletes. The inclusion of the legal literature is meant to adhere to the intellectual and methodological origins of critical race theory and to demonstrate how educational differences are institutionalized through coercion and ideology. This article concludes with a discussion on the interest-convergence principle to explain the educational process of African-American male student athletes and suggest an alternative strategy to improve their academic outcomes.

Popular perceptions of sports, African-American male participation and intercollegiate athletics in the United States

Sport in America is generally seen 'as a positive and progressive racial force, an avenue of racial progress and an arena of racial harmony ... the great racial equalizer, and a leader in Civil Rights, if not a literal model for race relations in the United States' (see Hartmann, 2000, p. 232). For African-American males in particular, the dominant thought regarding their participation in sport is that it legitimately: (1) provides educational opportunities and social mobility both individually and collectively; (2) furnishes 'role models and heroes' for African-American youth, as well as leaders and spokespersons for the *race* (emphasis added); and (3) serves as a venue for 'social interaction and community building among African-Americans as well as an important symbol of racial accomplishment and a source of [racial] pride and collective identification' (Hartmann, 2000, p. 233).

Studies investigating African-American male participation in sport suggest that because of the legacy of racial discrimination in US education and occupational attainment, sports' ethos of merit and emphasis on egalitarian principles make it a more appealing and viable career option (see Rudman, 1986). Therefore, Black males participating in sports are more likely to possess aspirations for pursuing sports professionally than their white counterparts because they believe they will be treated fairly. As a result, African-American males will generally interpret their involvement in intercollegiate (and interscholastic) sports as a conduit for achieving their career aspirations.

Moreover, by being affiliated with a 'non-profit' institution like a college or university, intercollegiate athletics perpetuates the dominant perception of sport. This stands in contrast to professional athletics where money is an explicit motivating aspect (e.g., player's and coaches' salaries, and endorsements/marketing of products) on the part of all participants. Athletics connected to higher education projects 'patriotic views consistent with America's professed ideals of racial justice and equality of opportunity' because it is seen as a contributing to the school's mission of promoting physical fitness, learning the value of hard work and perseverance, and being goal-oriented (see Edwards, 1985, p. 373).

I submit that the popular perceptions of sport in the US, African-American male participation in athletics, and collegiate sports has precluded critical examinations into the possibility that these young men may be *exploited* for their athletic ability within the context of education. Usage of the term *exploited* is appropriate considering the fact that these young men are recruited and admitted to these institutions primarily because of their physical talent. Concomitantly, Black males dominate football, which in some instances generates enough revenue to financially underwrite non-revenue-producing athletic sports such as crew, swimming, tennis and golf that are overwhelmingly populated by white middle and upper class students. In other words, sports, and intercollegiate athletics in particular, have not been viewed as mechanisms that can work against the academic advancement of African-American males. It is this construction of underachievement that I explore in this article.

I contend that for African-American males who possess the physical potential or talent to participate at the level of Division IA football, education no longer only serves their interests. Rather, the Black male student athletes' educational interests converge with the interests of other individuals and his institution. In other words, while a Black male football student athlete may be interested in receiving a college education and graduating (or playing professional football), other educational stakeholders such as football coaches and institutions of higher education may be more interested in the personal (i.e., cash bonuses for meeting academic incentives) and institutional advancement gained through association with or exploitation of the physical talents of these student athletes.[7] Institutional advancement refers to the generation of revenue from the following sources: (1) television and radio contracts; (2) sale of merchandise with the institution's logo; (3) ticket sales and concessions; (4) corporate sponsorship for advertising space during events or within the stadium; and (5) rental fees charged from luxury skybox suites to wealthy fans/supporters. The advancement of a university with a highly competitive football program also translates into 'intangible benefits' such as increase in donations from alumni/a, and a rise in the number of student applications and enrollments.[8] In other words, the more successful a football program is, the more that institution is able to enhance its image and market itself as a first-rate university.

Traditional theoretical approaches to understanding the education of African-American male student athletes

Conflict theory

Traditionally, researchers have employed a conflict theoretical perspective to addresses the larger social structures within which college athletics and student-athletes operate and to explain the academic outcomes of student athletes. Conflict theorists specifically cite the commercialization of college football as the reason for the low graduation rates of Black scholarship football student-athletes (Eitzen, 2001; Gerdy, 2000; Patterson, 2000). This position asserts that the significant sums of money involved with the cost of operation and generation of revenue has created a 'win at any cost' ethos. To illustrate, the 2002–2003 total expenses for football at The Ohio State University was $14,728,966, while their total revenue for football was $52,742,278 (OSU Department of Athletics, 2003). Subsequently, the win at any cost ethos creates a culture within these athletic programs that leads coaches to place pressure on student athletes to dedicate the majority of their time to sports instead of academics. During the football season, a student athlete's weekly schedule (in addition to taking a full-time student course load) includes mandatory activities such as: practice, weight training, team meetings, position meetings, film study, treating injuries, team dinner, and travel for away events. According to Harris (2000), most participants of major intercollegiate athletics spend approximately '28 hours per week on their sport alone, 12 hours attending class per week and an additional 12 hours preparing for class per week' (p. 48).[9]

Consequently, the institutional pressure to compete annually for prestige and revenue not only defines a student athlete's existence on campus; it explicitly tells him where to concentrate his energies for the next four to five years. Furthermore, the pressure to field a successful team contributes to the academic underachievement of student athlete because it leads to the recruitment and enrolment of student athletes who may not meet the minimum academic requirements for admission. For instance, it is not uncommon for student athletes in major football programs to be admitted with SAT scores that are 200 points lower than those of their non-athletic peers (Lapchick, 1996; Eitzen, 1999). The following universities have had a student athlete to non-student athlete SAT score discrepancy of 200 points or greater: (1) Clemson University at 271; (2) Duke University at 304; (3) the University of Colorado-Boulder at 216; (4) Rice University at 382; (5) the University of Michigan-Ann Arbor at 364; (6) UCLA at 229; (7) Stanford University at 298; (8) the University of Arizona-Tucson 213; and (9) the University of Florida-Gainesville at 319 (Eitzen,

1999, p. 109). As a result, these student athletes are 'specially' admitted to universities and encouraged to enrol in 'easy' courses caught by 'sympathetic' professors who may not expect much intellectually and are more inclined to provide a less rigorous curriculum.

The conflict position also points out that in extreme instances the pressure to win has led to the outright manipulation of a student athlete's education. For example, in October of 2000, the University of Minnesota-Twin Cities athletics counselling office was found guilty by the NCAA of 'preparing approximately 400 pieces of course work at various lengths, including theme papers, homework assignments and take-home exams, for at least 18 men's basketball student–athletes' from 1994 to 1998 (Friedenthal, 2000, p. 2). The National Collegiate Athletic Association also cited the University of Southern California of engaging in 'unethical conduct-academic fraud' from the summer of 1996 to March 1998. Personnel employed in the Office of Student Athlete Academic Services, including the coordinator of tutor services, 'knowingly committed academic fraud by conducting research and substantially composing and typing portions of a paper submitted by a football student–athlete' (Friedenthal, 2000, p. 2).

Social psychological theory

The social psychological framework on the other hand, addresses the micro-level issues affecting the education of African-American male football student athletes in its acknowledgment of the role(s) of racial, gender and athletic identity. The emphasis on identity is useful because it not only speaks to the formation and uniqueness of the *athletic* identity, it also acknowledges the potential conflict between student and athletic roles. The social psychological perspective is primarily concerned with knowing 'under what social circumstances people behave in predictable ways', rather than how individuals contribute to or influence a situation (Eitzen & Sage, 1997, p. 6). As such, social psychologists contend student participants of major college sports experience a set of challenges distinct from their non-athletic peers upon matriculating to campus (Snyder, 1985; Hughes & Coakley, 1991; Parham, 1993; Watt & Moore III, 2001; Howard-Hamilton & Sina, 2001). Parham (1993) identifies the following challenges as unique to student athletes:

> (a) learning to balance academic and athletic pursuits; (b) adapting to a certain degree of isolation from social and more 'mainstream' activities; (c) managing success or lack thereof; (d) attending to their own physical health in a more deliberate way so as to minimize injury and subsequent rehabilitation; (e) satisfying multiple relationships, including those having to do with coaches, parents, friends and community; and (f) terminating an athletic career and finding other activities in which participation will bring about a very similar, if not a more heightened level of satisfaction. (p. 412)

Summarily, the social psychological framework focus is on the behaviours and attitudes of individuals who share common characteristics (Eitzen & Sage, 1997). The use of identity is an attempt to understand the similarities among student athletes regarding their academic outcomes.

Critique of traditional theories

As useful as these dominant theoretical perspectives have been for providing some understanding of the issues that contribute to the academic shortcomings of student participants in high profile football programs, the conflict and social psychological frameworks do not consider the historical and contemporary status of being the Other and an athlete in the education of African-American male student athletes. In the instance of conflict theory, its causal explanation does not reveal how Black student athletes and other educational stakeholders' (i.e., teacher, parents, peers and coaches) conscious and/or unconscious subscription to the dominant ethos of sport may contribute to academic underachievement. According to Edwards (1984):

> …as soon as someone finds that a particular [B]lack youngster can run a little faster, throw a little harder, or jump a little higher than all of his grammar school peers, that kid becomes-something 'really special'. What this usually means is that, beyond sports excellence, from that point on little else is expected of him. (p. 9)

Conflict theory's deterministic focus on the commercialization of intercollegiate football renders it unable to articulate instances in which student athletes are academically successful in spite of the pressure for athletic success.

Similarly, the social psychological framework's emphasis on sameness prohibits exploration or consideration of difference within this marginalized group. For example, because the majority of African-American student athletes that participate in Division IA football come from urban areas and lower socioeconomic backgrounds, the social psychological perspective postulates their chances at academic success are less likely. Moreover, social psychologists do not critically employ race to investigate why major college football programs heavily recruit and admit student athletes from 'property-poor' school districts that have historically failed to meet the educational needs of African-Americans (Harris, 2000, p. 47).

Furthermore, both the conflict and social psychological frameworks do not critically examine how the student athlete himself and other educational stakeholders may view the social experience of being an athlete as an adequate accomplishment. Finally, both theoretical frameworks position the student athlete as passive rather than as an active agent in the education process, therefore framing the educational experience as a static instead of a dynamic phenomenon.

A critical race theoretical approach

Critical race theory (CRT) is a theoretical position that challenges mainstream notions of race, racism and racial power in American society. Originating in part from the American critical legal studies paradigm, CRT is an intellectual and methodological perspective grounded in the particulars of social reality based on an individual's lived experiences, and his or her racial group's collective historical experiences within the US. Critical race theory rejects the following entrenched positions on racism:

> ... [colour]'blindness' to race will eliminate racism ... racism is a matter of individuals, not systems ... one can fight racism without paying attention to sexism, homophobia, economic exploitation and other forms of oppression or injustice. (Valdes *et al.*, 2002, pp. 1–2)

Critical race theory situates race at the center of its critique through the following analytical and methodological strategies: (1) incorporating the absolute centrality of history and context (Crenshaw *et al.*, 1995); (2) rejecting notions of objectivity and neutrality; (3) recognizing that racism is endemic within US society (Bell, 1995a); (4) employing a variety of theoretical traditions including feminism, Marxism, post-structuralism, and critical legal studies in order to provide a more complete analysis of raced people (Matsuda *et al.*, 1993); (5) incorporating an individual's 'experiential knowledge' in order to posit that 'reality' is situational and socially constructed (Ladson-Billings, 1998, p. 11); and (6) working towards the elimination of racial oppression, with the goal of ending all forms of oppression (Matsuda *et al.*, 1993).

What this means is that race is more than categorical differences in phenotype, motivation, attitude or socioeconomic status. CRT treats race as a social construct situated in the lived experiences of a group of people with a common history and ancestry (Haney Lopez, 1996). The reliance upon a group's historical and current social standing is essential to explaining racial inequity both collectively and individually. Critical race theory also 'provides an entrance into how large political structures [schools, universities, and sports] influence opportunity without minimizing the role of individuals as important actors in the access and opportunity process' (Tate, 2003, p. 122). According to Harrison and Malia Lawrence (2003) CRT 'exposes the inherent racism in sports and institutions of higher education' (p. 376). In short, critical race theory contends that modern racism does not occur indiscriminately (see Derrick Bell, 1999). Instead, modern racism and racial inequity is systematic because it privileges and normalizes 'cultural messages and institutional policies and practices' that function to advantage whites—both directly and indirectly.

Moreover, critical race theory provides a more thorough explanation of the complex ways one's everyday experiences as a racialized Other are permanently designed. In summary, critical race theory is able to destabilize fixed, biologically determined notions of race in legal discourse by 'privileging contextual and historical description over transhistorical or purely abstract ones' (Matsuda *et al.*, 1993, p. 3)

CRT in education

In education, scholars and researchers using critical race theory have specifically questioned the manner in which race, racism and racial power function in the schooling of African-Americans and other students of colour. For example, Ladson-Billings and Tate (1995)—the first to introduce CRT to education—posit that, unlike the theoretical considerations of gender and class which have 'proliferated [and] continue to merit considerations as theoretical models for understanding social inequity', race has been 'untheorized [and] not been systematically employed in the analysis of educational inequality' (Ladson-Billings & Tate, 1995, pp. 49–51).

Yet, Ladson-Billings and Tate (1995) point out that class and gender separately or in conjunction cannot 'account for the extraordinarily high rates of school ... failure among African-American ... males' (Ladson-Billings & Tate, 1995, p. 51).

Likewise, Parker and Lynn (2002) comment that educational research that focuses on students of colour has traditionally: (1) ignored historically marginalized groups by simply not addressing their concerns; (2) relied heavily on genetic or biological determinist perspectives to explain away complex social educational problems; and (3) 'epiphenomenized' or de-emphasized race by arguing that the problems minority students experience in schools can be understood via class or gender analyses that do not fully take race, culture, language and immigrant status into account (p. 13). For Parker and Lynn (2002), methodological questions regarding race have 'often remained unaddressed or become shrouded in a language that fails to address important questions regarding the origins, uses, and abuses of social scientific inquiry and the importance of minority representation in this enterprise' (p. 13). In instances of epistemological biases in qualitative research, CRT raises 'important questions about the control and production of knowledge—particularly knowledge about people and communities of color' by asking the researcher to reveal his or her political, intellectual/academic and personal viewpoint(s) (Ladson-Billings, 2000, p. 272).

Still in the formative stages, critical race theory in education is not about 'coloring scholarship' or replacing one discourse for another (Ladson-Billings, 2000, p. 271). Like their legal colleagues, critical race scholars in education are committed to promoting social justice in the form of equitable access to quality educational opportunities for *all* students of colour. Unfortunately, many studies in education that employ critical race theory have been totally reliant on narrative methodologies to explain the material inequities and outcome disparities in the education of African-American and other students of colour. Absent from these critical race studies is the legal literature. Inclusion of this literature would not only adhere to the roots of CRT but would also provide a richer context for explaining the educational experiences of African-American student athletes in major college sports.

The legal literature and the educational experiences of African-American male student athletes in major college sports

The American legal literature is able to provide a fuller understanding of the educational experiences of African-American male Division IA football student athletes in two ways. The first is by contextualizing their relationship to an institution of higher education and the athletic department specifically. The second is by presenting examples of personal and institutional practices that influence their educational opportunities. The American judicial system recognizes the relationship between a university or college and enrolled students as contractual (Orenstein, 1996). An institution's course catalogues, bulletins, class schedules, codes of conduct, financial aid awards, degree requirements and other policies or regulations represent contracts between the student and the university (Hilbron, 1995). Student athletes, however, have a 'special relationship' with a post secondary institution because they have been actively recruited to perform a specific function (see Johnson, 1985; Hilbron, 1995; Davis, 1996; Ornstein, 1996; Emerick, 1997; Grant, 2003). This special relationship is governed by the terms and conditions stipulated in the National Letter of Intent (NLI) and an athletic scholarship as determined by the Collegiate Commissioners Association (CCA) and the NCAA. The National Letter of Intent is an independent program recognized by the NCAA as certification of a student athlete's intent to enrol at a specific college or university for the upcoming fall academic term. Similar to the NCAA, institutions voluntarily participate in the NLI.[10]

The National Letter of Intent is a 'binding agreement' between a prospective student-athlete and a university that has offered admission in exchange for their participation in athletics for one year (CCA, 2004). A purpose of the NLI is to ensure that the signing student athlete receives financial support for their participation in intercollegiate sports. Under CAA (2004) and NCAA (2004) guidelines a student athlete is found in 'breach' of the agreement by either not attending the signing institution or enrolling at another university that participates in the National Letter of Intent program. Consequently, the student athlete is penalized by preclusion from athletic competition and is required to complete course work in residence at the latter institution for two calendar years.[11] The NLI not only compels the student athlete to attend the named institution for the forthcoming academic year or term, it also legally insures and protects the school's interest because it prohibits other universities from contacting the signed student athlete. Furthermore, if the student athlete decides to transfer to another institution, both NCAA (2004) and CCA (2004) regulations require the athlete to obtain a Qualified Release Agreement, to abrogate the binding arrangement under the NLI.

Accompanying the National Letter of Intent is a financial aid agreement or athletic scholarship denoting the specific monetary amount and instalments to be awarded upon matriculation. An athletic scholarship stipulates that in exchange for athletic participation, the institution/athletic department agrees to pay for tuition, housing, meals, books and fees of the student athlete (NCAA, 2004). The NCAA bylaws governing the administering of athletic scholarships limits its award annually or on a term-by-term basis depending on institutional policy. In other words, unlike traditional scholarships, an athletic scholarship is not automatically renewed and not allowed to exceed an academic year. This financial 'agreement' between an institution and a student athlete is non-negotiable. Of greater import is that ensuing scholarship awards are contingent upon the student athlete's physical performance, meaning that a college or university is not financially obligated to a student–athlete if an injury inhibits their participation in athletics. In essence, both the National Letter of Intent and the athletic scholarship 'impose rules and regulations upon the student athlete in excess of those ordinarily implicit in the relationship between the university and the non-athlete student' (Johnson, 1985, p. 4). Moreover, because a student athlete is bounded to a stricter contract than non-student athletes, under the expressed terms, the student athlete's physical talent and ability are the property of the institution.

Treatment of both the National Letter of Intent and an athletic scholarship as a contractual relationship between a student athlete and a university legally establishes a set of 'expressed' and 'implied' duties between both groups. Under the terms and conditions expressed by both documents the expectations for the student athlete and university are made explicit. In return for their participation in athletics the institution agrees to bear related costs. The legal case responsible for establishing this understanding as precedent is *Taylor vs Wake Forest University* of 1972.

Taylor vs Wake Forest University

In *Taylor vs Wake Forest University*, Gregg Taylor, a former football player brought suit against the school alleging breach of contract. The basis of Taylor's lawsuit was that the teams' practice interfered with his academic progress. According to the case, Taylor's grade point average at the end of the Fall semester of 1967 (which coincided with the conclusion of the football season) was a 1.0 on a 4.0 scale (p. 3). At the time of his enrolment, Wake Forest required the following grade point average(s) for enrolled students: (1) 1.35 grade point average after a student's first year; (2) 1.65 after their sophomore year; and (3) 1.85 at the end of their junior year (p. 3). Subsequently, Taylor informed the football coach that he would no longer participate in practice the following spring until his grades improved. Taylor left the football program his junior year after earning a 2.4 grade point average. As a result of Taylor's decision, the athletic department terminated his scholarship, forcing him to bear the financial expenses to continue his enrolment.

Upon earning an undergraduate degree in 1971, Taylor brought his suit against Wake Forest University citing wrongful termination of scholarship and sought recovery for the educational expenses incurred. It was Taylor's contention that the university had orally agreed that 'in the event of any conflict between educational achievement and athletic involvement, participation in athletic activities could be limited or eliminated to the extent necessary to assure reasonable academic progress' (*Taylor vs Wake Forest*, Opinion, p. 2). Unfortunately, Taylor's case was dismissed with the opinion:

> Gregg Taylor, in consideration of the [athletic] scholarship award agreed to maintain his athletic eligibility and this meant both physically and scholastically. As long as his grade average equalled or exceeded the requirements of Wake Forest, he was maintaining his scholastic eligibility for athletics. Participation in and attendance were required to maintain his physical eligibility. When he refused to do so in the absence of any injury or excuse other than to devote more time to studies, he was not complying with his contractual obligations. (*Taylor vs Wake Forest*, Opinion, p. 5).

Taylor vs Wake Forest is significant for several reasons. First, the American court system recognized the written and signed communications between a student athlete and a post secondary institution as an 'express contract', in which both parties must meet the stated obligations (Johnson, 1985, p 6). Second, as an educational matter, this case demonstrates an instance where a student athlete's educational opportunity was adversely affected by the affirmative conduct and competing interests on the part of the athletic department. In addition, it points out the mediocre academic expectations student athletes in major college sports are held to by their 'biggest' supporters. Finally, this case is useful because it illustrates how a student athlete participating in a major collegiate sport can be academically successful despite the competitive interests of the institution. Unlike the majority of students participating in Division IA football, Taylor was able to recognize that his educational interests did not converge with the competitive interests of Wake Forest University's athletic department.

Unfortunately most African-American males involved in big time college sports are unable to share Taylor's experience, because they either ignored or could not identify a convergence of interest until their contract expired. Former Creighton University basketball player Kevin Ross personifies this point.

Ross vs Creighton University

Ross vs Creighton University, 1990, is a legal case that speaks to the issue of an 'implied duty' on the part of university regarding a student athlete. Ross, a former basketball player for Creighton University, filed a lawsuit against the institution for alleged educational malpractice. Similar to medical and legal malpractice lawsuits, educational malpractice claims assert that educational institutions have an obligation to educate students in such a manner as to impart a minimum level of competence in basic subjects (Sobocinski, 1996). Underpinning a plaintiff's assertion of educational malpractice is an institution's *moral* obligation to provide an education, hence justification for the term 'implied duty'. In other words, the plaintiff's actions are peripheral in the court's determination of the quality of education offered by the college or university. Ross sued on the grounds that the university 'injured him by recruiting him to attend the school on a basketball scholarship' (p. 1).

At the time of his matriculation in 1978, the average American College Test (ACT) score for students admitted to Creighton was 23.2 points, Ross scored '9 points out of a possible 36' on the exam (p. 1). According to the complaint, Creighton knew he was not prepared academically to handle college level coursework, 'but still kept him eligible for the basketball team by recommending that he enrol in "bonehead" courses such as ceramics, marksmanship and the respective theories of basketball, track and field, and football' (p. 1). The complaint further points out that:

> Under its rules, the university would have never accepted the pursuit of this esoteric curriculum by a non-athlete. After four years, when his basketball eligibility expired, Ross had earned only 96 of the 128 credits required to graduate, maintaining a 'D' average. His reading skills were those of a seventh grader; his overall language skills, those of a fourth-grader. In order to get Ross remedial education, representatives of Creighton made arrangements for Ross to attend Chicago's Westside Preparatory School. (pp. 1–2)

Unfortunately, like the Taylor case, Ross' suit against his former institution was unsuccessful. According to the court:

> Education is an intensely collaborative process requiring the interaction of student with teacher. A good student can learn from a poor teacher; a poor student can close his mind to a good teacher. Without effort by a student, he cannot be educated. (p. 6)

In short, the court viewed Ross as integral to his education. *Ross vs Creighton*, however, is able to provide a richer or more complete understanding of the educational experiences of African-American student athletes. It reveals that, like all students, these students believe educational institutions have an obligation to educate them. This was the basis of Ross' educational malpractice claim. According to Davis (1992) educational malpractice is premised on the notion that:

> ... academic institutions have a legal obligation to instruct students in such a manner as to impact a minimal competence in basic subjects. The theory behind educational malpractice has also been described as placing a duty on schools to provide that standard of education appropriate for the particular student. (p. 61)

Finally, *Ross vs Creighton* is an illustration (albeit extreme) of how a Black male's physical talent and academic development can be manipulated for the competitive interests of other educational stakeholders.

Unlike conflict and social psychological theoretical frameworks, a critical theoretical framework rooted in the legal literature is better equipped to highlight the synergistic nature of education. In both law cases discussed, the legal literature was able to identify systematically the practices that contribute to academic shortfalls of Black male participants in intercollegiate athletics. The utility of the legal literature is derived from establishing a pattern, and providing insight into strategies that seek redress. Nevertheless, when dealing with issues of race, racism and racial power, traditional mechanisms such as the law by themselves are insufficient. The emphasis of traditional American legal discourse on equality preserves the status quo, because its purpose is to recreate and legitimate the myth of individual merit. As a result, the impact of judicial remedies is never understood in collective terms.

Critical race scholars have pointed out that American jurisprudence has historically played and continues currently to play a determinate role in much of social inequity that exists among racial groups. Moreover, race is a central force shaping the dynamics of American law. Therefore, theories that employ analytical lenses such as the market system, the pluralist tradition, identity, social role conflict, and classical and neoliberalism cannot provide a complete assessment of social disparities that impact the lived experiences of nonwhites absent a consideration of race. Thus, applying the CRT framework to the case of student athletes is informative. In particular, evaluating the educational experiences of African-American male student athletes through the interest-convergence construct is useful in investigating institutions such as universities and athletics because it exposes their limitations and contradictions. An interest-convergence examination of these *neutral* spaces also demonstrates how the low academic outcomes for this group of African-American students are not fortuitous.

The interest-convergence principle

Interest-convergence is a mode of explanation within critical race theory conceived by legal scholar and social activist Derrick Bell (the founding father of CRT). The interest-convergence principle is an analytical construct that considers the motivating factors for laws and social policies established to eradicate racial discrimination or provide remedies for racial injustice on the basis of 'merit' and 'colour-blindness'. In addition, this analytical viewpoint suggests that terms such as merit and colour-blindness serve as code words for laws and policies that secure and advance the political and economic interests of upper class whites. The interest-convergence principle is premised on a racial groups' legal history within the US. This legal history serves as a precedent or social context for demonstrating how judicial relief for racism only occurs when it directly or indirectly furthers the best interest of the nation rather than the group that suffered the injustice. Bell (1992b) contextualizes and defines the interest-convergence construct as a phenomenon that occurs:

> In the absence of overt racial discrimination of a character that shocks the public conscience, the Fourteenth Amendment, standing alone, will not authorize judicial relief providing an effective remedy for [B]lacks where the remedy sought threatens the superior societal status of middle and upper class whites. It follows that the availability of Fourteenth Amendment protection in racial cases is not actually determined by the character of harm suffered by [B]lacks or the quantum of liability against whites. Rather, racial remedies are the outward manifestations of unspoken and perhaps unconscious judicial conclusions that the remedies, if granted, will secure or advance societal interests deemed important by the upper class. Racial justice or its appearance may, from time to time, be counted among the interests deemed important by the courts and the society's policymakers. (p. 646)

Bell, a former attorney with the National Association for the Advancement of Colored People (NAACP) Legal Defense Fund during the *Civil Rights*-Desegregation-Movement, employed the interest-convergence construct to explain how the US Supreme Court reached its decision in the *Brown vs Board of Education* case of 1954 (1992a, 1993, 1995a, 2004). Bell (1992a, 1993, 1995b, 2004) argued that the *Brown* decision was not the result of America coming to terms with its democratic ideals or moral sensibilities. According to Bell (1992b):

> The *Brown* decision represented an unstated understanding that legally-sanctioned segregation no longer furthered and in fact was now harmful to the interests of those whites who make policy for the country ... The greater receptivity of the Court to the plaintiffs' arguments in *Brown* can't be explained ... by the evidentiary record in the school cases of harm done to [B]lacks by segregated schools. That evidence was controverted by experts for the states. Until *Brown*, [B]lack claims that segregated public schools were inferior had been met by orders requiring merely that facilities be made equal. Courts had been unwilling to substitute their judgments for those of the legislatures as to the wisdom of school segregation policies. The decision in *Brown* to break with its long-held position on these issues, despite the language of the opinion, can't be understood without some consideration of the decision's impact on interests other than those of long-suffering [B]lack children and their parents. *Brown*, while taking from whites the benefits of segregation...has proved a greater value to whites than [B]lacks. Certainly, it has been a great blessing to whites in policy-making positions able to benefit from the economic and political advances at home and abroad that followed abandonment of apartheid in our national law. (pp. 639–640)

For Bell (1995b), the Supreme Court was more *interested* in providing 'immediate credibility to America's struggle with communist countries to win the hearts and minds of emerging third world people' than in doing what was morally right (p. 233).

Bell contends further, that public schools were purposely selected, because they 'represented a far more compelling symbol of the evils of segregation and a far more vulnerable target than segregated railroad cars, restaurants, or restrooms' (Bell, 1995b, p. 229). Thus, under the interest-convergence principle, passage of *Brown* is best understood as 'progress' requiring the coincidence of a pressing issue, more than a commitment to justice.

Law professor Mary L Dudziak (1988) conducted a historical document analysis of formerly confidential Supreme Court memos and other classified government materials to test the validity of the interest-convergence principle, and concurred with Bell that *Brown's* passage occurred more as a matter of national interest on the part of America, rather than a remedy for past social wrongs based on race. According to Dudziak (1988):

> In the years following World War II, racial discrimination in the Unites States received increasing attention from other countries. Newspapers throughout the world carried stories about discrimination against non-white visiting foreign dignitaries, as well as against American blacks. At a time when the US hoped to reshape the postwar world in its own image, the international attention given to racial segregation was troublesome and embarrassing. The focus of American foreign policy at this point was to promote democracy and to 'contain' communism. However, the international focus on US racial problems meant that the image of American democracy was tarnished. The apparent contradictions between American political ideology and practice led to particular foreign policy difficulties with countries in Asia, Africa and Latin America. US government officials realized that their ability to sell democracy to the Third World was seriously hampered by continuing racial injustice at home

In essence, the interest-convergence construct—as articulated by Bell (1992b) and substantiated by Dudziak (1988)—not only illustrates how practices, policies, and laws designated to provide equal access and fair opportunities benefit the dominant class more than the group that suffered the racial injury. The interest-convergence principle articulates how race is an underwriting factor in most political, social and educational decisions.

Interest-convergence and African-American student athletes

Law Professor Timothy Davis (1995) applied Bell's (1992b) interest-convergence principle to explain the integration of African-Americans into major college sports. According to Davis (1995) during the early 1900s, prior to World War II, '[B]lack athletes who played for white institutions were channelled into sports such as track and field', because they did not involve the type of 'intimate physical contact' football and basketball required (p. 8). However, by the end of World War II, the practice of racial exclusion changed as a result of economic factors both inside and outside of college athletics and higher education that led to the integration of football and men's basketball. Davis (1995) posits:

> Increased commercialization of college sport was one of the most significant intrinsic factors. It resulted in African-American student–athletes gaining greater access to

> opportunities to compete. Commercialization enhanced the pressure on colleges to field winning teams. This, in turn, propelled colleges to recruit and obtain the services of the most talented student–athletes regardless of their color. While moral desire to end segregation may have prompted many to seek the integration of organized collegiate sport, the economic interests of others may have been of primary importance. (p. 100)

Assertions on the recent participation of Black males in American sports are not new. Dyson (1993) argues:

> The prohibition of athletic activity by [B]lack men in mainstream society severely limited publicly acceptable forms of displaying [B]lack physical prowess, an issue that had been politicized during slavery and whose legacy extended into the middle of the twentieth century. Hence, the potentially superior physical prowess of [B]lack men validated for many by the long tradition of slavery that built American society, helped to reinforce racist arguments about the racial regimentation of social space and the denigration of the [B]lack body as an inappropriate presence in traditions of American sport. (p. 66)

These explanations regarding African-American male involvement in collegiate sports are noteworthy, for like the Taylor and Ross cases they suggest that the reasons for the presence of African-American males are not empathic or altruistically motivated. Although there are high-profile Division IA football programs with a legacy of displaying a commitment to the academic achievement of their African-American student athletes, (e.g., The Pennsylvania State University) for the majority of Black males who participate in major football programs either earning a college degree or developing a strong academic skill-set in technology, literacy, science, numeracy, history and the humanities is unlikely.

Therefore, the application of the interest-convergence construct to examine the educational experiences of these collegiate students is timely. The interest-convergence principle in this instance is advanced as a way to highlight the past and current educational location of African-American male student-athletes. Critical race studies using the interest-convergence construct acknowledge and make linkages to the ways through which secondary education may affect the collegiate setting with regard to student academic outcomes. According to Benson (2000), much of the data on the under-achievement of African-American male football student athletes has focused on either the deficit perspective or on the 'problems within society at large suggesting that these students' underachievement may be caused in part by the way schools are structured to maintain the prevailing social and economic order' (p. 223). A greater value in using the interest-convergence construct to examine the educational experiences and academic outcomes of these Black students is learning how they make sense of their educational experience. In other words, it is a 'culturally sensitive' methodology because it pays strict attention to the internal and external processes responsible for the construction and deployment of their interests (Tillman, 2002, p. 3). Benson's (2000) study of African-American football scholarship student athletes at a Division I program reveals that the 'marginal academic performance' of the participants was a 'phenomenon created by a series of interrelated practices engaged in by all significant members of the academic setting' (e.g., peers, coaches, advisors, teachers/professors, and the student-athlete) (p. 226).

Similarly, the interest-convergence construct accounts for and incorporates the differences that exist among Black student-athletes. Thus, it provides a way of understanding differing experiences and outcomes within this particular racial group.

Concurrently, the interest-convergence principle provides proactive strategies for Black scholarship student athletes in order to align their educational interests with the self-interests of other individuals. An approach under this principle is for student athletes to acknowledge their 'property interests' in their physical ability and athletic talent. Again, the legal literature is helpful, because the US courts have acknowledged the opportunity to participate in intercollegiate athletics, specifically at the Division I level, as property. In *Regents of the University of Minnesota vs National Collegiate Athletic Association*, 1976, the United States District Court for the District of Minnesota, Fourth Division found that the NCAA did not afforded three basketball players due process. According to the case, University of Minnesota's basketball players, Philip Saunders, Michael Thompson and David Winey were found in violation of NCAA eligibility rules. The university afforded the three basketball players a due process hearing that found that they did not violate NCAA rules and should not be declared ineligible. Based on these findings, the University of Minnesota-Twin Cities refused to declare the three players ineligible. As a result, the NCAA placed the university's entire athletic department, including all teams on probation.

It was the university's contention that it had a 'superior legal duty which ... prevents it from fulfilling its [contractual] duty to the NCAA. That superior legal duty is its constitutional obligation to afford its students the rights guaranteed to them by the Fourteenth Amendment's due process clause' (p. 3). According to the University of Minnesota's *amicus* brief:

> Because participation in the basketball program at the University of Minnesota may lead to a career in professional basketball and because this participation is an important part of the student-athlete's education, the court is satisfied that if the Minnesota Supreme Court were presented with this issue it would conclude that the interest in question is a substantial property right ... The court is convinced that, on this rationale alone, the Minnesota Supreme Court would conclude that this interest is a substantial property interest ... In summary, the opportunity to participate in intercollegiate basketball at the University of Minnesota is a property right entitled to due process guarantees.

The court agreed with the university, citing that 'Minnesota would be irreparably harmed' and directed the NCAA to remove its sanctions against all University of Minnesota's teams. In this case, the university based its argument on the premise that its economic interests and those of the student athletes who participate in big-time college sports such as basketball are a form of property.

Although participation in athletics is not a constitutional right (see *Albach vs Odle*, 1976), a student is entitled to public education as a property interest that is protected by the US Constitution (see *Goss vs Lopez*, 1975). In addition, attending an institution of higher education is a property right (see *Hall vs University of Minnesota*, 1982). Simply accepting that one has entered into a binding contract with an institution is insufficient. African-American student athletes in Division IA football must recognize their 'property rights' in participation and place education at the fore. This intersection of race and property in education contributes to a better understanding of the educational experiences of these particular students. For instance, encapsulated within the 'intersectionality' of race and property is *the right to use and enjoyment* (Crenshaw, 1995; Ladson-Billings & Tate, 1995). For student athletes of African descent, rights to use and enjoyment illustrate who is most likely to reap the benefits of their participation in sport at all levels not just college. Reputation and status property refers to the practices of major football programs that exclude African-American student athletes from the larger collegial setting of the university through in-season and 'off-season' activities that diminish their status as a student.

Conclusion

Unfortunately, the majority of critical race studies in education are too preoccupied with 'telling a story' to explain the educational experiences and outcomes of African-Americans and other students of colour. The omission of the legal literature by these studies reduces their ability to identify how difference is systematically created through coercion and ideology with the participants acting either consciously or unwittingly. Exclusion of the legal literature also limits these critical race studies' capacity to ascribe a richer context because they cannot make linkages to similar social institutions. In the case of African-Americans, the legal literature is able to articulate their structural and epistemic position in American society. For example, Derrick Bell's postulation that the *Brown* decision was the result of a convergence of interest is supported by the following legal incidents that were motivated by race and white supremacy: (1) the justifications for the enslavement of Africans; (2) the US Constitutional interpretation of citizens of African descent; (3) universal white male suffrage; (4) *Dred Scott vs Sandford* 1856; and (5) the Hayes-Tilden compromise in 1876 (Bell, 2004).

More importantly, the legal literature is complementary to a narrative approach because it substantiates the 'stories' being told. Finally, the inclusion of the legal literature adheres to the intellectual and methodological origins of critical race theory. That said, critical race theory and interest convergence are intellectual and political endeavours that ask and attempt to answer the following questions surrounding access to and equity in the distribution of social resources such as education: Who gets what (e.g., placement in advanced courses)? How and why do they get these advantages? Why did someone else or another group not receive the same benefits? Why does the same group continue *not* to benefit when all things are 'equal'? Is this a historical pattern or an isolated case?

At a time when the majority of African-American males are under some form of control by the US judicial system and American society constructs and transmits the image of the Black male athlete (and entertainer) as the highest form of racial achievement (Western *et al.*, 2003), educational researchers and other social scientists need to ask new questions—questions such as how and why it is that these 'chosen' individuals collectively are under-achieving academically. Given that the majority of

African-American males that participate in Division IA football will not play the sport professionally, earning a college degree is paramount for basic social and economic participation in technological and science-based fields such as 'computers, biochemistry, food technology, bio-genetics, communications and electronics [which represent] the new sites of power, control and wealth' in an increasingly post-industrial America (Madhubuti, 1998, p. 5). Critical race theory offers a means to better recognize and more fully understand the forces that have constructed a system in which African-American athletes are cheered on the field by wealthy alumni and powerful fans while at the same time denied opportunities to earn the degree that could lead to wealth and power of their own.

Acknowledgements

A portion of this article was presented at the 2004 Annual Meeting of the American Educational Research Association in San Diego, CA, USA. The author would like to thank Gloria Ladson-Billings and William F Tate, IV for their thoughtful comments on earlier drafts of this manuscript, and also Adrienne D Dixson and Celia K Rousseau for the opportunity to contribute to this special issue of REE.

Notes

1. From henceforth referred to as interest-convergence.
2. Division IA (and Division I) is term used to classify colleges and universities that participate at the highest level of athletic performance, as well as to demarcate institutional prestige. In a more technical sense, Division IA group institutions of higher education are able to meet the following criteria as stipulated by the governing body of intercollegiate athletics in the United States—the National Collegiate Athletic Association (NCAA) (2004): (1) Provide at minimum '76.5% of the 85 grant-in-aid' to football over a 'rolling two-year period'; (2) 'Annually participate in a minimum of five regular-season home contests against Division IA opponents'; (3) 'Sponsor a minimum of 16 varsity sports with a minimum of six varsity sports for men and a minimum of eight varsity sports for women';(4) 'Annually offer a minimum of 200 athletics grant-in-aid to student athletes'; and (5) 'Be able to demonstrate on a yearly average attendance of 15,000 for all home games' (p. 4).
3. The National Collegiate Athletic Association is the governing body for America's intercollegiate programs at both public and private four-year institutions of higher education. It is responsible for establishing requirements regarding athletic scholarships, recruitment of athletes, and student athlete academic eligibility. The membership of the NCAA is divided into three categories: (1) Division I; (2) Division II; and (3) Division III. Institutions with football programs are subdivided into Division IA and Division IAA. Division IA represents highest level in terms of prestige and competition. I will use the terms Division I and Division IA interchangeably only to report statistical findings as reported by the NCAA.
4. The graduation rates for football student–athletes at less prestigious colleges and universities, and lower level(s) of athletic competition are as problematic. For example, the graduation rate for Division II African-American male football players is 34% and 45% for his White counterpart (NCAA, 2003).
5. Graduation rates are considered as an indication of the quality of education and educational opportunity provided to enrolled students (see Smith & Walker, 2001).

6. A student athlete is eligible for a fifth year of financial support if he has not played in a game during his freshmen year (red-shirt), or is able to apply for a medical, military or religious exemption.
7. For example, Ohio State University's football coach Jim Tressel's contract for the 2002 season contained scheduled payments for reaching the following academic incentives: (1) $30,000 for a graduation rate of 50%; (2) $50,000 for a graduation rate of 60%; and (3) $100,000 for a football student–athlete graduation rate of 70% (Miller, 2002). The same contract rewarded Tressel if the following percentage of scholarship athletes had a cumulative grade point average (GPA) of 3.0 or higher: (1) $20,000 for 25%; (2) $35,000 for 40%; and $50,000 for 60% (Miller, 2002). Finally, Jim Tressel's 2002 contract contained a scheduled bonus payout based on the following percentage of scholarship athletes that had annual cumulative increases: (1) $10,000 for 70%; (2) $15,000 for 80%; and (3) $25,000 for 90% (Miller, 2002).
8. Although there is no proof that substantiates that fielding a successful football team contributes to these occurrences, there is very little empirical data that completely dispels this commonly held belief.
9. Others have put the amount of time student athletes spend on athletically related activities closer to 60 hours, once 'voluntary' commitments are included.
10. Interestingly enough 57 collegiate conferences and 560 institutions—including all Division IA football programs—are members of the program (CCA, 2004).
11. According to CCA (2004) over 50 conferences and 500 institutions of higher education participate in the NLI program.

References

Albach vs Odle, 531 F.2d 983 (United States Court of Appeals for the Tenth Circuit 1976).

Bell, D. (1972) Integration: a no win policy for blacks? *Integrated Education,* September–October, 32–45.

Bell, D. (1983) Time for the teachers: putting educators back into the Brown remedy, *The Journal of Negro Education,* 52(3), 290–301.

Bell, D. (1987) *And we are not saved: the elusive quest for racial justice* (New York, Basic Books).

Bell, D. (1992a) *Faces at the bottom of the well: the permanence of racism* (New York, Basic Books).

Bell, D. (1992b) *Race, racism and American law* (Boston, Little, Brown).

Bell, D. (1995a) Racial realism, in: K. W. Crenshaw, N. Gotanda, G. Peller & K. Thomas (Ed.) *Critical race theory: the key writings that formed the movement* (New York, The New Press), 302–312.

Bell, D. (1995b) Serving two masters: integration ideals and client interests in school desegregation litigation, in: R. Delgado (Ed.) *Critical race theory: the cutting edge* (Philadelphia, Temple University Press), 228–238.

Bell, D. (1999) Revocable rights and a peoples' faith: Plessy's past in our future, *Rutgers Race & the Law Review,* 1(347), 1–9 (retrieved 1 December 2002 from LexisNexis).

Bell, D. (2000) *Brown vs Board of Education:* forty-five years after the fact, *Ohio Northern Law Review,* 26(171), 1–171 (retrieved 30 November 2002 from LexisNexis).

Bell, D. (2004) *Silent covenants: Brown vs Board of Education and the unfilled hopes for racial reform* (New York, Oxford University Press).

Benson, K. F. (2000) Constructing academic inadequacy: African-American athletes' stories, *The Journal of Higher Education,* 71(2), 223–246.

Braddock, J. H. (1979) *Academics and athletics in American high schools: some further considerations of the adolescent subculture hypothesis* (Baltimore, MD, The John Hopkins University).

Braddock, J. H. (1981) Race, athletics and educational attainment: dispelling the myths, *Youth & Society,* 12(3), 335–350.

Braddock, J. H. (1982) Academics and athletics in American high schools: some further considerations of the adolescent subculture hypothesis, *Journal of Social and Behavioral Sciences,* 28(4), 88–94.

Crenshaw, K. W. (1995) Mapping the margins: intersectionality, identity politics and violence against women of color, in: N. G. K. Crenshaw, G. Peller & K. Thomas (Ed.) *Critical race theory: the key writings that formed the movement* (New York, The New Press), 357–383.

Crenshaw, K. W., Gotanda, N., Peller, G. & Thomas, K. (1995) Introduction, in: K. W. Crenshaw, Gotanda, N., Peller, G. & Thomas, K. (Ed.) *Critical race theory: the key writings that formed the movement* (New York, The New Press), xiii–xxxii.

Davis, T. (1992) Examining educational malpractice jurisprudence: should a cause of action be created for student–athletes?, *Denver University Law Review,* 69(1), 57–96.

Davis, T. (1995) The myth of the superspade: the persistence of racism in college athletics, *Fordham Urban Law Journal,* 22, 615.

Davis, T. (1996) College athletics: testing the boundaries of contract and tort, *UC Davis Law Review,* 29, 971.

Dudziak, M. L. (1988) Desegregation as a cold war imperative, *Stanford Law Review,* 41(61), 1–61.

Dyson, M. E. (1993) *Reflecting Black: African-American cultural criticism* (Minneapolis, University of Minnesota Press).

Edwards, H. (1984) The Black 'dumb jock': an American sports tragedy, *The College Board Review,* 131, 8–13.

Edwards, H. (1985) Educating Black athletes, in: D. Chu, J. U. Segrave & B. J. Becker (Eds) *Sport and higher education* (Champaign, IL, Human Kinetics), 373–384.

Eitzen, D. S. (1999) *Fair and foul: beyond the myths and paradoxes of sport* (Lanham, MD, Rowman & Littlefield).

Eitzen, D. S. (2001) Big-time college sports: contradictions, crises and consequences, in: D. S. Eitzen (Ed.) *Sport in contemporary society: an anthology* (New York, Worth), 201–212.

Eitzen, D. S. & Sage, G. H. (1997) *Sociology of North American sport* (Boston, WCB McGraw-Hill).

Emerick, M. L. (1997) The university/student-athlete relationship: duties giving rise to a potential educational hindrance claim, *UCLA Law Review,* 44, 865.

Foster, M. (1997) *Black teachers on teaching* (New York, The New Press).

Friedenthal, J. H. (2000) *University of Minnesota, Twin Cities public infractions report.* National Collegiate Athletic Association. Available online at: www.ncaa.org/releases/makepage.cgi/infractions/2000102401in.htm (accessed 4 December 2002).

Friedenthal, J. H. (2001) *University of Southern California public infractions report.* National Collegiate Athletic Association. Available online at: www.ncaa.org (accessed 14 December 2002).

Gerdy, J. R. (2000) College athletics as good business?, in: J. R. Gerdy (Ed.) *Sports in school: the future of an institution* (New York, Teachers College Press), 42–54.

Goss vs Lopez, 419 U.S. 565 (Supreme Court of the United States 1974).

Grant, O. B. (2003) African-American college football players and the dilemma of exploitation, racism and education: a socio-economic analysis of sports law, *Whittier Law Review,* 24, 645.

Gregg F. Taylor & George J. Taylor v. Wake Forest University, 191 S.E.2d 379; 1972 N.C. App. Lexis 1651 (Court of Appeals of North Carolina 16 N.C. App. 117).

Hall v. The University of Minnesota, 530 F. Supp. 104 (United States District Court for the District of Minnesota, Fourth Division 1982).

Haney Lopez, I. F. (1996) *White by law: the legal construction of race* (New York, New York University Press).

Harris, O. (1991) Athletics and academics: contrary or complementary activities?, in G. Jarvie (Ed.) *Sport, racism, and ethnicity* (London, Falmer Press), 124–149.

Harris, O. (1998) Race, sport and future orientations, in: G. A. Sailes (Ed.) *African-Americans in sport* (New Brunswick, NJ, Transaction), 241–260.

Harris, O. (2000) African-American predominance in sport, in: D. Brooks & R. Althouse (Eds) *Racism in college athletics: the African-American athlete's experience* (Morgantown, WV, Fitness Information Technology), 37–52.

Harrison, C. K. & Malia Lawrence, S. (2003) African-American student athletes' perception of career transition in sport: a qualitative and visual elicitation, *Race ethnicity and education,* 6(4), 373–394.

Hartmann, D. (2000) Rethinking the relationships between sport and race in American culture: golden ghettos and contested terrain, *Sociology of Sport Journal,* 17, 229–253.

Hilbron, H. B. (1995) Student–athletes and judicial inconsistency: establishing a duty to educate as a means of fostering meaningful reform of intercollegiate athletics, *Northwestern University Law Review,* 89(741).

Howard-Hamilton, M. F. & Sina, J. A. (2001) How college affects student athletes, *New Directions for Student Services,* 93, 35–45.

Hughes, R. & Coakley, J. (1991) Positive deviance among athletes: the implication of overconformity to the sport ethic, *Sociology of Sport Journal,* 8, 307–325.

Johnson, D. Q. (1985) Educating misguided student athletes: an application of contract theory, *Columbia Law Review,* 85, 1–38 (retrieved 16 February 2003 from LexisNexis).

Kevin Ross vs Creighton, 740 F. Supp. 1319; 1990 U.S. Dist. Lexis 7354 (United States District Court for the Northern District of Illinois, Eastern Division 1990).

Ladson-Billings, G. (1994) *The dreamkeepers: successful teachers of African-American children* (San Francisco, Jossey-Bass Publishers).

Ladson-Billings, G. (1998) Just what is critical race theory and what's it doing in a nice field like education? *Qualitative Studies in Education,* 11(1), 7–24.

Ladson-Billings, G. (2000) Racialized discourses and ethnic epistemologies, in: N. K. Denzin & Y. S. Lincoln (Ed.) *Handbook of qualitative research* (Thousand Oaks, CA, Sage), 257–277.

Ladson-Billings, G. & Tate IV, W. F. (1995) Toward a critical race theory of education, *Teachers College Record,* 97(1), 47–68.

Lapchick, R. E. (1996) Race and college sports: a long way to go, in: R. E. Lapchick (Ed.) *Sport in society: equal opportunity or business as usual?* (Thousand Oaks, CA, Sage), 5–18.

Madhubuti, H. R. (1998) Cultural work: planting new trees with new seeds, in: M. J. Shujaa (Ed.) *Too much schooling, too little education: a paradox of Black life in White societies* (Trenton, NJ, Africa World Press), 1–6.

Matsuda, M., Lawrence III, C. R., Delgado, R. & Crenshaw, K. W. (1993) Introduction, in: M. Matsuda, C. R. Lawrence III, R. Delgado & K. W. Crenshaw (Eds) *Words that wound: critical race theory, assaultive speech and the first amendment* (Boulder, CO, Westview Press), 1–17.

Meggyesy, D. (2000) Athletes in big-time college sport, *Society,*March/April, 24–28.

Miller, R. (2002) *Successful year for Buckeyes pays off for Tressel.* Available online at: www.centralohio.com/ohiostate/stories/20021218/football/601444.html (accessed 3 February 2003).

National Collegiate Athletic Association (2003) Graduation-rates report: Division IA. Available online at: www.ncaa.org/ (accessed 8 September 2003).

Ornstein, J. K. (1996) Broken promises and broken dreams: should we hold college athletic programs accountable for breaching representations made in recruiting student-athletes?, *Seton Hall Journal of Sport Law,* 6, 641.

Parham, W. D. (1993) The intercollegiate athlete: a 1990s profile, *The Counseling Psychologist,* 21(3), 411–429.

Parker, L. & Lynn, M. (2002) What's race got to do with it? Critical race theory's conflict with and connections to qualitative research methodology and epistemology, *Qualitative Inquiry,* 8(1), 7–22.

Patterson, C. M. (2000) Athletics and the higher education marketplace, in: J. R. Gerdy (Ed.) *Sports in school: the future of an institution* (New York, Teachers College Press), 119–127.

Regents of the University of Minnesota vs National Collegiate Athletic Association, 422 F. Supp. 1158 (United States District Court for the District of Minnesota, Fourth Division 1976).

Rudman, W. J. (1986) The sport mystique in Black culture, *Sociology of Sport Journal,* 3, 305–319.

Siddle Walker, V. (1996) *Their highest potential: an African-American school community in the segregated south* (Chapel Hill, NC, The University of North Carolina Press).

Smith, R. K. & Walker, R. D. (2001) From inequity to opportunity: keeping the promises made to big-time intercollegiate student-athletes, *Nevada Law Journal,* 1(160), 1–45.

Snyder, E. E. (1985) A theoretical analysis of academic and athletic roles, *Sociology of Sport Journal,* 2, 210–217.

Sobocinski, E. J. (1996) College athletes: what is fair compensation?, *Marquette Sports Law Journal,* 7, 257–294.

Tate, W. (2003) The 'race' to theorize education: who is my neighbor?, *Qualitative Studies in Education,* 16(1), 121–126.

The Ohio State University (2002–2003) Reporting of institutional information concerning intercollegiate athletics programs. Available online at: http://ohiostatebuckeyes.collegesports.com/genrel/EADA/eada-2000.html (accessed 1 May 2004).

Tillman, L. C. (2002) Culturally sensitive research approaches: an African-American perspective, *Educational Researcher,* 31(9), 3–12.

Trent, W. T. (1982) Contributions of athletic participation in high school to adult outcomes for college and non-college trained young men, *Journal of Social and Behavioral Sciences,* 28(4), 104–112.

Valdes, F., McCristal Culp, J. & Harris, A. P. (2002) Introduction: battles waged, won and lost: critical race theory at the turn of the millennium, in: F. Valdes, J. McCristal Culp & A. P. Harris (Ed.) *Crossroads, directions and new critical race theory* (Philadelphia, Temple University Press), 1–6.

Watt, S. K. & Moore III, J. L. (2001) Who are student athletes?, *New Directions for Student Services,* 93, 7–18.

Western, B., Schinaldi, V. & Ziedenberg, J. (2003) *Education and incarceration* (Washington, D.C., Justice Policy Institute).

Winant, H. (2001) *The world is a ghetto: race and democracy since World War II* (New York, Basic Books).

Interest-divergence and the colour of cutbacks: race, recession and the undeclared war on Black children

David Gillborn

Drawing on Critical Race Theory (CRT) and illustrating with examples from the English system, the paper addresses the hidden racist dimension to contemporary education reforms and argues that this is a predictable and recurrent theme at times of economic crisis. Derrick Bell's concept of 'interest-convergence' argues that moments of racial progress are won when White power-holders perceive self-interest in accommodating the demands of minoritised groups; such moments are unusual and often short-lived. Presently, we are witnessing the reverse of this process; a period of pronounced *interest-divergence*, when White power-holders imagine that a direct advantage will accrue from the further exclusion and oppression of Black groups in society. Behind rhetoric that proclaims the need to improve educational standards for all and celebrates a commitment to closing the existing achievement gaps; in reality education reforms are being enacted that systematically disadvantage Black students and demonstrably widen educational inequalities.

Introduction

> A woman in her 30s, who was involved in the riots in north London, said: 'I think some people were there for justice for that boy who got killed. And the rest of them because of what's happening: the cuts, the government not doing the right thing. No job, no money. And the young these days need to be heard. It's got to be justice for them. (Newburn, Lewis, Addley, & Taylor, 2011)

> For me it is clear that the root cause of this mindless selfishness is the same thing that I've spoken about for years. It is a complete lack of responsibility in parts of our society. People allowed to feel that the world owes them something, that their rights outweigh their responsibilities, and that their actions do not have consequences. Well, they do have consequences. (Cameron, 2011c[1])

In August 2011, major cities in England witnessed prolonged periods of urban unrest variously described as 'uprisings' by activists but dismissed as 'mindless' violence and 'riots' by media and politicians (John, 2011). The events began – as they often have in the past – after police action left a Black man dead in the street. Legitimate and peaceful family led protests were treated with disdain; frustration led to more violent protests and disturbances spread, at first throughout London and, eventually, across England (BBC News, 2011a). Subsequent research with participants confirmed what many argued at the time that the escalation reflected widespread anger and resentment towards authority, not least because of the racist use of stop-and-search police powers and the government's withdrawal of the Educational Maintenance Allowance, a welfare payment that had helped fund disadvantaged students to stay in education beyond the legal minimum (Harrison, 2012; Lewis, Newburn, Taylor, & Ball, 2011; Newburn et al., 2011).

On occasion such extreme events can bring about a pause, even a reversal of policy as policy-makers realise that things have gone too far and that it is in everyone's interest to at least be seen to take some action to curb the extremes of racial injustice. This is what the CRT scholar Derrick Bell (1980a) described as 'interest-convergence'. Such situations are rare. Following the 2011 uprisings, policy-makers *accelerated* their reforms and used the 'riots' as yet more evidence that dramatic (Rightist) change was needed. This paper argues that the situation can be characterised as 'interest-divergence', that is, a period where White power-holders perceived an advantage in even greater race inequity. I further contend that this is a predictable and historically familiar process at times of major economic crisis, such as the global downturn sparked by the market collapse of 2008. The paper explores the nature of interest-divergence in education by examining the English case, where contemporary education reforms are having a direct and demonstrably negative impact on Black students.[2] In the first section, I outline the CRT concepts of interest-convergence and -divergence.

Policy in whose interests?

Traditional mainstream approaches to education policy tend to imagine a series of incremental steps leading towards improved attainments and ever greater degrees of equity and social inclusion. In recent decades, however, critical perspectives have become prominent, placing policy within a wider political context, often as part of a global neoliberal project of late capitalism (Apple, Kenway, & Singh, 2005; Ball, 2006; Rizvi & Lingard, 2009). Critical Race Theory (CRT) takes a complementary approach but, rather than emphasising a dominant role for social class inequities, CRT focuses primarily (though by no means exclusively) on the *racial* dynamics of social inequities and the political process. From its origins in radical US legal scholarship of the 1970s and 1980s, CRT has grown into a cross-disciplinary international movement of scholars united by their focus on understanding and resisting the operation of White supremacy as a global political force (Crenshaw, Gotanda, Peller, & Thomas,1995; Delgado & Stefancic, 2001; Zamudio, Russell, Rios, & Bridgeman, 2011). In this perspective, White supremacy is understood not in terms of the crude and obvious fascistic groups that operate at the fringe of capitalist societies but as a system of taken-for-granted beliefs and practices that saturate the everyday mundane reality of society, supporting and extending the dominant position of White people (Delgado & Stefancic, 1997; Gillborn, 2005; Leonardo, 2009):

> White supremacy is the unnamed political system that has made the modern world what it is today … the most important political system of recent global history – the system of domination by which white people have historically ruled over and, in certain important ways, continue to rule over nonwhite people – is not seen as a political system at all. It is just taken for granted; it is the background against which other systems, which we *are* to see as political, are highlighted. (Mills, 1997, pp. 1–2, original emphasis)

Interest-convergence

One of the most influential concepts in the CRT canon addresses the means by which policy is re/made through a process that balances the interests of White elites against the dangers of pushing minoritised groups to the point of rebellion. Coined by the late

African American legal scholar Derrick Bell, the concept of 'interest-convergence' can be summarised as follows:

> The interests of blacks in achieving racial equality have been accommodated only when they have converged with the interests of powerful whites. (Taylor, 1998, p. 123)

Interest-convergence points to the political and power dimensions involved in bringing about racial justice. Active and organised resistance to White supremacy plays a major role in changing the context within which White power-holders make calculations about how much race inequity is sustainable. However, the concept also highlights the uncertain nature of even the most impressive-looking victories. For example, when reviewing the key civil rights decisions of the US Supreme Court, Bell (1980a) shows how, in retrospect, these famous victories can be seen to have operated in much more complex (and ambivalent) ways than is popularly imagined. Hailed as epochal victories that would change the social landscape forever, Bell argues that their progressive impact was not only uncertain and short-lived but that, in the long run, their consequence may be to further protect the racial status quo. Bell argues (and subsequent examination of the public record supports the view) that the famous *Brown vs Board of Education* legal decision, which was hailed as ending segregated education, served the interests of the White elite by removing the most obvious and crass forms of Apartheid-style public segregation while leaving the fabric of *de facto* economic, residential and educational segregation largely untouched (Bell, 1980a; 1980b, Dudziak, 2000). In this way, the USA could continue to present itself globally as the home of democracy while engaged in a cold war struggle with the Soviet Union to win economic and political allies in Africa.

The interest-convergence principle is probably the most frequently cited concept in CRT, but it is prone to a great deal of misunderstanding. In particular, it is vital to remember that interest-convergence, as set out by Bell, does *not* envisage a rational and balanced negotiation between minoritised groups and White power-holders (where change is achieved through the mere force of reason and logic). History suggests that advances in racial justice must be won through political protest and mobilisation that create a situation where – for White interests – taking *some* action against racism becomes the lesser of two evils because an even greater loss of privilege might be risked by failure to take any action at all. For example, the Brown decision may have served certain White interests, but it is inconceivable that there would have been any such change without the civil rights protests that brought the issue to the top of the international news agenda.

Interest-divergence

It is perhaps surprising that so much attention has focused on interest-convergence (which describes an exceptional set of social and political conditions) rather than its reverse, the much more common position, where racial interests are assumed to diverge. In fact, Bell wrote of the dangers of interest-divergence in the same *Harvard Law Review* article that launched the concept of interest-convergence (Bell, 1980a). It was Lani Guinier (2004), however, who placed interest-divergence at the centre of analysis when she addressed the reasons for the failure of the Brown decision to lead to long-lasting change. Guinier argues that interest-divergence holds the key to understanding 'racism's ever-shifting yet ever-present structure' (p. 100). She views it as a powerful explanatory device in understanding how White supremacy is protected and emboldened (through the creation and manipulation of apparent interest-divergence between racial groups):

> Those most advantaged by the status quo have historically manipulated race to order social, economic, and political relations to their benefit… The racialized hierarchies that result reinforce divergences of interest among and between groups with varying social status and privilege, which the ideology of white supremacy converts into rationales for the status quo. Racism normalizes these racialized hierarchies; it diverts attention from the unequal distribution of resources and power they perpetuate. Using race as a decoy offers short-term psychological advantages to poor and working-class whites, but it also masks how much poor whites have in common with poor blacks and other people of color. (Guinier, 2004, p. 114)

Although the concept has received less attention, the global economic crisis that began in 2008 points to the particular dangers of interest-divergence, by which I mean 'a situation where White people imagine that some benefit will accrue from the further marginalization and oppression of racially minoritised groups'. Just as Bell (1980a) and Guinier (2004) highlight the important psychological benefits that poor Whites draw from their sense of racial superiority (despite their own continued economic marginalisation), so periods of economic downturn make interest-divergence an even greater threat to racial justice. When economic conditions become harder, we can hypothesise that White elites will perceive an even greater need to placate poor Whites by demonstrating the continued benefits of their whiteness (as a means of securing their loyalty to the existing structures of race and class inequality).

This form of interest-divergence is clearly evident on both sides of the Atlantic. In the UK, recent years have witnessed a campaign by politicians and the media to present the true racial victims in education as 'white working-class' children, especially boys (see Gillborn, 2010; Sveinsson, 2009). As a direct result, multicultural education programmes have been cut and special programmes targeted at supporting 'poor' white students have multiplied across the country (Gillborn, 2010). The most obvious example of interest-divergence in the USA concerns recent developments in Arizona; here the state has moved to outlaw a Raza Studies programme that demonstrated significant advances in the educational attainments of Latino/students:

> … students have outperformed all other students on the state's high stakes graduation exam and have graduated at a higher rate than their Anglo peers. In addition… students have matriculated to college at rate that is 129% greater than the national average for Chicana/o students. (Romero & Arce, 2010, p. 181)

Despite – or possibly *because* – of these outcomes, there was a vociferous campaign against multicultural education in the state. The campaign received national attention, and Raza Studies was demonised as stirring up trouble and resentment against White people:

> … when an ethnically based education, which is bad enough, transmogrifies into an ethnically based education of grievance and oppression that vilifies the United States and anyone with white skin – well, this is simply untenable. And yet this product is exactly that which goes by the name Raza Studies … (Julian, 2009)

The banning of all ethnic studies programmes in Arizona, and related moves to increase the surveillance and routine harassment of people of colour (based on the need to demonstrate their legal immigration status), amount to what Richard Delgado (1996, 2007) describes as a new form of colonialism; a policy aimed at securing ever greater control over the Latino population as a means of preventing political control shifting away from Whites as they become a numerical minority in certain states. Legal theorist George Martinez has taken these insights to a further level in the development of his 'state of nature theory' of racial oppression (2010):

> This theory posits that the dominant group tends to relate to racial minorities as if it were in a state of nature – i.e., there is a tendency to act as if there were no legal or moral constraints

> on their actions or to move to a situation where there are fewer constraints in contexts in which it deals with racial minorities. (p. 202)

According to Martinez's theory, the actions of White power-holders can be understood – and predicted – on the basis that they will tend to act in relation to their perceived 'self-interest or self-preservation' and to adopt 'an amoral perspective' when deciding on the most advantageous course of action (2012, p. 195). Hence, both interest-convergence and -divergence are wrapped together in a theory that makes sense of policy as a never-ending campaign to secure ever greater control and benefit to White power-holders. In this context, periods of economic decline and hardship represent a particular threat to the interests of racial justice; as White interests are threatened, we can predict that minoritised ethnic groups will be in the firing line. In the next section of this paper, I explore the empirical evidence that indicates the operation of interest-divergence in the past and present.

Race, recession and white supremacy

> The job losses that came with the onset of the current crash hit black and ethnic minorities harder than the national average worker. (Dorling, 2009, p. 1)

> The recession is having a further impact on the BME sector and increasing inequalities. (East of England Black and Minority Ethnic Network, n.d.)

Recessions are bad news for most people, but periods of economic hardship and contraction are especially bad news for minority ethnic groups. A clear pattern has emerged in previous recessions that is being replicated in the post-2008 downturn: historically minoritised groups suffer the negative impacts of recessions earlier, deeper and longer than the White population. This pattern is clear in unemployment data for both the USA and the UK. Black unemployment in the UK, for example, rose by more than *twice* the rate for Whites between 2008 and 2009:

> Members of the Caribbean and African community have seen unemployment levels rise by 6.9 per cent – from 13.2 per cent in the first quarter of 2008, to 20.1 per cent in the third quarter of 2009. This compares with a 2.8 per cent rise in white unemployment, up from 4.8 per cent to 7.6 per cent, over the same period. (Equality & Human Rights Commission, 2009)

These patterns of racialised economic inequalities are especially pronounced in the USA. For example, an analysis of US unemployment during recessions over the last three decades shows that White unemployment at the *worst* of times is rarely as high as Black unemployment at the *best* of times:

> The Applied Research Center analyzed statistics from the Current Population Survey over a 37-year period and found that unemployment for people of color rarely fell below even the highest, recession-level rates of white unemployment. Black unemployment was at least double that of whites for all but five of those years. (ARC, 2009, p. 14)

In one sense, therefore, Black unemployment in the States is permanently at (the equivalent of White) recession levels, and race inequities become even worse at times of widespread economic hardship. These patterns are well known and clearly supporta CRT analysis of White supremacy in general and, in particular, the operation of interest-divergence at times of economic crisis. We might predict, therefore, that a similar set of pressures would be at work in the field of education. The following sections explore this question with reference to the situation in contemporary England.

Interest-divergence and the attack on multiculturalism

> The interests of the white working class are habitually pitched against those of minority ethnic groups and immigrants, while larger social and economic structures are left out of the debate altogether ... Instead, there is a fairly consistent message that the white working class are the losers in the struggle for scarce resources, while minority ethnic groups are the winners – at the *direct expense* of the white working class. (Sveinsson, 2009, p. 5, original emphasis)

The attacks of September 2001 have had a profound effect on virtually every aspect of governmentality in societies such as the USA and the UK. In the USA, for example, Pauline Lipman (2004) has noted the use of accountability measures in education to close down critical debate and enforce a limited understanding of democracy and civic education (see also Delgado, 2003). In the UK, these processes have been given an added impetus by the London bombings of 2005. Subsequent policy has adopted an aggressively majoritarian stance that portrays minority communities as a potentially destructive influence and emphasises the need for minorities to 'integrate' while minimising disruption for the White majority (Gillborn, 2008, pp. 81–86). This shift in policy was already well underway before the 2010 general election which resulted in a Conservative/Liberal Democrat Coalition – the UK's first coalition government since the Second World War. The right-wing Conservative Party has determined the majority of the coalition's policy priorities, and the prime minister made clear his position in a speech to the Munich Security Conference. One section of the speech was widely reported in TV news broadcasts:

> Under the doctrine of state multiculturalism, we have encouraged different cultures to live separate lives, apart from each other and apart from the mainstream ... We've even tolerated these segregated communities behaving in ways that run completely counter to our values. So, when a white person holds objectionable views, racist views for instance, we rightly condemn them. But when equally unacceptable views or practices come from someone who isn't white, we've been too cautious frankly – frankly, even fearful – to stand up to them. (Cameron, 2011b)

This sound-bite neatly combined the image of 'different cultures' living outside the mainstream alongside the idea that White people are somehow the victims of a double-standard that judges them more harshly than minoritised groups. The total inaccuracy of this assertion is exposed by the fact that Cameron made no mention of a demonstration that *same day* by the English Defence League (EDL) – a violently anti-Muslim organisation – which brought the town of Luton (30 miles north of London) to a total standstill. Despite the scale of the disruption and the threatening and offensive nature of the demonstration – which, for example, included placards reading 'Disgusting pedophile (sic) Islamist sex gangs deliberately share, molest and rape our daughters' – a senior government figure dismissed the suggestion that Cameron might have tempered his speech simply 'because some people have chosen to march down a street' (BBC News, 2011b).

Education, economy and the widening of achievement gaps

> This policy is driven, like all our education policy, by our guiding moral purpose – the need to raise attainment for all children and close the gap between the richest and poorest. (Gove, 2010)

> I am disgusted by the idea that we should aim for any less for a child from a poor background than a rich one. I have contempt for the notion that we should accept narrower horizons for a black child than a white one. (Cameron, 2011a)

These quotations could not be clearer in stating the government's high aspirations for all and, in particular, their commitment to address existing achievement gaps. Despite this soaring rhetoric, however, the coalition's policies follow a path that *increases* disparities of achievement and, in the case of race inequity, amount to a war on Black children. Beneath a colour-blind rhetoric of high standards for all, the government's reforms pursue strategies that are demonstrably weighted against the interests of Black children. In this section, I will outline two of the key changes, involving reforms of school governance (the expansion of 'Academy' schools) and the assessment system (the introduction of the 'English Baccalaureate').

The academies programme

Alongside a small market in private education, schooling in England has traditionally been delivered to the vast majority of children through schools that are administered by the local authority (which answers to locally elected councillors); education funding mostly comes to authorities as a grant from central government. Successive national governments, however, have reformed educational governance to continually remove powers and funding from local authorities. The most dramatic change has come since the 2010 Conservative/Liberal Democrat Coalition came to power. The coalition has sought to rapidly expand the number of 'academy schools' to a point where they become the dominant form of schooling within the state-funded system.[3]

Academy schools were introduced by a Labour Government in 2000 (Lipsett, 2007). They are funded by a combination of private sponsorship and direct resourcing from central government. Academies have more control over their curriculum, stand entirely outside local democratic control and usually receive greater funding than comparable local schools (because their income is not top-sliced by the Local Authority in order to provide shared services such as provision for students designated as having 'special educational needs'). Originally academies were focused on areas of considerable social and economic disadvantage, but the coalition has made the expansion of academies a priority for existing schools with good inspection reports. This is highly significant because the government's own data suggest that Black students do not draw equitable rewards from attending academy schools; to add insult to injury the data were made public in the 'Equalities Impact Assessment' for the Academies Bill, that is, in the document intended to show that the reforms would *not* have an adverse equalities impact (DfE, 2010a); perhaps predictably, a subsequent reform removed the requirement to conduct such assessments (BBC News, 2012).

Figure 1 compares the achievement in the first 63 academies alongside the national average for students in each of the crude ethnic groups described in official statistics,[4] plus attainment in a specially selected 'comparison group' of schools. The Education Department describes this group of 310 local authority schools as 'in similar circumstances to Academies in that they have pupils with similar levels of prior attainment and are in similar areas of social deprivation' (DfE, 2010a, para. 10).

It is not surprising that students in academies are less likely to attain the benchmark level of achievement than their peers nationally; as already noted, the first academies served areas of higher than average social disadvantage (where achievement is generally

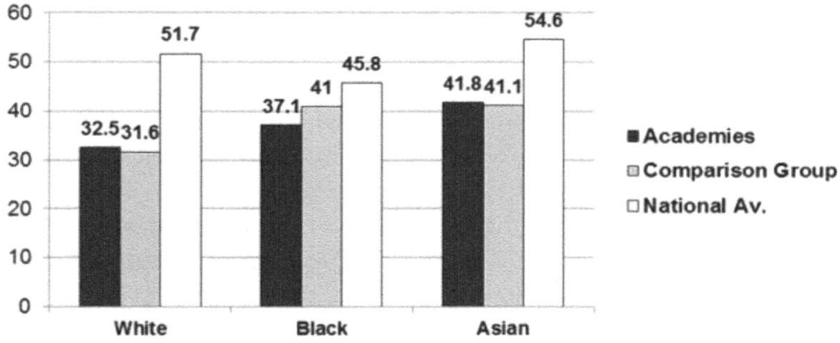

Figure 1. Achievement by Ethnic Group in Academies, Comparison Schools and Nationally: England, 2009 (percentages).
Source: Adapted from DfE (2010a: Table 2).

lower). Turning to the 'comparison group', Figure 1 shows that White and 'Asian' students were marginally more likely to attain the benchmark in academies (the difference was less than 1% point in both cases). For Black students, however, the academy students were 3.9% points *less* likely to reach the benchmark than their peers in the 'comparison group'. According to a comparison crafted by the Education Department itself, therefore, the best available evidence suggests that for Asian and White students the advantage of attending an academy is negligible, while for Black students there appears to be a clear disadvantage. Despite this shocking finding, the academy reforms went ahead unchanged.

The English Baccalaureate: how changing the assessment widens the gaps

The coalition's first set of education reform proposals, published in November 2010, introduced the 'English Baccalaureate' as a new summary measure of achievement for students at the end of their compulsory schooling. To qualify students need higher grade General Certificate of Secondary Education (GCSE) passes in a specific range of subjects: English, maths, two sciences, a modern or ancient foreign language and a humanity (history or geography).[5] The stated rationale was 'to encourage schools to offer a broad set of academic subjects to age 16, whether or not students then go down an academic or vocational route' (DfE, 2010b, p. 11). The composition of the 'E.Bacc', as it has become known, gives immediate cause for concern because only a minority of students even *enter* the requisite subjects, let alone gain pass grades in them.

According to official statistics (DfE, 2012), only around one student in five (21.6%) sit examinations in all the subjects required to qualify for the E.Bacc. These include high-status subjects (such as separate sciences) which schools often restrict to the students they judge to be 'most able'. Sometimes these judgments reflect genuine differences in achievement, but research (both quantitative and qualitative) has consistently shown that teachers' preconceptions about certain groups also play an important role, especially in relation to ethnic origin (Araujo, 2007; Bradbury, 2011; CRE, 1992; Gillborn, 2008; Gillies & Robinson, 2012; Hallam, 2002; Hallam & Toutounji, 1996; Rollock, 2007; Strand, 2012; Sukhnandan & Lee, 1998; Tikly, Haynes, Caballero, Hill, & Gillborn, 2006). Put simply, teachers' expectations of Black students tend to be systematically lower than warranted by their performance in class. These stereotypes exert a powerful influence on students' opportunities to succeed, making it less likely that they gain access to high-status courses and resulting in their being disproportionately placed in the lowest teaching groups (where they cover less of the curriculum and have a reduced chance of achieving the highest grades). As a result, all children do not have an equal chance of attaining an E.Bacc. Whereas 32.8% of Indians and 21.5% of White British students entered the full range of E.Bacc subjects, this was true of 17.3% of Pakistani and only 13% of Black Caribbean students (DfE, 2012, Table 2a).

The same stereotyping processes that restrict access to high-status courses for some groups, also depress their overall levels of attainment. Consequently, the patterns of differential access are compounded by differences in attainment. The introduction of the E.Bacc, therefore, has immediately widened inequalities of achievement between certain ethnic groups.

Figure 2 shows the different levels of achievement for students measured alternatively by the previous benchmark (five or more higher grade GCSEs including English and maths) and by the E.Bacc. The illustration shows the overall achievements of students in the largest ethnic groups, accounting for around 90% of the student population.[6] Students in every group are much less likely to attain the E.Bacc than the GCSE measure. Considering all students in state-maintained schools in 2011, the proportion of academically successful young people shifts from the previous dominant measure (overall 58.2% achieve the GCSE benchmark) to the new measure (15.4% achieved the E.Bacc). At a stroke, therefore, overall levels of achievement have been slashed from a target achieved by more than half of students to a new level achieved by less than one in six.

As Figure 2 illustrates, the impact of introducing the E.Bacc is not equally harsh on all groups. This can be seen more clearly in Table 1, which calculates the cost of the E. Bacc to each group: what we might think of as an *E.Bacc penalty* (column D). It is clear that the shift to the E.Bacc has a particularly racialised impact: the highest penalties are suffered by Black Caribbean students (where 84.3% of students successful under the old measure are excluded from E.Bacc success), followed by Bangladeshi students (83.4%), dual heritage students with White and Black Caribbean parents (81.2%) and Black African students (80.6%).

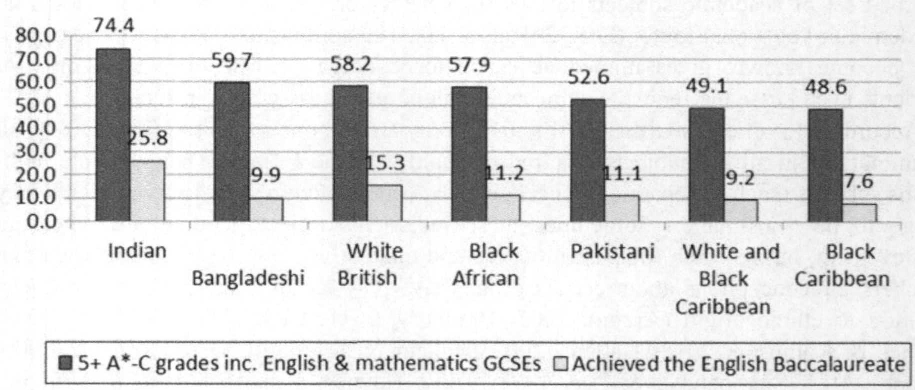

Figure 2. Two measures of pupil achievement compared: England 2011 by Ethnic Origin (percentages), all state-maintained schools.
Source: Adapted from DfE (2012: Table 1).

Table 1. The *E.Bacc Penalty*: England, 2011, by ethnic origin.

	[A] 5+ A*–C grades inc. English and maths GCSEs (%)	[B] Achieved the English Bacc. (%)	[C] Percentage point difference between GCSE and E.Bacc benchmarks	[D] E.Bacc Penalty ('C' as% of 'A')	[E] odds ratios for GCSE benchmark	[F] Odds ratios for English Bacc. benchmark
Ethnic origin						
White British	58.2	15.3	42.9	73.7	–	–
Indian	74.4	25.8	48.6	65.3	2.09	1.92
Bangladeshi	59.7	9.9	49.8	83.4	1.06	0.61
Black African	57.9	11.2	46.7	80.6	0.99	0.70
Pakistani	52.6	11.1	41.5	78.8	0.80	0.69
Mixed: White and Black Caribbean	49.1	9.2	39.9	81.2	0.69	0.56
Black Caribbean	48.6	7.6	41.0	84.3	0.68	0.46
All pupils	58.2	15.4	42.8	73.5		

Source: Data in columns 'A' and 'B' from DfE (2012: Table 1).
Note: Total for 'all pupils' includes those in ethnic groups that are not shown in the table.

Differences in achievement can also be expressed as an Odds Ratio (OR). This shows the odds of academic success for one group of students relative to the odds for another group. If the figure is *greater* than 1, the first group is *more* likely to succeed, but if the figure is *less* than 1, it indicates how much *less* likely the first group is to succeed. Table 1 details the OR for the GCSE benchmark (column E) and for the E.Bacc (column F) for each minoritised group relative to White British students. The results are clear: in each case the odds of success for minoritised groups get worse in the E.Bacc. Black Caribbean students, for example, are only around half as likely to achieve the E.Bacc as their White British counterparts.

The introduction of the E.Bacc. as an indicator of success, therefore, has a significant regressive impact on race equality in the English educational system. This move disproportionately penalises minoritised groups, especially Black Caribbean and Bangladeshi students. The prime minister's 'contempt' for those who 'accept narrower horizons for a black child than a white one' (quoted earlier) obviously does not extend to those who champion policy changes that institutionalise lower achievement for Black children compared to White ones. It could be argued, of course, that the government's 'horizons' (their *aspirations*) for Black children are as high as anyone's despite their *actions* having a clear discriminatory impact on Black youth. But these inconsistencies between policy rhetoric and policy impacts are not new, and they should not surprise us. The present government is by no means the first administration to proclaim a set of goals that are not reflected in the real-world impact of their decision-making, and we need to view this as something more significant than a case of mere hypocrisy or faulty policy-making. The reforms – by increasing the scale of race inequity in education – serve White interests and represent a clear case of interest-divergence in action.

Conclusions

> [The riots of 2011 were] an explosion of anger to police and authority in general who have let them down. Possibly the only way to be heard when they feel no one listensor does anything about their problems. (Community stakeholder, Salford. Quoted in Report for the Cabinet Office, Morrell, Scott, McNeish, & Webster, 2011, p. 33)

> We've had 50 years of carrot… Now it's time for some stick.

> We have had 50 years of the carrot – welfare, rehabilitation, social conscience and rights. It has not worked. It is now time for the stick – law, justice, discipline, individual conscience and responsibilities. (*Mail on Sunday*, 14 August 2011)

One of the most frequently cited concepts in CRT is the notion of interest-convergence, where apparently progressive reforms come about because White power-holders become convinced of a White advantage to some modicum of greater racial equality (Bell, 1980a). In this paper, I have argued for attention to be focused on the CRT concept of interest-divergence, where White power-holders perceive an advantage in pursuing even greater race inequalities in society (Bell, 1980a; Guinier, 2004). I have argued that this concept has wide application in understanding the routine shape of policy-making in societies, like the USA and UK, that are structured in racial domination. The concept has particular relevance at times of perceived threats to the well-being of White people, especially during economic downturns. On both sides of the Atlantic, Black people are known to experience the effects of economic depressions more quickly and deeply than the ethnic majority. I hypothesised that interest-divergence would also be present in education policy-making and have traced evidence of this in recent reforms to the English education system.

The widespread civil unrest in English cities during August 2011 made headline news around the world. Subsequent studies, both independently organised and government funded, undermined the official interpretation of the events as 'criminality, pure and simple' (Cameron, 2011c). But despite growing awareness of the anger and resentment that lay behind the disturbances, the government's response has been to push ahead with an educational reform programme wrapped in the rhetoric of high standards for all, but delivering even greater inequalities of achievement between White and Black students. This experience is mirrored in the economy, where Black unemployment rates have risen at twice the White unemployment rate. These patterns have clear historical precedents, and their contemporary incidence is neither accidental nor coincidental. The coalition's approach to English education reform reflects the wider processes of interest-divergence, i.e. its actions appear to embody a belief among White power-holders that a direct benefit can be drawn from even greater exclusion and oppression of minoritised groups. The quotation from the *Mail on Sunday*, above, is highly relevant. The *Mail* is the country's second largest-selling daily newspaper and by far, its most politically influential. The assertion that 'it's time for some stick' encapsulates the aggressive mood among the political elite; a mood reflected in the prime minister's assertion that White people are held to a higher moral standard than minorities, and his rejection of the 'doctrine of state multiculturalism'. At this time, the interests of minoritised groups in general, and Black people in particular, appear to be wilfully sacrificed by reforms that extend academy schools (despite their negative impact on Black student achievement) and by the introduction of a new measure of attainment, the E.Bacc., which demonstrably worsens inequality of achievement. Although these developments have occurred within the English system, there is at least *prime facie* evidence to suggest they operate internationally also. This suggests that the concept of interest-divergence has potential to inform our analysis of current inequities and our struggles to achieve greater race equity in the future.

Notes

1. Verbatim transcript, by the author, from BBC News night, TV broadcast.
2. By 'Black' I mean people who would generally self-identify in relation to that term, especially where they identify their family origins as – at least in part – in Black Africa and/or the Caribbean. In UK census categories, this would include 'Black Caribbean', 'Black African', 'Mixed: White and Black Caribbean', and 'Any Other Black' Group.
3. Although the majority of funding for academies comes directly from the national government, they enjoy freedoms usually associated with private schools and are entirely independent of local authority control. The number of academies has risen from 203 in May 2010 (when the coalition came to power) to 2309 just over two years later (BBC News, 2013).
4. The general category 'Asian' became much less prominent in official statistics from the late 1990s until the coalition's election in 2010. The category is especially unhelpful because it lumps together particularly diverse demographic groups (Indian, Pakistani, Bangladeshi) whose political, economic, cultural and educational profiles are markedly different. Indian students, for example, generally achieve above the national average, whereas Pakistani students tend to achieve below the average. For an extended analysis of Indian students' educational experiences and achievement, see Gillborn (2008), especially Chapter 7.
5. The GCSE is the dominant form of assessment for young people in England at the end of compulsory schooling, aged 16. Students are assessed for separate GCSEs in each curriculum subject that they follow throughout their secondary schooling.
6. These are the distinct ethnic census categories with a minimum of 5000 students in the annual cohort: together they account for 89.7% of the student population in 2010–2011.

References

Apple, M. W., Kenway, J., & Singh, M. (Eds.). (2005). *Globalizing education: Policies, pedagogies, and politics*. New York: Peter Lang.

Applied Research Center (ARC). (2009). *Race and recession: How inequity rigged the economy and how to change the rules*. Oakland, CA: Author.

Araujo, M. (2007). Modernising the comprehensive principle: Selection, setting and the institutionalisation of educational failure. *British Journal of Sociology of Education*, *28*(2), 241–257. doi:10.1080/01425690701192752

Ball, S. J. (2006). *Education policy and social class*. London: Routledge.

BBC News. (2011a). *England riots: Maps and timeline*. Retrieved from http://www.bbc.co.uk/news/uk-10321233

BBC News. (2011b). *Row over David Cameron multiculturalism speech timing*. Retrieved from http://www.bbc.co.uk/news/uk-politics-12376304

BBC News. (2012). *Cameron 'calls time' on labour's equality impact assessments*. Retrieved from http://www.bbc.co.uk/news/uk-politics-20400747

BBC News. (2013). *Academies could 'fuel social segregation'*. Retrieved from http://www.bbc.co.uk/news/education-20960500

Bell, D. (1980a). Brown v. Board of Education and the Interest-Convergence Dilemma. *Harvard Law Review*, *93*(3), 518–533. doi:10.2307/1340546

Bell, D. (1980b). *Race, racism and American law*. Boston, MA: Little Brown.

Bradbury, A. (2011). *Learner identities, assessment and equality in early years education* (Unpublished doctoral dissertation). Institute of Education, University of London.

Cameron, D. (2011a). *Leadership for a better Britain, Speech to the Conservative Party Conference*. London: Conservative Party. Retrieved from http://www.conservatives.com/News/Speeches/2011/10/David_Cameron_Leadership_for_a_better_Britain.aspx

Cameron, D. (2011b). *PM's speech at Munich Security Conference*. Retrieved from http://www.number10.gov.uk/news/speeches-and-transcripts/2011/02/pms-speech-at-munich-security-conference-60293

Cameron, D. (2011c). *Prime Minister's Statement to the House of Commons, 11 August 2011*. Hansard. Retrieved from http://www.publications.parliament.uk/pa/cm201011/cmhansrd/cm110811/debtext/110811-0001.htm

Commission for Racial Equality (CRE). (1992). *Set to fail? Setting and banding in secondary schools*. London: Commission for Racial Equality.

Crenshaw, K., Gotanda, N., Peller, G., & Thomas, K. (Eds.). (1995). *Critical race theory: The key writings that formed the movement*. New York: New Press.

Delgado, R. (1996). *The coming race war? And other apocalyptic tales of America after affirmative action and welfare*. London: New York University Press.

Delgado, R. (2003). *Justice at war: Civil liberties and civil rights during times of crisis*. New York: New York University Press.

Delgado, R. (2007). Rodrigo's corrido: Race, postcolonial theory, and US civil rights. *Vanderbilt Law Review*, *60*, 1689–1745.

Delgado, R., & Stefancic, J. (1997). *Critical white studies: Looking behind the mirror*. Philadelphia: Temple University Press.

Delgado, R., & Stefancic, J. (2001). *Critical race theory: An introduction*. New York: New York University Press.

Department for Education (DfE). (2010a). *The importance of teaching white paper equalities impact assessment*. London: Author.

Department for Education (DfE). (2010b). *The importance of teaching: The Schools White Paper 2010*. London: Author.

Department for Education (DfE). (2012). *GCSE and equivalent attainment by student characteristics in England, 2010/11*. London: Author.

Dorling, D. (2009). Race and the repercussions of recession. *Bulletin: Runnymede Quarterly*, 1–3.

Dudziak, M. L. (2000). Desegregation as a Cold War imperative. In R. Delgado & J. Stefancic (Eds.), *Critical White studies: Looking behind the mirror* (pp. 106–117). Philadelphia, PA: Temple University Press.

East of England Black & Minority Ethnic Network. (n.d.). *The regional race equality council partnership (RRECP)*. Retrieved from http://www.menter.org.uk/content/regional-race-equality-council-partnership-rrecp

Equality & Human Rights Commission. (2009). *Commission and GEO research shows impact of recession on equality groups*. EHRC press release. Retrieved from http://www.equalityhumanrights.com/news/2009/december/commission-and-geo-research-shows-impact-of-recession-on-equality-groups

Gillborn, D. (2005). Education policy as an act of white supremacy: Whiteness, critical race theory and education reform. *Journal of Education Policy*, *20*(4), 485–505. doi:10.1080/02680930500132346

Gillborn, D. (2008). *Racism and education: Coincidence or conspiracy?* London: Routledge.

Gillborn, D. (2010). The White working class, racism and respectability: Victims, degenerates and interest-convergence. *British Journal of Educational Studies*, *58*(1), 3–25. doi:10.1080/01425690701192752

Gillies, V., & Robinson, Y. (2012). 'Including' while excluding: Race, class and behaviour support units. *Race Ethnicity & Education*, *15*(2), 157–174. doi:10.1080/13613324.2011.578126

Gove, M. (2010, June 16). *Michael Gove to the National College Annual Conference, Birmingham*. DfE Speeches. Retrieved from http://www.education.gov.uk/inthenews/speeches/a0061371/michael-gove-to-the-national-college-annual-conference-birmingham

Guinier, L. (2004). From racial liberalism to racial literacy: Brown v. Board of Education and the interest-divergence dilemma. *Journal of American History*, *91*(1), 92–118. doi:10.2307/3659616

Hallam, S. (2002). *Ability grouping in schools: A literature review*. London: Institute of Education, University of London.

Hallam, S., & Toutounji, I. (1996). *What do we know about the grouping of pupils by ability? A Research Review*. London: Institute of Education, University of London.

Harrison, A. (2012). *More teenagers Neet – not in work or education*. Retrieved from http://www.bbc.co.uk/news/education-18623398

John, G. (2011). *Black, Asian, minority ethnic communities and inner city riots*. Retrieved from http://www.gusjohn.com/2011/11/black-asian-minority-ethnic-and-refugee-communities-and-inner-city-riots/

Julian, L. (2009). 'Raza studies' defy American values, *CBS News Opinion*. Retrieved from http://www.cbsnews.com/2100-215_162-4227721.html

Leonardo, Z. (2009). *Race, Whiteness, and education*. London: Routledge.

Lewis, P., Newburn, T., Taylor, M., & Ball, J. (2011, December 5). Rioters say anger with police fuelled summer unrest: Reading the riots. *The Guardian*. Retrieved from http://www.guardian.co.uk/uk/series/reading-the-riots

Lipman, P. (2004, March). Education accountability and repression of democracy Post-9/11, *Journal for Critical Education Policy Studies*, *2*(1), 1–39. Retrieved from http://www.jceps.com/?pageID=article&articleID=23

Lipsett, A. (2007, November 13). What are academy schools? *The Guardian*, http://www.guardian.co.uk/education/2007/nov/13/newschools.schools

Mail on Sunday (2011, August 14). We've had 50 years of carrot … Now it's time for some stick. Retrieved from http://www.dailymail.co.uk/debate/article-2025816/UK-riots-Weve-50-years-carrot–time-stick.html

Martinez, G. A. (2010). Race, American law and the state of nature. *West Virginia Law Review*, *112*, 799–838.

Martinez, G. A. (2012). Arizona, immigration, and Latinos: The epistemology of Whiteness, the geography of race, interest convergence, and the view from the perspective of critical theory. *Arizona State Law Journal*, *44*, 175–211.

Mills, C. W. (1997). *The racial contract*. London: Cornell University Press.

Morrell, G., Scott, S., McNeish, D., & Webster, S. (2011). *The August riots in England: Understanding the involvement of young people*. Report for the Cabinet Office. London: NatCen.

Newburn, T., Lewis, P., Addley, E., & Taylor, M. (2011). 'David Cameron, the Queen and the rioters' sense of injustice': Reading the Riots. *The Guardian*. Retrieved from http://www.guardian.co.uk/uk/2011/dec/05/cameron-queen-injustice-english-rioters

Rizvi, F., & Lingard, B. (2009). *Globalizing education policy*. London: Routledge.

Rollock, N. (2007). *Failure by any other name? Educational policy and the continuing struggle for Black academic success*. London: Runnymede Trust.
Romero, A., & Arce, M. S. (2010). Culture as a resource: Critically compassionate intellectualism and its struggle against racism, fascism, and intellectual apartheid in Arizona. *Hamline Journal of Public Law and Policy, 31*, 179–217.
Strand, S. (2012). The White British–Black Caribbean achievement gap: Tests, tiers and teacher expectations. *British Educational Research Journal, 38*(1), 75–101. doi:10.1080/01411926.2010.526702
Sukhnandan, L., & Lee, B. (1998). *Streaming, setting and grouping by ability*. Slough: NFER.
Sveinsson, K. P. (Ed.). (2009). *Who cares about the White working class?* London: Runnymede Trust.
Taylor, E. (1998). A primer on critical race theory. *The Journal of Blacks in Higher Education, 19*, 122–124. doi:10.2307/2998940
Tikly, L., Haynes, J., Caballero, C., Hill, J., & Gillborn, D. (2006). *Evaluation of aiming high: African Caribbean achievement project*. Research Report RR801. London: DfES.
Zamudio, M. M., Russell, C., Rios, F. A., & Bridgeman, J. L. (2011). *Critical race theory matters: Education and ideology*. London: Routledge.

"I don't think I'm a racist": Critical Race Theory, teacher attitudes, and structural racism

Sabina E. Vaught and Angelina E. Castagno

This article is an ethnographic examination of teacher attitudes towards race, racism, and White privilege in response to anti-bias in-service trainings in two major U.S. urban school districts through the theoretical lens of Critical Race Theory. We employ the analytic tools of Whiteness as property to make sense of the messages teachers perceived and developed about race and racism. Further, we examine what teacher attitudes reveal about the structural dimensions of racial inequity in schooling and achievement. We argue that the racial attitudes expressed by teachers in this study are illustrative of larger structural racism that both informs and is reinforced by these attitudes and their manifestation in practice.

In attempting to understand the racialized components of schooling and achievement, scholars have recently examined teacher attitudes in relation to race (Kailin 1999; King 1991; Ladson-Billings 2000a). To complement and extend this good work, we examine teacher attitudes towards Whiteness and White privilege in two major urban school districts through the theoretical lens of Critical Race Theory. Specifically, we focus on the racialized responses of both White teachers and teachers of color to anti-bias or anti-racist in-service teacher trainings in both districts. In this context, we ask the following questions: (1) what messages about the nature of race and racism did teachers take from the trainings, (2) what structural limitations do these messages reflect, and (3) how does Harris' (1993) concept of Whiteness as property illuminate the relationship between the individuals and the structure, between equality and equity? Our data indicated that the messages teachers took and also created from the trainings were grouped under three interconnected themes: White privilege, individualism, and cultural awareness. So, in response to our questions, we argue that these thematically-grouped racial attitudes expressed by teachers in this study are illustrative of larger structural racism that both informs and is reinforced by these attitudes and their manifestation in practice. Importantly, we will share and analyze teachers' reactions to the trainings; we are not making evaluative claims about the effectiveness of the trainings from our own perspectives. Here, we are mainly interested in teachers' perceptions of the trainings and how teachers, as agents of action in the classroom and with children, reacted in racialized ways to what they perceived they learned in the trainings. In leveling a structural critique through analysis of teacher reactions, we do not imply that teachers should not be accountable for creating equitable classrooms, nor do we suggest that there is no room for investigating both best (Ladson-Billings 1994) and worst practices (Ferguson 2001;

Valenzuela 1999). Rather, the purpose of this article is twofold: first, to employ the analytic tools of Whiteness as property to make sense of the messages teachers perceive about race and racism; and, second, to examine what teacher attitudes reveal to us about the structural dimensions of racial inequity in schooling and achievement (Gillborn, 2005).

Critical Race Theory, Whiteness, and structural racism

We turn shortly to a description of the district trainings and to teacher responses to these trainings in order to engage a Critical Race Theory (CRT) structural analysis of racism. First, however, we introduce CRT, our general theoretical framework, and specifically Harris' concept of Whiteness as property, which we use to analyze our data. Critical Race Theory operates on three basic premises: that racism is pervasive; that racism is permanent; and that racism must be challenged (Bell 1992; Bernal 2002; Crenshaw, Gotanda, Peller, and Thomas 1995; Delgado and Stefancic 2001; Ladson-Billings and Tate 1995; Lynn, Yosso, Solórzano, and Parker 2002; Tate 1997). Central to CRT is the notion that racism is a pervasive, systemic condition, not merely an individual pathology. Racism is a vast system that structures our institutions and our relationships. Second, racism adapts to socio-cultural changes by altering its expression, but it never diminishes or disappears. Finally, critical race theorists hold that scholarship that challenges social inequities must take into account systemic racism and must counter positivist notions of neutral, colorblind inquiry. Throughout this article, we will frame the teacher and administrator responses to the district trainings with CRT in order to examine the ways in which participants' reactions to the concepts promoted in the trainings *both* illuminated their understandings and experiences of race and racism *and* reflected the larger socio-cultural racial structures that informed their thinking (Ladson-Billings 2000b).

Although a number of analytic tools have developed out of CRT (i.e. interest convergence, empathic fallacy, and so on), we draw specifically on the concept of Whiteness as property (Harris 1993). Harris explains Whiteness as property as, in part, the 'legitimation of expectations of power and control that enshrine the status quo as a neutral baseline, while masking the maintenance of white privilege and domination' (p. 1715). Whiteness as property is a concept that reflects the conflation of Whiteness with the exclusive rights to freedom, to the enjoyment of certain privileges, and to the ability to draw advantage from these rights. As Harris explains, it came to be that individuals owned their Whiteness and the associated rights of freedom and privilege, both of which were expected and protected by the structural collapse of property and rights. She describes this collapse by noting that 'to be identified as white' was 'to have the property of being white. Whiteness was the characteristic, the attribute, the property of free human beings' (1993, 1721). This characteristic was transformed by legal and societal structural practice: 'According whiteness actual legal status converted an aspect of identity into an external object of property, moving whiteness from privileged identity to a vested interest' (1993, 1725). In this way, individual White persons came to exercise, benefit from, and mutually create and recreate a larger structural system of collective, institutional White privilege. The societal systems that sustain the reign of White race privilege are peopled and the concurrent, interactive acts of individuals and systems inexorably reinforce and entrench pervasive racial power across institutions, sites, and events.

Methodologies and research contexts

The data for this article are drawn from two separate ethnographic studies. During the 2002–2003 school year, Vaught undertook a multi-site ethnographic study of racism and the achievement gap in a West Coast urban district she calls Jericho (Vaught 2006). And, in

2004–2005, Castagno conducted a multi-sited ethnographic investigation of multicultural education in Zion, an urban district located in the Rocky Mountain region (Castagno 2006). Data for both studies were collected through formal and informal interviews, observation, and participation in Jericho and Zion. For the purposes of this article, we draw primarily on interview data with teachers and administrators across the districts. It is important to note that we not only identified participants racially, but were raced by participants in the context of these interviews and observations. Castagno was consistently raced White, while Vaught was raced in shifting ways depending on the racial, cultural, and political locations of the participant. Significanlty, White participants regularly assumed a shared racial identity with Vaught.

Both studies draw on critical methodologies (Anderson 1989; Anyon 1997; Carspecken and Walford 2001; Fine and Weis 1998) and critical feminist approaches (Foster 1996; Luttrell 1997; Stacey 1988) to ethnography, which make central to their practice and purpose the challenging of societal power inequities. In particular, many scholars from these theoretical and methodological traditions have suggested that ethnographic scholarship tells the story of a particular, local setting, but that it also has implications for the larger, national, cultural system from which the localized practices emerge. This attention to the reinforcing processes between individual actions and expressions and societal structures is essential to our work for two reasons: first, we are able to ethically challenge racist structures without suggesting that local individuals or organizations are unique or are simply and singularly culpable; and, second, we are able to adhere to the core assertion of CRT that racism is not merely an individual pathology, but a cultural system which is played out in our institutions – here, schools (Lawrence 1993).

The Jericho and Zion Public School districts are two large urban systems with racially diverse student populations. The racial breakdown of the student population in the Jericho Public School district was as follows: 23% African American; 40% White; 23% Asian American/Pacific Islander; 11% Chicano/a and Latino/a; and 3% First Nation. The certified staff in Jericho were: 10% African American; 78% White; 9% Asian American/Pacific Islander; 2% Chicano/a and Latino/a; and 1% First Nation. In Zion 4% of students were African American, 48% were White, 10% Asian American/Pacific Islander, 35% were Chicano/a and Latino/a, and 2% were First Nation.[1] While over 50% of students in Zion are students of color, less than 10% of the certified staff in the district identify as such. In both Jericho and Zion there were persistent racialized achievement gaps. In the spring of 2003 in Jericho, that achievement gap appeared as follows: while over 70% of White students were passing the single, high-stakes test soon to be tied to graduation, 92% of African American children were failing it; on a 9th grade standardized test used as a student competency measure of the district's high-stakes standards, 51% of Black, 66.7% of Samoan, and only 9.8% of White children were below standard; and the expulsion rate for Black students was triple that for Whites. In Zion, similar gaps existed. While White and Asian American students scored over 80% on the district's Criterion Reference Test in both Math and Language Arts, for example, all other racialized student groups scored an average of below 60%. In both districts, there existed vast racialized differences in GPA, enrollment in honors, graduation rates, SAT scores, and disciplinary action.

Partly in response to these gaps and to the attendant publicity and pressure, both districts adopted professional developments aimed at increasing racial, ethnic, and cultural awareness among teachers and administrators in hopes of alleviating the achievement gap. In the 2002–2003 school year, Jericho Public School's senior leadership contracted an outside organization to deliver a district-wide, anti-bias, teacher and administrator training. Like many districts nationwide, Jericho Public School was under pressure both from federal policy mandates and public concern to raise test scores and close the proverbial achievement gap. The intention of the program, as explained by the central leadership of Jericho Public School, was to address the racialized achievement gap by creating greater awareness and understanding of race, racism, and cultural difference amongst teachers and administrators. Although participation was not mandated through negotiations with the teachers' union, all teachers were asked to attend and were offered typical in-service compensation. Attendance was high and widespread throughout the year. The training in Zion was developed and delivered by a different organization than the one in Jericho, but it was similar in that it focused on cultural difference and awareness. The Zion district administration implemented this professional development training as part of a multicultural education policy, which was created largely in response to community pressure to better meet the needs of students of color in the district. The training was voluntary and participation was not expected; consequently, very few teachers throughout the district attended.

Because these training programs were not unlike many other 'diversity' workshops implemented in other districts across the country and aimed at altering teacher bias, participant responses reveal critical insight not only into the particular workings of these trainings, but into the dilemma of districts relying on professional development to close a racialized achievement gap that is structural in nature. In other words, we suggest that there is an inherent and problematic tension in attempting to address a systemic and structural problem (in this case, the achievement gap) solely through individual transformation. A Whiteness as property analysis of participant responses to the trainings allows those responses to serve as a window through which to view the tension between the individual and structural in efforts to challenge racism. As will become clear through our data analysis and discussion, this awkward pairing of a structural problem with an individual solution is *both* illustrative of the entrenchment of race and racism in the United States *and* fails to result in greater equity in schools.

In the following pages, we examine a range of participant narratives and begin to connect them to the structural dimension of racial awareness and understanding. First, we explore data that narrate participant self-perceptions as both individuals and members of racial groups, highlighting the structural implications of divergent self-perceptions. Second, we examine teacher responses to the concept of White privilege. And, third, we highlight the messages teachers took from the trainings regarding the importance of cultural awareness. Throughout this discussion, our data will reveal the specific components of Whiteness as property. We close with a discussion of the implications of using teacher attitudes as a window onto structural racial inequity and, specifically, the role of White privilege and awareness in challenging structural inequities.

'That wasn't the point': White privilege and individualism

In Jericho, many participants responded to the trainings by talking about the concept of White privilege (Fine 1997; Lee 2005; McIntosh 1988). Among White participants, definitions of White privilege varied. One typical understanding of the concept is captured in the conversation that follows. In this conversation, a White female teacher was discussing her ancestors and their role, or lack thereof, in slavery:

> Teacher: So, I'm sorry that that happened. I'm sorry that in Bosnia, when the Croatians and the Serbians and all those people were fighting that they were committing genocide, but you know what? Just because I'm of those nationalities, doesn't mean that I did it. Or that I believe in it any more than they personally believe in it. Ok. Now they would say that's White denial. That's me not, just not acknowledging that I have White privilege, because I am White.

Vaught: How do you see that privil—
Teacher: White privilege is being able to go into a restaurant ... and not even care who's in the restaurant cause you know nobody's gonna be attacking your race.

Significantly, in this exchange this teacher initially dismantled the structural component of White privilege by defining White privilege as an individual benefit drawn only from individual actions. The teacher positioned race, ethnicity, and national origin as interchangeable. Then she suggested that the resulting conglomerate identity accrued power (and so responsibility) through action and history. Being of Slavic decent, she argued, did not make her any more culpable of atrocities in Serbia than being White made her accountable for slavery. Here, she cast race as historical and national (Gotanda 1995; Winant 2001) and as such defined a Whiteness that only benefited from privilege resulting from direct participation in historical atrocities. By doing so, she distanced herself from the larger societal power structures that continuously (as opposed to historically) and mutually reinforce the privileges of individual Whites. When Vaught began to ask her about her mention of White privilege, she illustrated it as the ability to function freely in society. While this statement acknowledged more explicitly that there are differences in experience based on race, which are not bound by personal choices to participate in genocide, for example, it still perpetuated a normative notion of individual Whiteness. She did not suggest, for example, who might be in a restaurant attacking a person of color on the basis of race. Instead, Whites are positioned as free of attack. This is the discursive extent of their privilege. Similarly, other White teachers discussed not being followed by security or clerks in department stores as illustrative of the benefits of White privilege. While these examples were perhaps accurate, they were limited to a narrow understanding of stereotypes and how those stereotypes affected individuals. But more importantly, these understandings of White privilege simply addressed the ability to be free of scrutiny and did not capture even a nascent understanding of the ways in which power over others (not freedom from attack) benefits Whites individually and collectively.

As Vaught spoke with White teachers at Martin Luther King High School (MLKHS) about the training in Jericho, 'White privilege' consistently emerged as a catchphrase for their understanding of the awareness they should have around issues of racism. In her characterization of White privilege, McIntosh (1988) acknowledges that racism is not defined singularly by personal bias or hostility, but by systemic, 'arbitrarily-awarded' (p. 12) privilege unrecognized by benefiting Whites. However, the central thrust of McIntosh's oft-cited piece is awareness. Whether her intention or not, the common use of White privilege now makes salient two characteristics: its purported invisibility; and, the importance of being *individually aware* of privilege. In the context of this study, these definitional emphases were expressed repeatedly in White teacher conceptualizations of White privilege. Because so many White teachers consistently relied on such definitions, racial power (and so racism) was never truly engaged as a structural phenomenon. Relegated to the personal, White racial privilege failed to conceptually shift the focus to racial power inequities that structure institutions of schooling and the racial pattern of student school failure.

The concept of White privilege did not even enter the discourse of White teachers in Zion. The ways in which they articulated their understanding of the achievement gap and multiculturalism stopped with cultural difference and did not extend to conversations about racial power and privilege. Significantly, there was no evidence that White teachers in Zion were familiar with notions of White privilege or power. Out of the many teachers and administrators Castagno interviewed, only one teacher, a male teacher of color, referenced the notion of White privilege. He explained that the concept arose in education courses he took with other district teachers at the local university:

> I mean I noticed a lot of, well, I mean, a lot of our teachers here are Caucasian. Um, they were very resistant to some of the ah, I can't remember what it was called. They were offended by ah, I think it was White privileges is how it was ah, termed … Oh, but yeah, there were some good, I thought interesting things that came up but we kind of just glossed over them because they offended people or they got, you know, they wouldn't accept that is the way things are. They said, I'm not like that. And that wasn't the point … it's the point that you have to understand that is how some people feel.

His primary perception was that White teachers were resistant to notions of their own racialized power. Notably, White teachers' objections that they were 'not like that' obscured the structural nature of White privilege, even as those White teachers exercised tremendous collective power in shutting down a conversation about race.

According to many teachers in Jericho, the notion of White privilege was central to much of the anti-bias professional development training; consequently, it became a common topic during interviews. While a couple of White teachers in Jericho communicated to Vaught a desire to understand and embrace the racial power concepts they described as learning through the trainings, most White teachers expressed a resistance to the concept of White privilege. The following conversation between Vaught and a White, female teacher focused explicitly on one of the recent trainings this teacher had attended. The teacher raised the issue of White privilege and Vaught asked if that teacher believed she experienced White privilege within Martin Luther King High School:

> Absolutely not … if I discipline a student, and they know it's [me]. If [I] had Black skin they would just say, okay, this is correct. [I don't] have Black skin, so they wonder what went on. And second guess me.

In a separate interview about the concepts related to the training, a different White, female teacher echoed this idea that White privilege did not function within the high school:

> I think it's probably because there's actually no, there's no power here. You know what I mean? In other words, like I'm not, I mean, by power I mean like, really power power … Like, you're outta here. Bye. Type power that I'm talkin' about. And I don't think that there's that type of of power here.

A third teacher, a White male teaching in the same high school, also repeated this perception of White privilege. When Vaught asked if he thought White privilege operated within Martin Luther King High School, he replied:

> Oh, oh. Uhm, I, I'd be surprised. Uhm, and not through my perception. You know, I mean, it's like, you know, we're, they're more White teachers here than other teachers. *But*, we're in a school which is mostly minority – Afro-American, Samoan, you now, uh, Asian. Uhm, and, being in such a school, with, uhm, the emphasis being on, uhm, Afro-American kids, minority, things like that, I don't see that as prevalent as maybe in a, an all-White school with, you know, token Black teachers there, or something.

These denials of the existence or function of White privilege – of systemic, racialized power not solely individually created and enacted – were common among many White teachers at MLKHS. Significantly, embedded in these dismissals of systemic race privilege was a belief that racial dynamics were defined by the isolated numerical presence of one race or another in a specific location, not on societal power, and motivated by nothing more than sheer volume. These assumptions illuminate the complexity of addressing racial power in our cities' most struggling schools, which are often peopled predominantly by students of color and White teachers. Unable to recognize that White racial power permeates every institution, teachers fail to understand how race and racism inform low student achievement, among other factors.

This perception was echoed in Zion, where a White female teacher discussed with Castagno her belief that the absence of institutionalized racism at her school had to do with the numerical majority of students of color in the building:

> [Birch] is maybe not the interesting place to be, to find out a take on ethnicity and views of ethnicity. Perhaps the place to be is a place where – well, like minorities are a majority here. Maybe here is not the place to reveal institutional racism. Because it's not um, if there is institutional racism going on, it wouldn't reveal itself in a school where the minority are the majority. It would reveal itself in a school where the minority are the minority. The minority *are* the minority. Because it's a Federal designation of what minority is. In fact I freaked out the first time when I looked at um, there's a column that the Federal Government tracks and it says the language claimed is the first language and then on the spreadsheet it says whether they are a minority or they are not a minority. And then I went, wait, ok so minority means non-white? That's what minority means. Ok, I kind of freaked out on that.

White privilege, and institutionalized racism, was understood by teachers in Jericho and Zion as contingent upon local context and so was cast as an entirely individual experience. They communicated no recognition that their privilege moved with them from context to context and that their authority as White teachers of children of color was highly powerful and determinative (Delpit 1988). And, they seemed unaware of the fact that White institutions create power hierarchies with or without the immediate presence of White students (Fine 1997; Fordham 1996; Lipman 2004). As one mixed White/First Nation female teacher suggested to Vaught, 'I think that all Whites don't understand the fact that they're privileged because they are White.'

Using Whiteness as property (Harris 1995) as a theoretical lens through which to examine the concept of White privilege helps us to understand why the concept of White privilege is limited and perhaps ineffective. Harris explains that historically Whiteness became conflated with property in a legal and societal system in which rights were achieved through individual ownership. Whiteness has become singularly inseparable from humanity, individuality, and personal freedom. Accordingly, these White teachers understood White privilege as singularly an individual experience and failed to recognize its systemic, structural component. While they recognized the existence of White privilege, they did not acknowledge its distribution across Whites and across settings.

Whiteness and 'the continued right to determine meaning'

One component of Whiteness as property that is critical to our understanding of teacher constructions of White privilege and race power is 'the continued right to determine meaning' (Harris 1993, 1762). The teachers above engaged in this right by taking the concept of White privilege presented in the trainings and adopting and adapting elements of the concept in ways that fit a pre-existing racial framework. Our data suggest that the framework within which they were working was that racism and White privilege are inextricable, and that they are exclusively individual issues. As critical race theorists point out, racism is not an individual pathology, rather it is a systemic structural problem that is constructed and maintained by the collective acts of many individuals, but which is larger and far more powerful than any individual (Crenshaw 1997; Guinier and Torrres 2002; Ladson-Billings and Tate 1995; Parker and Lynn 2002). What is important here, then, is that these teachers were not just individually but simultaneously creating meaning themselves; they were tapping into and recreating meanings that already existed within the district's structural practices and within the larger society. For example, teachers we interviewed and observed consistently and separately determined the meaning of racial power and privilege as a numbers issue. In other words, they explicitly linked the absence of their own racial privilege with participation in a localized numerical majority (read: 'a Black school'). These definitions revealed the ways in which the districts, as an institution of Whiteness, engaged in the White property practice of normalizing structures and isolating individual behaviors. As Harris notes, one of the attendant rights of Whiteness as a property is the right to retain and protect individualism. She defines rights as 'shields from interference' (1993, 1778). This protection and the inherent dismissal of collective racial rights means that 'existing inequities are obscured and rendered nearly invisible' (1993, 1777). Therefore, these teachers' and their White colleagues' responses to and understandings of White privilege reveal not merely an individual misconception to be understood and addressed as individual teachers' racism, but in fact a collective misconception enacted by those individual teachers both in creation of and response to the larger, collective structural practices of the district.

Understood through the lens of Whiteness as property, the fact that many White teachers defend themselves as not being implicated in racism or White privilege is a logical consequence and expression of their epistemological frame (Ladson-Billings 2000b). Because Whiteness as property assumes the salience of the individual, to accept personal accountability for race privilege would position these White teachers as ultimately culpable instead of as participants in a larger structure that they can collectively challenge and change, or be asked to change. What this means is that individual White teachers may perceive that they are being asked to individually carry the burden of a problem that is structural, systemic, and collective. Training individuals to question and challenge their own experiences of White privilege without training them to understand how individual experiences and behaviors are both drawn from and constituent of structural privilege and power assumes that change can occur effectively on the individual level. However, Whiteness as property clearly challenges this assumption. We suggest that although understanding White privilege must be an element of teacher training – as individuals certainly must understand and make efforts to change their own practices – it should be reframed through the lens of Whiteness as property in order to counter the appropriation of White privilege into the individualistic and unaccountable White epistemological race paradigms that our data reveal. This is particularly important as districts attempt to utilize individual concepts of race and privilege to address major racial structural issues, such as the achievement gap. The structural force of racism obviates the possibility that individual training alone could remedy the racialized achievement gap.

Because Jericho and Zion Public Schools did not address the achievement gap as a structural issue, they allowed an individualized understanding of the sources of the gap to persist. For example, neither district incorporated racialized analyses of policies or organizational practices at the central administrative and school levels. Teachers and principals were neither encouraged nor invited to think about how classroom practice, school structure, and district policies might be interconnected forms of White race power that function in concert to perpetuate schools' failure to adequately educate children of color. In addition, the districts confused what they projected as the individual source of the achievement gap – teachers in classrooms – with an overtly individualized racism defined by attitude, not power. District administrators shared that they felt many teachers simply carried misunderstandings of their students' 'cultures' or that they did not have proper training in teaching 'different' students. However, the teachers above explained that because they worked in diverse schools, and so did not believe they had *privilege* (conflated here with attitude, not power) within the schools, they were thus not implicated in the problem. So, in the absence of an explicitly structural understanding of racism, many White teachers drew on the propertied right to determine meaning to construct a definition of White privilege devoid of attention to structural power. In so doing, these White teachers ironically exercised their real White privilege – the propertied right to determine racial meaning – to deny their individual participation in the collective, structural racism that perpetuates racialized student failure. This is an exclusive right only engaged by the dominant racial group. Significantly, these meaning making practices exclude definitions of White privilege that account for collective power.

'I don't feel like I'm racist': individualism and formal equality

Evidence that White property is individualized by Whites and White institutions and not recognized as collective emerged in our interviews. This section focuses on stories from teachers and administrators that illustrate how they viewed themselves as either individuals or as members of groups. We begin with narratives of White participants and later juxtapose those with narratives by teachers and administrators of color.

A White male member of the Jericho Public Schools senior leadership discussed the impetus behind the in-service, anti-bias training sponsored by the district and the source of inequities in school achievement:

> One of the great motivators of [this training] … And, uh, that is so critical for, ah, finding a way to take – we have thirty-seven hundred teachers – to move them to a space where they will be fluent in connecting with kids whose cultural context is deeply different [long pause] from theirs … [W]e're asking a set of people that, uhm, have not had much history [pause] in dealing with low income kids, African American kids, being able to build strong and compelling personal relationships with, starting to create an environment where they can learn.

Notably, this senior district administrator located the source of the achievement gap and the impetus for the training to help remedy this gap with teachers. His characterization was of racially un-marked White teachers who must change their pedagogical and personal style to reach 'low income kids', whom he defined as 'African American kids' (a category which, across the district, included Pacific Islander children). Though he identifies both class and race, which reflect deep structural components, he glosses over this possibility and focuses on 'culture' and 'personal relationships' in this culturally defined framework. This 'deeply different' culture was the focus for many participants and was often used in place of explicit reference to race. This substitution of culture was significant, as participants did not conceive of cultures as differentially powered or in power relationships with one another. Cultural misunderstandings, rather than racism, occurred between individual teachers and groups of students, were devoid of power, and could be remedied through individual teacher understanding. In fact, when Vaught shared with a White female school board member that she had heard from many people that Jericho Public Schools had problems with racism amongst its teachers, she said, 'Oh golly. You know, as much as I hate to admit it, I'm sure we do. We have three thousand teachers.' However, she quickly explained what the district was doing to remedy this possible problem: the training program. She elaborated that the training was all about cultural awareness for individual (read: White) teachers. Because culture was used in place of race in part to individualize the structural problem of racialized achievement and cast it as the isolated struggles of individual teachers working with 'different' students, the racialized structural barriers that informed, maintained, and entrenched individual practice went unnoticed. Focusing on culture provides a way to deflect power. While addressing the notion of culture might appear to be a recognition of collective identity, when it is approached in a structural vacuum, it is only a recognition of the collective identity of the Other. Students of color are recognized only as members of collectives while teachers are afforded the propertied right of individualism. Talking about cultural difference maintains the status quo and makes it look neutral, embodying the neutrality central to Whiteness as property (Harris 1993). This focus falsely defines the playing field and ensures that there will be no understanding of power as structural. One material manifestation of this emphasis on culture in both Zion and Jericho was the development and use of 'culture capsules' and 'culture grams'. In Jericho, the district was following up on the anti-bias training by developing what one school board member called 'culture capsules'. Though she had not yet seen one, she said they were 'kind of like little vignettes of different cultures. You know, like Cliff's Notes for different cultures that teachers can look at'. In Zion, the culture grams were nearly identical. They were explained to Castagno as online summaries of specific ethnic groups (without reference to race) that teachers were encouraged to use to learn about the 'culture' of their students. Because the achievement gaps in Jericho and Zion were so glaringly evident, it was in the interest of the White leadership of both districts to acknowledge difference. The focus on difference in the form of culture conveniently converged with their common worldview that celebrating and overcoming difference *defined* American equality and *gave legitimacy* to meritocracy (Crenshaw 1997; Kennedy 1995). The use of culture as a substitute for race not only elided the enormous racial disparities across measures in both districts, but drew on a romanticized, dominant narrative notion of the history of cultural assimilation in the US – one that functioned on the basis of collective and individual merit – ostensibly experienced by Italians or Irish, for example. Several participants in fact drew on their own White family histories to emphasize this cultural ideology and to give it supremacy over the role, function, and existence of race. In this way, participants used their own or family members' success to legitimate meritocracy and deny structural models of understanding power difference.

However, along with the propertied right to define Whites as individuals and Others as members of cultural groups is attached individualized blame. Without acknowledgement of the collective White structure of school districts as institutions, individual teachers are singled out as having personal difficulties when in fact their difficulties are drawn from and reflect (and reproduce) the structural nature of White property. Further, the relegation of students of color to cultural groups both denies their individuality (a quality revered under the system of propertied rights) and reduces their collective identity to a simplistic, unified whole, thus setting up individual White teachers in opposition to large groups of reductively racialized students. In the discursive representations of central administration and in the districts' rationale for instituting the anti-bias trainings, White teachers were positioned as hyper-individualized. As a consequence, many White teachers revealed that they therefore perceived themselves as singularly blamed for the racialized achievement gap. This perception, in unfortunate concert with the construction of students of color as cultural groups alone, resulted in a backlash that entrenched pre-existing racism. White teachers, feeling overwhelmingly defensive, denied White power, while they simultaneously appropriated an understanding of culture that reduced students of color in the districts to static, stereotypical collectives – dehumanized wholes, denied the property of rights which inheres only in individuals.

Expressing individuality is an ultimate freedom in a society based on property. By focusing on the individual and by seeing teachers solely as individuals instead of different and overlapping groups, districts fail to recognize the structural and systemic elements of racism. And, by attempting to promote structural change through individuals who are entrenched in a system of heightened individualism, districts put teachers on the defensive.

A common expression of this defensiveness is to engage narratives that heighten the individual/collective dichotomy.

When Vaught asked one White male teacher if he thought the training was a worthwhile program for the district to have adopted and what he considered the aim of it to be, he replied:

> Well, I mean, I think, for me, ah, again this is gonna sound probably like an ignorant response, but, I mean I don't feel like I'm racist, so I don't think it's gonna have as much impact on me, cause I'm teaching at [Martin Luther King] … And, uhm, and, so for me it doesn't, I think for other people it, who might not be associated with these students, uhm, a lot of Afro-American or Hispanic or Samoan kids, I think it could be beneficial, if they're kind of isolated in their cubicle, you know.

Like a strikingly large number of his White colleagues, this teacher illogically collapsed the fact of his teaching at a predominantly Black school with the unlikelihood or impossibility of personal racism (Kailin 1999). In his new awareness, he did not conceive of himself as a structural player, nor did he understand racism as a systemic, institutional dynamic (Bell 1987; Guinier 1994; Hacker 1995; Omi and Winant 1994; West 2004); rather, he understood himself to be free of what he embraced as an individual pathology (Ladson-Billings and Tate 1995). Importantly, this White teacher conflated his lack of structural awareness and understanding with his individual sense that his willing association with students of color made him a non-racist. He reifies the belief promoted by the district and embedded in the individualism of the property of Whiteness that racism is a function of individual perception – a conceptualization of racism bereft of collective power dynamics.

A White female teacher from MLKHS responded to Vaught's questions about the training by saying they were not useful and that race was not one of the school's 'real issues'. She characterized the trainings as a 'band-aid' for other problems, such as individuals' poor teaching in the building. When Vaught asked what this teacher felt should be discussed, she replied:

> It's hard to say. I think. I think it's more, to me it's more of an individual problem than a, than a school problem … I don't look at it as a conspiracy against *me* because of my color. I, I look at certain individuals and say, 'Gosh, this person's a jerk, that person's a jerk.' And I know that because, uhm, because I am coming from a White background that I don't take that as, as a, I don't take it as because of my race. And I know that if it was reversed, uhm, because, if somebody's been discriminated against their whole lives, they're gonna see that as having to do with race; whereas, I don't.

This particular teacher was able to recognize that people of color experience discrimination constantly. In spite of that recognition, she asserted that racism was not a problem within her school. The problem, she claimed, inhered in individuals alone. While acknowledging her White frame of reference, she nonetheless explained the Black frame of reference as equally influenced by experience. Further, she characterized both frames of reference as affected by common, if not collective, intra-group experiences, but as defined by the individual experience. This adaptation of the propertied rights of individual Whiteness to the discourse around culture and race reflects what Harris (1993) suggests is the ability of White property to constantly modify itself to fit shifting societal expectations and contexts. This teacher embraced difference as explaining the differing outcomes of personal experience, informed by societal patterns such as race discrimination. Her adaptation of a frame of difference emerged throughout the conversation as she simultaneously acknowledged and articulated the facets of White privilege and relegated racism to individual purveyors and, notably, *recipients*.

This semiotic tip of the hat reflects a new ritual of White property: to ostensibly name itself as a means of asserting indirect authority and control over meaning-making. In the data excerpted above and in the larger interview conversation, this teacher comfortably suggested that the experience of racism was possibly concocted in the minds of individuals as a response to their different experiences. A person of color, she claimed, is going to experience an individual being a 'jerk' as 'having to do with race'. Most tellingly, she juxtaposed that understanding with her assertion that she would not perceive an individual's behavior as a reflection of 'race' (read: racism). So, while she acknowledged, to some degree, the fact that people of color experience racism, she followed immediately with an ostensibly sympathetic assessment that suggests the judgment of people of color is qualified by their experience of racism. Significantly, she never responded to the initial question posed to her. Her position was not unlike that of many White teachers interviewed, who repeatedly cast people of color as reactive in their understandings of interactions and relationships. This understanding, however, was, with few exceptions, stated as a form of understanding 'difference'. This position actually reiterates with striking resonance one of the purposes of the training articulated by one member of the Jericho Public School senior leadership above. Rather than have White teachers understand racism, the leadership hoped to have them understand the *different* perceptions, or worldviews, of 'culturally' (i.e. racially) different people.

One male teacher of color in Zion offered a critique of these individualized self-narrations of race as property, and of the conflation of race and culture; he instead posited a more collective understanding of experience:

> But there are certain things that you might take for granted if you are White, which is not even a culture, I hate saying White, but you know, people were amazed that I felt sometimes some hesitancy about doing certain things because I'm not White. They were amazed by that. And I told the incident of where I came home one day and there was a rock thrown through my window. And I said most people would say that was just kids, if you were White you would say that is just kids fooling around, but I have to think about is it just kids fooling around or is it somebody that doesn't like me because of my ethnicity? Is it ah, somebody is targeting me? When I go to a store sometimes to return items, I get a little bit worried that they are going to say, that they are going to reject my return, they are not going to trust me, it doesn't happen but it's always in the back of my mind. I mean, I don't just go walk in there with confidence and think that they are going to just let me have what I want.

Embedded in this narrative is a critique of the individualization of propertied race rights. This teacher of color rejected the 'culture' model of race in favor of 'ethnicity' race, defined here by the presence or absence of privilege. In doing so, he drew on personal experiences such as vandalism and shopping to illustrate his statement that White teachers in the trainings did not understand or were surprised by his race-based feelings. However, he framed these anecdotes as representative of a larger system of race power and privilege – an individual-centered analysis of structural phenomenon. Because racist vandalism is still quite real across the US and because customer service is still frequently tied to the race of the customer, this teacher explains how these structural realities shape not just his perceptions, but also his knowledge, his choices, and his freedom. Countering the White teacher above who believed that people of color often had skewed perceptions because of individual encounters with racism, this teacher of color explained to Castagno that his perceptions were based on an awareness of a larger system of racism.

Expanding on this critique of the individualization of racial power, a principal of color in Jericho spoke about the district's approach to addressing racial inequities in school and his feeling that he was left alone to fend for his own students, overwhelmingly students of color. When Vaught asked him if there was any way he alone could fight racism effectively on behalf of his students and create equity within his school, he replied, 'I can't. Cause I think it's a collective effort. Not only is there a collective effort, but I also believe that there has to be a collective *will* to undo what is wrong.' That 'collective will' is reference to a larger, structural shift that would need to occur in conjunction with the dismantling of individualized White property rights. Importantly, both people of color and Whites who expressed critical insight into the structural underpinnings of racially inequitable schooling and achievement never directed *blame* to individual teachers or suggested that a remedy be sought singularly through the improvement of individual teachers' attitudes. Instead, they spoke of collective accountability. While they consistently affirmed the importance of the responsibility of individual teachers to equity, they articulated the path to that responsibility as one that included collective transformation. These participants captured what Lawrence (1993) writes so poignantly:

> The institutionalization of white supremacy within our culture has created conduct on the societal level that is greater than the sum of individual racist acts. The racist acts of millions are mutually reinforcing and cumulative because the status quo of institutionalized white supremacy remains long after deliberate racist actions subside (p. 61).

On the other hand, those Whites and people of color who did not level structural critiques were stuck blaming teachers because locating the problem on an individual level was the only explanation available to them within a system of Whiteness as property. This reflects the district's liberal interest (Guinier 2004) in promoting a discursively moral critique of racism, but maintaining the larger structures that fail to promote true equity for children of color. In other words, the liberal interest is defined by working within and relying upon existing structures, and assuming that those structures are just and equitable. In Jericho and Zion Public Schools, this would imply that the structure of the school systems is good, but that changes need to be made within individuals who reside inside that structure. This new racism (Giroux 1994) adopts the liberal discourse but avidly supports the legitimation (Crenshaw 1995) of the system as a whole and positions individual teachers as culprits.

This legitimation is a function of Whiteness as property that, like hegemony (Gramsci 1971), reifies the status quo by appearing to extend privileges and rights to non-dominant members of the society. For example, Black children were extended the right to attend historically all-White schools. However, this right did not include the structural changes to these institutions which would have been necessary for providing equitable educational experiences for these Black children (Bell 1995, 2004; Guinier 2004). Legitimation, then, is the outcome of what Harris (1995) defines as 'formal equality'. 'Formal equality,' she writes, 'overlooks structural disadvantage and requires mere non-discrimination or 'equal treatment'' (p. 289). The essential flaw and primary purpose of formal equality is that it protects and perpetuates the property vested in Whiteness and not only falls shy of, but blights equity. A mixed White/First Nation teacher in Jericho, referring to the racialized achievement gap and addressing the training undertaken by the district, explained succinctly:

> And, you can't take equality and make things equal, because they're not equal. They never have been equal. They're not equal now … So, it's racism by privilege. It's White privilege. It's not overt. It's very underneath. Ok. That's what's goin' on here.

'One of the great cop outs': the pitfalls of awareness

Strikingly, acknowledging a kind of White privilege is a form of entrenching White property by extending formal equality through the hyper-individualized discourse of liberal self-awareness. This self-awareness is limited, however, because it is not accompanied by a structural awareness. The very nature of legitimation is that it is deceptive. The formal equality that legitimates systems confuses superficial change at the individual level with structural transformation.

Teachers and administrators in both Zion and Jericho Public Schools characterized the trainings as focusing on awareness and some questioned that focus in the absence of action. A White female central office administrator told Castagno that in terms of training the teachers get in the Zion district, it makes them 'sensitive and aware' but the 'in depth training is not there'. A White female teacher in Zion said, 'I think it gives you awareness but I don't feel like either of them gives you um, ah, you're in the classroom right now, what are you going to do about it.' This disconnect between awareness and change was also captured by an African American principal in Jericho, who said:

> I just believe that [this training] just created greater awareness, just awareness. But it didn't change behavior. Because one would actually have to examine themselves and that is a hurting process. To admit, to have to admit, not to others, but just to yourself, that what I do brings harm to children. That hurts ... That's *not* gonna happen.

As this administrator identified, individual awareness alone did not bring about transformation. His critique suggests again that the myopic focus on individual teachers was unsuccessful because it 'hurt' to be held singularly responsible for harming children – in this case, causing the racialized achievement gap. With discerning acuity, he described one of the reactions of many White teachers to the trainings in Jericho: they were 'hurt' and defensive, and so rejected not only their own race privilege but also any potentially modest recognition of structural racial power inequities. Echoing the Jericho administrator above, a White male teacher in Zion critiqued his district's training as 'very surface level' and explained that it dealt only with cultural awareness. In response, he decided to develop trainings which dealt specifically with 'power and privilege'. He created these in collaboration with the Zion Public Schools and the Zion teachers' union and posted them on the district's professional development website. Because there was very low enrollment for this series of trainings, he was forced to cancel the offerings. In other words, an attempt to shift the focus of professional development away from awareness and towards structural issues was not widely viewed as important, interesting, or relevant.

Our findings indicated that within the American system of pervasive racism (Bell 1992), *awareness* was collapsed with *transformation*. This collapse illustrated the larger districts' legitimation of their inequitable structures. However, this use of awareness and focus on cultural difference resulted in a backlash. For those teachers who perceived difference as deficit, there was a slippery slope from the non-judgmental approach of awareness of cultural difference to the highly judgmental ideology of cultural, and so racial, deficiency (Sleeter and Grant 2003; Winant 2001). This was bolstered by the emphasis on White privilege and the understandable defensiveness of being individually implicated in structural racial inequities in schooling. The following White female teacher from Jericho discussed her perceptions of participating in the trainings with her school's Black administrators:

> Teacher: Because one of the great cop outs when you're in a setting like this [training] is anything that I do to you is based on race, even if it isn't. I was angry with [the African American principal] because she lied to me, it's not because she's who she is, racially ... But on the other hand I think they're getting – I'm trying to teach them a better perspective on who a White teacher is. So anyway, I go to these meetings and ... if I raise my hand, he doesn't call me right, well so what. I don't raise

my hand that much in this group. And uhm, he'll come up and talk to [a Black teacher from the same school], a buddy kind of thing, and just completely ignore, because I'm a White (inaudible). That's my first instinct. Whether that's true or not, I don't know. But it feels like that. Especially in this setting [the training].

Vaught: That you're being ignored on the basis of race?

Teacher: It's like it's like, turnabout is fair play and now I'm here and because I look Aryan, if you will, I'm going to be treated like a racist when I don't think I am.

Significantly, this teacher responded to the trainings with a troubling combination of defensiveness and hostility. Instead of applying an understanding of racial power dynamics to her interactions with her Black colleagues and supervisors, she instead was threatened by what she perceived as the denial of her individuality – an absolute, inalienable right of White property – and as treatment as a member of a racial collective. A collective identity against which she balked. She argued to Vaught that pulling 'the race card' is a 'cop out' when done by people of color, yet she pulled the same card to explain what she perceived as her mistreatment by people of color. Within this framework of Whiteness as property, Whites are seen as individuals merely by virtue of being White and discrimination is only acknowledged when it occurs against Whites, as individuals. Thus, according to this rationale, if members of racialized groups are getting something, it is always and only on the basis of group identification. This teacher's own heightened awareness of individual Whiteness, without any awareness of structural racism, placed her squarely against people of color. By co-opting White privilege into an individualistic paradigm of Whiteness as property, this teacher entrenched the property of her own racial power by denying the individual experiences of people of color and erasing the collective power of Whites.

Her attitudes and comments were not unlike those of many White participants in the trainings in Jericho and Zion. To varying degrees, these teachers articulated an awareness of difference in place of differential power. Minus an attention to power, this defensiveness often degenerated into hostility and a sense of indignation at what they perceived as the lack of gratitude for their sacrifices (Gallagher 1997; Kincheloe and Steinberg 1998; Ross 1997). This reflected that within a White property system, the districts' encouragement of individual awareness of difference was in fact inseparable from a denial of real and annihilative racial power. Worse, it sometimes promoted heightened animosity. In many cases 'awareness' created a racialized backlash veiled in the deceptive progress of formal equality.

The lack of structural change in both Zion and Jericho Public Schools was significant. The structural changes necessary to address racial inequity ran the gamut from funding to governance. Here, we offer two examples shared by a teacher and administrator. A very successful White male teacher at MLKHS in Jericho questioned the funding of these trainings in light of the marked absence of monies for technology at his school:

Teacher: [The training is] a waste; it's a waste of time.

Vaught: It's a waste of time? What do you think – ?

Teacher: That money should be more utilized and – perfect example, we have, I have what, twenty kids in my class? We only have fifteen computers that work. It had meat globs on their software. Ok, that hundred or million dollars you spent, you could spread that around. [Medgar Evers High School] and them have labs that are functional, but if you just spread it to [Thurgood Marshall High School], here, some of the middle schools, elementary schools, you gonna, you gonna serve more rights.

This teacher points to what he perceives as the problematic nature of the trainings in contrast with the structural, material realities of Black and Blackened (Ong 2000) student failure in his school. By sharing this data, we do not suggest that the structural racial inequities we discuss are singularly material. Instead, we are offering one teacher's illustration of one particularly tangible facet of structural domination. An African American principal in another low-performing, predominantly Black high school shared a similar critique. She described how her entire high school was to be displaced for the second time in five years, ultimately in order to placate White communities' demands for certain buildings:

> We want to eliminate the gap, but you want to displace the students who are entrapped in the gap? That to me says that eliminating the gap is truly not our intent. Now, it may sound good, it is good. But our *practice* is not good.

This principal went on to describe that 'practice' as the district's consistent failure to support students, teachers, administrators, and schools of color. Both of these participants were critical of the district efforts that offered formal equality through raising individual teacher awareness, but which failed to address the White propertied practices of perpetuating structural barriers to true racial equity.

Implications and conclusion

As we have shown, awareness did not lead to empathy amongst teachers, but resulted instead in a reinvention of meaning that reified existing, culturally constructed, racist frameworks. Further, these districts' lack of action in creating institutional change in conjunction with the trainings allowed the structural dimension of racism to persist unchallenged (Gillborn 2005), veiled as an individual pathology (Bell 1992; Crenshaw 1997; Harris 1995; Omi and Winant 1994) or worse, as formal equality. This suggests that barring structural transformation, racism adapts to any new ideology introduced, accommodating the discourse within a framework of continued racial supremacy. And, further, that by working within a White property framework, districts cannot address their own structural inequities.

By looking through the window of these teachers' attitudes onto the structural problems in the Jericho and Zion Public School districts, we see not only what is problematic, but a vision of what can be undertaken to begin to address the racialized achievement gap. Critical Race Theory offers a way to begin to address this through its own critique of Whiteness as property and the formal equality that undergirds and reproduces it. According to Harris (1993), the 'de-legitimation' of White property 'should be accomplished not merely by implementing equal treatment, but by equalizing treatment among the groups that have been illegitimately privileged or unfairly subordinated by racial stratification' (p. 1780). Harris offers a concrete conceptual means by which to approach this process of de-legitimation: 'distributive justice'. Distributive justice, she writes, is a conceptual frame in which both individuals and groups can make claim to the privileges or advantages they would have earned or received in an equitable context. Similarly, distributive justice 'also holds that individuals or groups may *not* claim positions, advantages, or benefits that they would *not* have been awarded under fair conditions' (p. 1784). Importantly, distributive justice 'does not focus primarily on guilt and innocence, but rather on entitlement and fairness' (p. 1783) and posits that, 'equal protection requires that individuals receive the share of the benefits they would have secured in the absence of racism' (p. 1783). Distributive justice speaks to the uneasy and clouded tension between equality and equity in the conflict between racial power and privilege as merely individual or collective, as defined by the interactions of individuals to create and recreate an institution larger than themselves. By moving beyond individual blame, distributive justice provides for structural understandings that require individual and collective accountability towards equity.

We suggest that in Zion and Jericho, distributive justice would include an emphasis on structural transformation. As Harris (1993) reminds us, 'what persists is the expectation of white-controlled institutions in the continued right to determine meaning – the reified privilege of power – that reconstitutes the property interest in whiteness in contemporary form' (p. 1762). Therefore, in both design and implementation, this transformation would necessarily include the distributive justice notion that groups within the districts contribute with the power and meaning-making authority they would have in the absence of existing structural racism. We also suggest that professional development is a healthy and essential part of change, if in fact that training focuses on the structural elements of racialized achievement inequities and gives all teachers tools to understand their position in structural systems and systemic change – positions that do not 'focus primarily on guilt and innocence' (p. 1783).

The responses of Zion's and Jericho's teachers and administrators to training programs touted by the districts as responses to the racialized achievement gaps in each district strongly indicate that, regardless of the merit of any one program, the collective, structural nature of Whiteness as property in schooling means that efforts at raising individual awareness cannot serve as the singular remedy for the achievement gap. The hegemonic, systemic interests of White property permits the co-optation of formal equality into racism. Awareness is collapsed with change. Difference is conflated with deficiency. Equality replaces equity. And, White privilege is countered by Black 'racism'.

The responses to the trainings catalogued in this article and the particular dynamics of racism which they reveal suggest (perhaps unsurprisingly) that without structural transformation, the fact and practice of racism will go unaltered and may become even further entrenched. These responses thus beg deeper questions of how to effectively challenge the achievement gap. What are the feasible structural changes that must be put in place to create true accountability to children of color? Is it truly necessary to focus on White privilege in order to create racially equitable achievement? How can distributive justice be effectively achieved within urban school systems?

Notes

1. While we stayed consistent with district-determined racial categories, we selected terms we felt most appropriate for those categories. For example, we replaced 'Hispanic' with 'Chicano/a and Latino/a'.

References

Anderson, G. 1989. Critical ethnography in education: Origins, current status, and new directions. *Review of Educational Research* 59: 3.

Anyon, J. 1997. *Ghetto schooling: A political economy of urban educational reform.* New York: Teachers College Press.

Bell, D. 1987. *And we are not saved: The elusive quest for racial justice.* New York: Basic Books.

———. 1992. *Faces at the bottom of the well: The permanence of racism.* New York: Basic Books.

———. 1995. Brown v. Board of Education and the interest convergence dilemma. In *Critical Race Theory: Key writings that formed the movement,* ed. K. Crenshaw, N. Gotanda, G. Peller and K. Thomas. New York: The New Press.

———. 2004. *Silent covenants: Brown v. Board of Education and the unfulfilled hopes for racial reform.* Oxford: Oxford University Press.

Bernal, D. 2002. Critical Race Theory, Latino critical theory, and critical raced-gendered epistemologies: Recognizing students of color as holders and creators of knowledge. *Qualitative Inquiry* 8, no. 1: 105–126.

Carspecken, P., and G. Walford, eds. 2001. *Critical ethnography and education.* New York: Routledge.

Castagno, A. 2006. Uncertain but always unthreatening: Multicultural education in two urban middle schools. Unpublished Dissertation, University of Wisconsin, Madison.

Crenshaw, K. 1995. Race, reform, and retrenchment: Transformation and legitimation in antidiscrimination law. In *Critical Race Theory: The key writings that formed the movement,* ed. K. Crenshaw, N. Gotanda, G. Peller and K. Thomas. New York: The New Press.

———. 1997. Race, reform, and retrenchment: Transformation and legitimation in antidiscrimination law. In *Critical Race Theory: Essays on the social construction of 'race',* ed. N. Gates, 85–141. New York: Garland Publishing.

Crenshaw, K., N. Gotanda, G. Peller, and K. Thomas, eds. 1995. *Critical Race Theory: The key writings that formed the movement.* New York: The New Press.

Delgado, R., and J. Stefancic, 2001. *Critical Race Theory: An introduction.* New York: New York University Press.

Delpit, L. 1988. The silenced dialogue: Power and pedagogy in educating other people's children. *Harvard Educational Review* 58: 3.

Ferguson, A. 2001. *Bad boys: Public schools in the making of Black masculinity.* Ann Arbor, MI: University of Michigan Press.

Fine, M. 1997. Witnessing whiteness. In *Off white: Readings on race, power, and society,* ed. M. Fine, L. Powell, L. Weis and L. Mun Wong, 57–65. New York: Routledge.

Fine, M., and L. Weis, 1998. *The unknown city: The lives of poor and working-class young adults.* Boston: Beacon Press.

Fordham, S. 1996. *Blacked out: Dilemmas of race, identity, and success at Capital High.* Chicago: University of Chicago Press.

Foster, M. 1996. Like us but not one of us: Reflections of a life history study of African American teachers. In *Unrelated kin: Race and gender in women's personal narratives,* ed. G. Etter-Lewis and M. Foster, 215–224. New York: Routledge.

Gallagher, C. 1997. White racial formation: Into the twenty-first century. In *Critical white studies: Looking behind the mirror,* ed. R. Delgado and J. Stefancic. Philadelphia: Temple University Press.

Gillborn, D. 2005. Education policy as an act of white supremacy: Whiteness, Critical Race Theory and education reform. *Journal of Education Policy* 20, no. 4: 484–505.

Giroux, H. 1994. *Disturbing pleasures: Learning popular culture.* New York: Routledge.

Gotanda, N. 1995. A critique of 'Our constitution is color-blind'. In *Critical Race Theory: Key writings that formed the movement,* ed. K. Crenshaw, N. Gotanda, G. Peller and K. Thomas, 257–275. New York: The New Press.

Gramsci, A. 1971. Selections from the prison notebooks. New York: International Publishers.

Guinier, L. 1994. *The tyranny of the majority: Fundamental fairness in representative democracy.* New York: The Free Press.

Guinier, L. 2004. From racial liberalism to racial literacy: 'Brown v. Board of Education' and the interest-divergence dilemma. *Journal of American History* 91, no. 1: 92–118.

Guinier, L., and G. Torrres, 2002. *The miner's canary: Enlisting race, resisting power, transforming democracy.* Cambridge: Harvard University Press.

Hacker, A. 1995. *Two nations: Black and white, separate, hostile, unequal.* New York: Ballantine Books.

Harris, C. 1993. Whiteness as property. *Harvard Law Review* 106, no. 8: 1707–1791.

———. 1995. Whiteness as property. In *Critical Race Theory: Key writings that formed the movement,* ed. K. Crenshaw, N. Gotanda, G. Peller and K. Thomas, 276–291. New York: The New Press.

Kailin, J. 1999. How white teachers perceive the problem of racism in their schools: A case study in 'liberal' Lakeview. *Teachers College Record* 100, no. 4: 724–750.

Kennedy, D. 1995. A cultural pluralist case for affirmative action in legal academia. In *Critical Race Theory: Key writings that formed the movement,* ed. K. Crenshaw, N. Gotanda, G. Peller and K. Thomas, 159–176. New York: The New Press.

Kincheloe, J., and S. Steinberg. 1998. Addressing the crisis of whiteness: Reconfiguring white identity in a pedagogy of whiteness. In *White reign: Deploying whiteness in America,* ed. J. Kincheloe, S. Sheinberg, N. Rodriguez and R. Chennault, 3–30. New York: St. Martin's Griffin.

King, J. 1991. Dysconscious racism: Ideology, identity, and the miseducation of teachers. *Journal of Negro Education* 60, no. 2: 133–146.

Ladson-Billings, G. 1994. *The dreamkeepers: Successful teachers of African American children.* San Francisco, CA: Jossey-Bass.

———. 2000a. Fighting for our lives: Preparing teachers to teach African American students. *Journal of Teacher Education* 51, no. 3: 206–214.

———. 2000b. Racialized discourses and ethnic epistemologies. In *Handbook of qualitative research* (2nd ed.), ed. Y. Lincoln and N. Denzin. Thousand Oaks, CA: Sage.

Ladson-Billings, G., and W. Tate. 1995. Toward a Critical Race Theory of education. *Teachers College Record* 97, no. 1: 47–64.

Lawrence, C. 1993. If he hollers let him go: Regulating racist speech on campus. In *Words that wound: Critical Race Theory, assaultive speech, and the first amendment,* ed. M. Matsuda, 53–88. Boulder, CO: Westview Press.

Lee, S. 2005. *Up against whiteness: Race, school, and immigrant youth.* New York: Teachers College Press.

Lipman, P. 2004. *High stakes education: Inequality, globalization, and urban school reform.* New York: Routledge Falmer.

Luttrell, W. 1997. *Schoolsmart and motherwise: Working-class women's identity and schooling.* New York: Routledge.

Lynn, M., T.J. Yosso, D.G. Solórzano, and L. Parker. 2002. Critical Race Theory and education: Qualitative research in the new millennium. *Qualitative Inquiry* 8, no. 1: 3–6.

McIntosh, P. 1988. White privilege and male privilege: A personal account of coming to see correspondences through work in Women's Studies. In *Critical White studies: Looking behind the mirror,* ed. R. Delgado and J. Stefancic, 291–299. Philadelphia: Temple University Press.

Omi, M., and H. Winant. 1994. *Racial formation in the United States: From the 1960s to the 1990s.* 2nd ed. New York: Routledge.

Ong, A. 2000. Cultural citizenship as subject making: Immigrants negotiate racial and cultural boundaries in the United States. In *Race, identity, and citizenship: A reader,* ed. R. Torres, L. Miron and J. Inda. Malden, MA: Blackwell.

Parker, L., and M. Lynn. 2002. What's race got to do with It? Critical Race Theory's conflicts with and connections to qualitative research methodology and epistemology. *Qualitative Inquiry* 8, no. 1: 7–22.

Ross, T. 1997. Innocence and affirmative action. In *Critical white studies: Looking behind the mirror,* ed. R. Delgado and J. Stefancic, 27–32. Philadelphia: Temple University Press.

Sleeter, C., and C. Grant. 2003. *Making choices for multicultural education: Five approaches to race, class, and gender,* 4th ed. New Jersey: John Wiley and Sons.

Stacey, J. 1988. Can there be a feminist ethnography? *Women's Studies International Forum* 11, no. 1: 21–27.

Tate, W. 1997. Critical Race Theory and education: History, theory, and implications. *Review of Research in Education* 22, no. 1997: 195–247.

Valenzuela, A. 1999. *Subtractive schooling: US-Mexican youth and the politics of caring.* Albany: State University of New York Press.

Vaught, S. 2006. *The peculiar institution: Racism, public schooling, and the entrenchment of Whiteness.* Unpublished Dissertation, University of Wisconsin, Madison.

West, C. 2004. Race matters. In *Race, class, and gender: An anthology,* ed. M. Andersen and P. H. Collins, 5th ed., 122–125. Australia: Wadsworth.

Winant, H. 2001. White racial projects. In *The making and unmaking of whiteness,* ed. B. Rasmussen, E. Klinenberg, I. Nexica and M. Wray. Durham: Duke University Press.

Whose culture has capital? A critical race theory discussion of community cultural wealth

Tara J. Yosso

This article conceptualizes community cultural wealth as a critical race theory (CRT) challenge to traditional interpretations of cultural capital. CRT shifts the research lens away from a deficit view of Communities of Color as places full of cultural poverty disadvantages, and instead focuses on and learns from the array of cultural knowledge, skills, abilities and contacts possessed by socially marginalized groups that often go unrecognized and unacknowledged. Various forms of capital nurtured through cultural wealth include aspirational, navigational, social, linguistic, familial and resistant capital. These forms of capital draw on the knowledges Students of Color bring with them from their homes and communities into the classroom. This CRT approach to education involves a commitment to develop schools that acknowledge the multiple strengths of Communities of Color in order to serve a larger purpose of struggle toward social and racial justice.

Introduction

> Theory, then, is a set of knowledges. Some of these knowledges have been kept from us—entry into some professions and academia denied us. Because we are not allowed to enter discourse, because we are often disqualified and excluded from it, because what passes for theory these days is forbidden territory for us, it is *vital* that we occupy theorizing space, that we not allow white men and women solely to occupy it. By bringing in our own approaches and methodologies, we transform that theorizing space. (Anzaldúa, 1990, p. xxv, emphasis in original)

In the epigraph above, Gloria Anzaldúa (1990) calls on People of Color to transform the process of theorizing. This call is about epistemology—the study of sources of knowledge. Scholars such as Gloria Ladson-Billings (2000) and Dolores Delgado Bernal (1998, 2002) have asked: whose knowledge counts and whose knowledge is discounted? Throughout US history, race and racism have shaped this epistemological debate (Scheurich & Young, 1997; Lopez & Parker, 2003). Indeed, it has been over a century since DuBois (1903, 1989) predicted that racism would continue to emerge as one of the United States' key social problems. Racism overtly shaped US social institutions at the beginning of the twentieth century and continues, although more subtly, to impact US institutions of socialization in the beginning of the twenty-first century. Researchers, practitioners and students are still searching for the necessary tools to effectively analyze and challenge the impact of race and racism in US society.

In addressing the debate over knowledge within the context of social inequality, Pierre Bourdieu (Bourdieu & Passeron, 1977) argued that the knowledges of the upper and middle classes are considered capital valuable to a hierarchical society. If one is not born into a family whose knowledge is already deemed valuable, one could then access the knowledges of the middle and upper class and the potential for social mobility through formal schooling. Bourdieu's theoretical insight about how a hierarchical society reproduces itself has often been interpreted as a way to explain why the academic and social outcomes of People of Color are significantly lower than the outcomes of Whites. The assumption follows that People of Color 'lack' the social and cultural capital required for social mobility. As a result, schools most often work from this assumption in structuring ways to help 'disadvantaged' students whose race and class background has left them lacking necessary knowledge, social skills, abilities and cultural capital (see Valenzuela, 1999).

This interpretation demonstrates Anzaldúa's point: 'If we have been gagged and disempowered by theories, we can also be loosened and empowered by theories' (Anzaldúa, 1990, p. xxvi). Indeed, if some knowledges have been used to silence, marginalize and render People of Color invisible, then 'Outsider' knowledges (Hill Collins, 1986), *mestiza* knowledges (Anzaldúa, 1987) and transgressive knowledges (hooks, 1994) can value the presence and voices of People of Color, and can re-envision the margins as places empowered by transformative resistance (hooks, 1990; Delgado Bernal, 1997; Solórzano & Delgado Bernal, 2001). Critical race theory (CRT) listens to DuBois' racial insight and offers a response to Anzaldúa's theoretical challenge. CRT is a framework that can be used to theorize, examine and challenge the ways race and racism implicitly and explicitly impact on social structures, practices and discourses.

Below, I discuss the ways CRT centers Outsider, *mestiza*, transgressive knowledges. After outlining the theoretical framework of CRT, I critique the assumption that Students of Color come to the classroom with cultural deficiencies. Utilizing a CRT lens, I challenge traditional interpretations of Bourdieuean cultural capital theory (Bourdieu & Passeron, 1977) and introduce an alternative concept called community cultural wealth. Then, I outline at least six forms of capital that comprise community cultural wealth and most often go unacknowledged or unrecognized. In examining some of the under-utilized assets Students of Color bring with them from their homes and communities into the classroom, this article notes the potential of community cultural wealth to transform the process of schooling.

Critical race theory in education

CRT draws from and extends a broad literature base of critical theory in law, sociology, history, ethnic studies and women's studies. Kimberlé Crenshaw (2002) explains that in the late 1980s, various legal scholars felt limited by work that separated critical theory from conversations about race and racism. Alongside other 'Outsider' scholars (Hill Collins, 1986) Crenshaw (2002) was 'looking for both a critical space in which race was foregrounded and a race space where critical themes were central' (p. 19). Mari Matsuda (1991) defined that CRT space as:

> ... the work of progressive legal scholars of color who are attempting to develop a jurisprudence that accounts for the role of racism in American law and that work toward the elimination of racism as part of a larger goal of eliminating all forms of subordination. (p. 1331)

In previous work, I describe a genealogy of CRT that links the themes and patterns of legal scholarship with the social science literature (Solórzano & Yosso, 2001). Figure 1 addresses some of this intellectual history.[1]

In its post-1987 form, CRT emerged from criticisms of the Critical Legal Studies (CLS) movement. CLS scholars questioned the role of the traditional legal system in legitimizing oppressive social structures. With this insightful analysis, CLS scholarship emphasized critique of the liberal legal tradition as opposed to offering strategies for change. Scholars such as Derrick Bell and Alan Freeman asserted that one reason why the CLS critique of the law could not offer strategies for social transformation was because it failed to incorporate race and racism into the analysis (Delgado, 1995a; Ladson-Billings, 1998). Not listening to the lived experiences and histories of those oppressed by institutionalized racism limited CLS scholarship. This argument had also been taking place in social science and history circles, specifically in ethnic and women's studies scholarship.

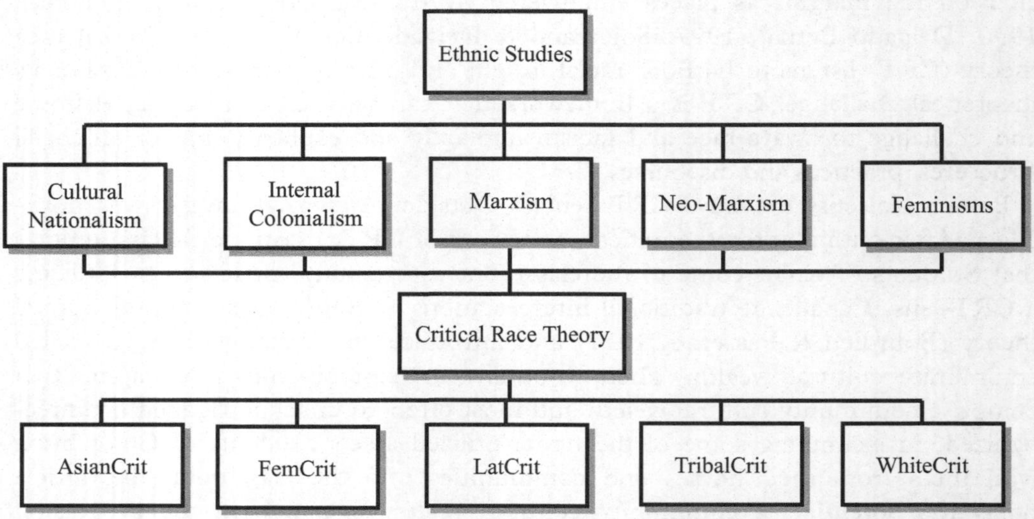

Figure 1. An intellectual genealogy of critical race theory

Critical race theorists began to pull away from CLS because the critical legal framework restricted their ability to analyze racial injustice (Delgado, 1988; Crenshaw *et al.*, 1995; Delgado & Stefancic, 2001; Crenshaw, 2002). Initially, CRT scholarship focused its critique on the slow pace and unrealized promise of Civil Rights legislation. As a result, many of the critiques launched were articulated in Black vs White terms. Women and People of Color who felt their gendered, classed, sexual, immigrant and language experiences and histories were being silenced, challenged this tendency toward a Black/White binary. They stressed that oppression in the law and society could not be fully understood in terms of only Black and White. Certainly, African Americans have experienced a unique and horrendous history of racism and other forms of subordination in the US. Other People of Color have their own histories that likewise have been shaped by racism and the intersecting forms of subordination (Espinoza & Harris, 1998). By offering a two-dimensional discourse, the Black/White binary limits understandings of the multiple ways in which African Americans, Native Americans, Asian/Pacific Islanders, Chicanas/os, and Latinas/os continue to experience, respond to, and resist racism and other forms of oppression.

For example, Latina/o critical race (LatCrit) theory extends critical race discussions to address the layers of racialized subordination that comprise Chicana/o, Latina/o experiences (Arriola, 1997, 1998; Stefancic, 1998). LatCrit scholars assert that racism, sexism and classism are experienced amidst other layers of subordination based on immigration status, sexuality, culture, language, phenotype, accent and surname (Montoya, 1994; Johnson, 1999). Indeed, the traditional paradigm for understanding US race relations is often a Black/White binary, which limits discussions about race and racism to terms of African American and White experiences (Valdes, 1997, 1998). Like Manning Marable (1992), who defines racism as 'a system of ignorance, exploitation and power used to oppress African Americans, Latinos, Asians, Pacific Americans, American Indians, and other people on the basis of ethnicity, culture, mannerisms, and color' (p. 5), CRT scholarship has benefited from scholarship addressing racism at its intersections with other forms of subordination (Crenshaw, 1989, 1993).

Over the years, the CRT family tree has expanded to incorporate the racialized experiences of women, Latinas/os, Native Americans and Asian Americans (see Figure 1). For example, LatCrit, TribalCrit and AsianCrit are branches of CRT, evidencing Chicana/o, Latina/o, Native American and Asian American communities' ongoing search for a framework that addresses racism and its accompanying oppressions beyond the Black/White binary (Ikemoto, 1992; Chang, 1993, 1998; Chon, 1996; Delgado, 1997; Williams, 1997; Brayboy, 2001, 2002). Women of Color have also challenged CRT to address feminist critiques of racism and classism through FemCrit theory (Caldwell, 1995; Wing, 1997, 2000). In addition, White scholars have expanded CRT with WhiteCrit, by 'looking behind the mirror' to expose White privilege and challenge racism (Delgado & Stefancic, 1997).

CRT's branches are not mutually exclusive or in contention with one another. Naming, theorizing and mobilizing from the intersections of racism, need not initiate some sort of oppression sweepstakes—a competition to measure one form of oppression against another. As Cherrie Moraga (1983) writes,

> The danger lies in ranking the oppressions. The danger lies in failing to acknowledge the specificity of the oppression. The danger lies in attempting to deal with oppression purely from a theoretical base. Without an emotional, heartfelt grappling with the source of our own oppression, without naming the enemy within ourselves and outside of us, no authentic, non-hierarchical connection among oppressed groups can take place. (pp. 52–53)

Indeed, racism and its intersections with other forms of subordination shape the experiences of People of Color very differently than Whites (Bell, 1986; 1998; Essed, 1991; Baca Zinn, 1989). Still, the popular discourse in the US, as well as the academic discourse, continues to be limited by the Black/White binary. CRT adds to efforts to continue to expand this dialogue to recognize the ways in which our struggles for social justice are limited by discourses that omit and thereby silence the multiple experiences of People of Color (Ellison, 1990).

As a student of Chicana/o Studies, the theoretical models informing my work included the Internal Colonial model (Bonilla & Girling, 1973; Blauner, 2001), Marxism (Bowles & Gintis, 1976; Barrera, 1979), Chicana and Black feminisms (Anzaldúa, 1987; hooks, 1990; Zavella, 1991; Hurtado, 1996; Hill Collins, 1998, 2000; Saldivar-Hull, 2000) and cultural nationalism (Asante, 1987). Even with all of their strengths, each of these frameworks had certain blindspots that limited my ability to examine racism. Now, as a professor of Chicana/o Studies, my work is informed by the hindsight of CRT and its genealogical branches. To document and analyze the educational access, persistence and graduation of underrepresented students, I draw on my interdisciplinary training and those theoretical models whose popularity may have waned since the 1960s and 1970s, but whose commitment to speaking truth to power continues to address contemporary social realities.

For the field of education, Daniel Solórzano (1997, 1998) identified five tenets of CRT that can and should inform theory, research, pedagogy, curriculum and policy:[2] (1) the intercentricity of race and racism; (2) the challenge to dominant ideology; (3) the commitment to social justice; (4) the centrality of experiential knowledge; and (5) the utilization of interdisciplinary approaches.

1. *The intercentricity of race and racism with other forms of subordination.* CRT starts from the premise that race and racism are central, endemic, permanent and a fundamental part of defining and explaining how US society functions (Bell, 1992; Russell, 1992). CRT acknowledges the inextricable layers of racialized subordination based on gender, class, immigration status, surname, phenotype, accent and sexuality (Crenshaw, 1989, 1993; Valdes *et al.*, 2002).
2. *The challenge to dominant ideology.* CRT challenges White privilege and refutes the claims that educational institutions make toward objectivity, meritocracy, colorblindness, race neutrality and equal opportunity. CRT challenges notions of 'neutral' research or 'objective' researchers and exposes deficit-informed research that silences, ignores and distorts epistemologies of People of Color (Delgado Bernal, 1998; Ladson-Billings, 2000). CRT argues that these traditional claims

act as a camouflage for the self-interest, power, and privilege of dominant groups in US society (Bell, 1987; Calmore, 1992; Solórzano, 1997).

3. *The commitment to social justice.* CRT is committed to social justice and offers a liberatory or transformative response to racial, gender and class oppression (Matsuda, 1991). Such a social justice research agenda exposes the 'interest-convergence' (Bell, 1987) of civil rights 'gains' in education and works toward the elimination of racism, sexism and poverty, as well as the empowerment of People of Color and other subordinated groups (Freire, 1970, 1973; Solórzano & Delgado Bernal, 2001).
4. *The centrality of experiential knowledge.* CRT recognizes that the experiential knowledge of People of Color is legitimate, appropriate, and critical to understanding, analyzing and teaching about racial subordination (Delgado Bernal, 2002). CRT draws explicitly on the lived experiences of People of Color by including such methods as storytelling, family histories, biographies, scenarios, parables, *cuentos, testimonios*, chronicles and narratives (Bell, 1987, 1992, 1996; Delgado, 1989, 1993, 1995a, b, 1996; Espinoza, 1990; Olivas, 1990; Montoya, 1994; Carrasco, 1996; Solórzano & Yosso, 2000, 2001, 2002a; Solórzano & Delgado Bernal, 2001; Delgado Bernal & Villalpando, 2002; Villalpando, 2003).
5. *The transdisciplinary perspective.* CRT goes beyond disciplinary boundaries to analyze race and racism within both historical and contemporary contexts, drawing on scholarship from ethnic studies, women's studies, sociology, history, law, psychology, film, theatre and other fields (Delgado, 1984, 1992; Olivas, 1990; Gotanda, 1991; Harris, 1994; Garcia, 1995; Gutiérrez-Jones, 2001).

These five themes are not new in and of themselves, but collectively they represent a challenge to the existing modes of scholarship. Informed by scholars who continue to expand the literature and scope of discussions of race and racism, I define CRT in education as a theoretical and analytical framework that challenges the ways race and racism impact educational structures, practices, and discourses. CRT is conceived as a social justice project that works toward the liberatory potential of schooling (hooks, 1994; Freire, 1970, 1973). This acknowledges the contradictory nature of education, wherein schools most often oppress and marginalize while they maintain the potential to emancipate and empower. Indeed, CRT in education refutes dominant ideology and White privilege while validating and centering the experiences of People of Color. CRT utilizes transdisciplinary approaches to link theory with practice, scholarship with teaching, and the academy with the community (see LatCrit Primer, 1999; Solórzano & Yosso, 2001).

Many in the academy and in community organizing, activism, and service who look to challenge social inequality will most likely recognize the tenets of CRT as part of what, why and how they do the work they do. CRT addresses the social construct of race by examining the ideology of racism. CRT finds that racism is often well disguised in the rhetoric of shared 'normative' values and 'neutral' social scientific principles and practices (Matsuda *et al.*, 1993). However, when the ideology of racism is examined and racist injuries are named, victims of racism can often find their voice. Those injured by racism and other forms of oppression discover that they are not alone and moreover are part of a legacy of resistance to racism and the layers of racialized oppression. They become empowered participants, hearing their own stories and the stories of others, listening to how the arguments against them are framed and learning to make the arguments to defend themselves.

Challenging racism, revealing cultural wealth

CRT's five tenets provide a helpful guiding lens that can inform research in Communities of Color. Looking through a CRT lens means critiquing deficit theorizing and data that may be limited by its omission of the voices of People of Color. Such deficit-informed research often 'sees' deprivation in Communities of Color. Indeed, one of the most prevalent forms of contemporary racism in US schools is deficit thinking. Deficit thinking takes the position that minority students and families are at fault for poor academic performance because: (a) students enter school without the normative cultural knowledge and skills; and (b) parents neither value nor support their child's education. These racialized assumptions about Communities of Color most often leads schools to default to the banking method of education critiqued by Paulo Freire (1973). As a result, schooling efforts usually aim to fill up supposedly passive students with forms of cultural knowledge deemed valuable by dominant society. Scholars Shernaz García and Patricia Guerra (2004) find that such deficit approaches to schooling begin with overgeneralizations about family background and are exacerbated by a limited framework to interpret how individual views about educational success are shaped by personal 'sociocultural and linguistic experiences and assumptions about appropriate cultural outcomes' (p. 163). Educators most often assume that schools work and that students, parents and community need to change to conform to this already effective and equitable system.

Indeed, García and Guerra's (2004) research acknowledges that deficit thinking permeates US society, and both schools and those who work in schools mirror these beliefs. They argue that this reality necessitates a challenge of personal and individual race, gender and class prejudices expressed by educators, as well as a 'critical examination of systemic factors that perpetuate deficit thinking and reproduce educational inequities for students from nondominant sociocultural and linguistic backgrounds' (p. 155). I believe CRT can offer such an approach by identifying, analyzing and challenging distorted notions of People of Color.

As part of the challenge to deficit thinking in education, it should be noted that race is often coded as 'cultural difference' in schools. Indeed, culture influences how society is organized, how school curriculum is developed and how pedagogy and policy are implemented. In social science, the concept of culture for Students of Color has taken on many divergent meanings. Some research has equated culture with race and ethnicity, while other work clearly has viewed culture through a much broader lens of characteristics and forms of social histories and identities. For my purposes here, culture refers to behaviors and values that are learned, shared, and exhibited by a group of people. Culture is also evidenced in material and nonmaterial productions of a people.

Culture as a set of characteristics is neither fixed nor static (Gómez-Quiñones, 1977). For example, with Students of Color, culture is frequently represented symbolically through language and can encompass identities around immigration status, gender, phenotype, sexuality and region, as well as race and ethnicity.

Looking through a CRT lens, the cultures of Students of Color can nurture and empower them (Delgado-Gaitan, 2001; Delgado Bernal, 2002). Focusing on research with Latina/o families, Luis C Moll, Cathy Amanti, Deborah Neff and Norma Gonzalez (1992), Carlos Vélez-Ibáñez and James Greenberg (1992) and Irma Olmedo (1997) assert that culture can form and draw from communal *funds of knowledge* (Gonzalez *et al.*, 1995; Gonzalez & Moll, 2002). Likewise, Douglas Foley (1997) notes research revealing the 'virtues and solidarity in African American community and family traditions' as well as the 'deeply spiritual values passed from generation to generation in most African American communities' (p. 123).

Taken together, the CRT challenge to deficit thinking and understanding of the empowering potential of the cultures of Communities of Color, leads me to the following description of cultural wealth. I begin with a critique of the ways Bourdieu's (Bourdieu & Passeron, 1977) work has been used to discuss social and racial inequity. In education, Bourdieu's work has often been called upon to explain why Students of Color do not succeed at the same rate as Whites. According to Bourdieu, cultural capital refers to an accumulation of cultural knowledge, skills and abilities possessed and inherited by privileged groups in society. Bourdieu asserts that cultural capital (i.e., education, language), social capital (i.e., social networks, connections) and economic capital (i.e., money and other material possessions) can be acquired two ways, from one's family and/or through formal schooling. The dominant groups within society are able to maintain power because access is limited to acquiring and learning strategies to use these forms of capital for social mobility.

Therefore, while Bourdieu's work sought to provide a structural critique of social and cultural reproduction, his theory of cultural capital has been used to assert that some communities are culturally wealthy while others are culturally poor. This interpretation of Bourdieu exposes White, middle class culture as the standard, and therefore all other forms and expressions of 'culture' are judged in comparison to this 'norm'. In other words, cultural capital is not just inherited or possessed by the middle class, but rather it refers to an accumulation of specific forms of knowledge, skills and abilities that are *valued* by privileged groups in society. For example, middle or upper class students may have access to a computer at home and therefore can learn numerous computer-related vocabulary and technological skills before arriving at school. These students have acquired cultural capital because computer-related vocabulary and technological skills are valued in the school setting. On the other hand, a working class Chicana/o student whose mother works in the garment industry may bring a different vocabulary, perhaps in two languages (English and Spanish) to school, along with techniques of conducting errands on the city bus and translating mail, phone calls and coupons for her/his mother (see Faulstich Orellana, 2003). This cultural knowledge is very valuable to the student and her/his family, but is not necessarily considered to carry any capital in the school context. So, are there forms of cultural capital that marginalized groups bring to the table that traditional cultural capital theory does not recognize or value? CRT answers, yes.

CRT shifts the center of focus from notions of White, middle class culture to the cultures of Communities of Color. In doing so, I also draw on the work of sociologists Melvin Oliver and Thomas Shapiro (1995) to better understand how cultural capital is actually only one form of many different aspects that might be considered valuable. Oliver and Shapiro (1995) propose a model to explain how the narrowing of the income or earnings gap between Blacks and Whites is a misleading way to examine inequality. They argue that one's income over a typical fiscal year focuses on a single form of capital and that the income gap between Blacks and Whites is narrowing over time. On the other hand, they examine separately the concept of wealth and define it as the total extent of an individual's accumulated assets and resources (i.e., ownership of stocks, money in bank, real estate, business ownership, etc). They then argue that while the income of Blacks may indeed be climbing and the Black/White income gap narrowing, their overall wealth, compared to Whites, is declining and the gap is diverging (see also Shapiro, 2004).

Traditional Bourdieuean cultural capital theory has parallel comparisons to Oliver and Shapiro's (1995) description of income. Both place value on a very narrow range of assets and characteristics. A traditional view of cultural capital is narrowly defined by White, middle class values, and is more limited than wealth—one's accumulated assets and resources. CRT expands this view. Centering the research lens on the experiences of People of Color in critical historical context reveals accumulated assets and resources in the histories and lives of Communities of Color.

Figure 2 demonstrates that community cultural wealth is an array of knowledge, skills, abilities and contacts possessed and utilized by Communities of Color to survive and resist macro and micro-forms of oppression.[3]

Indeed, a CRT lens can 'see' that Communities of Color nurture cultural wealth through at least 6 forms of capital such as aspirational, navigational, social, linguistic, familial, and resistant capital (see Delgado Bernal, 1997, 2001; Auerbach, 2001; Stanton-Salazar, 2001; Solórzano & Delgado Bernal, 2001; Faulstich Orellana, 2003).These various forms of capital are not mutually exclusive or static, but rather are dynamic processes that build on one another as part of community cultural wealth. For example, as noted above, aspirational capital is the ability to hold onto hope in the face of structured inequality and often without the means to make such dreams a reality. Yet, aspirations are developed within social and familial contexts, often through linguistic storytelling and advice (*consejos*) that offer specific navigational goals to challenge (resist) oppressive conditions. Therefore, aspirational capital overlaps with each of the other forms of capital, social, familial, navigational, linguistic and resistant. As Anzaldúa asserts, 'In our *mestizaje* theories we create new categories for those of us left out of or pushed out of existing ones' (Anzaldúa, 1990, p. xxvi, emphasis in original).

1. *Aspirational capital* refers to the ability to maintain hopes and dreams for the future, even in the face of real and perceived barriers. This resiliency is evidenced

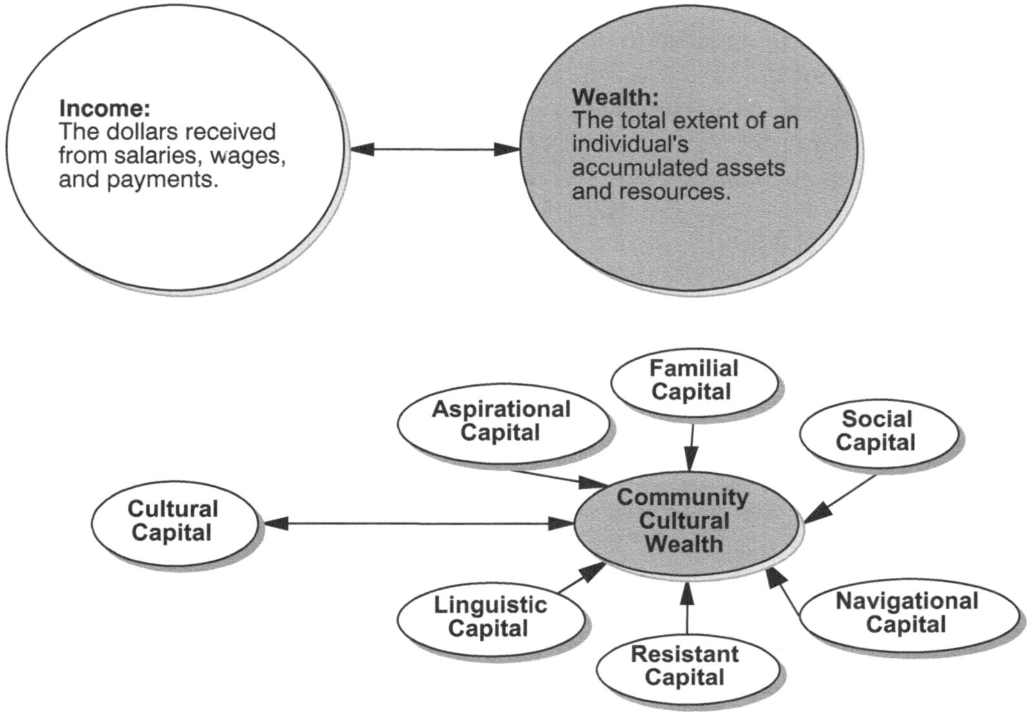

Figure 2. A model of community cultural wealth. Adapted from: Oliver & Shapiro, 1995

in those who allow themselves and their children to dream of possibilities beyond their present circumstances, often without the objective means to attain those goals. This form of cultural wealth draws on the work of Patricia Gándara (1982, 1995) and others who have shown that Chicanas/os experience the lowest educational outcomes compared to every other group in the US, but maintain consistently high aspirations for their children's future (Delgado-Gaitan, 1992, 1994; Solórzano, 1992; Auerbach, 2001). These stories nurture a culture of possibility as they represent 'the creation of a history that would break the links between parents' current occupational status and their children's future academic attainment' (Gándara, 1995, p. 55).

2. *Linguistic capital* includes the intellectual and social skills attained through communication experiences in more than one language and/or style (see Faulstich Orellana, 2003).[4] This aspect of cultural wealth learns from over 35 years of research about the value of bilingual education and emphasizes the connections between racialized cultural history and language (Cummins, 1986; Anzaldúa, 1987; Darder, 1991; García & Baker, 1995; Gutierrez *et al.*, 1995; Macedo & Bartolomé, 1999; Gutierrez, 2002). Linguistic capital reflects the idea that Students of Color arrive at school with multiple language and communication skills. In addition, these children most often have been engaged participants in a storytelling tradition, that may include listening to and recounting oral histories,

parables, stories (*cuentos*) and proverbs (*dichos*). This repertoire of storytelling skills may include memorization, attention to detail, dramatic pauses, comedic timing, facial affect, vocal tone, volume, rhythm and rhyme. Linguistic capital also refers to the ability to communicate via visual art, music or poetry.[5] Just as students may utilize different vocal registers to whisper, whistle or sing, they must often develop and draw on various language registers, or styles, to communicate with different audiences. For example, Marjorie Faulstich Orellana (2003) examines bilingual children who are often called upon to translate for their parents or other adults and finds that these youth gain multiple social tools of 'vocabulary, audience awareness, cross-cultural awareness, "real-world" literacy skills, math skills, metalinguistic awareness, teaching and tutoring skills, civic and familial responsibility, [and] social maturity' (p. 6).

3. *Familial capital* refers to those cultural knowledges nurtured among *familia* (kin) that carry a sense of community history, memory and cultural intuition (see Delgado Bernal, 1998, 2002). This form of cultural wealth engages a commitment to community well being and expands the concept of family to include a more broad understanding of kinship. Acknowledging the racialized, classed and heterosexualized inferences that comprise traditional understandings of 'family', familial capital is nurtured by our 'extended family', which may include immediate family (living or long passed on) as well as aunts, uncles, grandparents and friends who we might consider part of our *familia*. From these kinship ties, we learn the importance of maintaining a healthy connection to our community and its resources. Our kin also model lessons of caring, coping and providing (*educación*),[6] which inform our emotional, moral, educational and occupational consciousness (Reese, 1992; Auerbach, 2001, 2004; Elenes *et al.*, 2001; Lopez, 2003). This consciousness can be fostered within and between families, as well as through sports, school, religious gatherings and other social community settings. Isolation is minimized as families 'become connected with others around common issues' and realize they are 'not alone in dealing with their problems' (Delgado-Gaitan, 2001, p. 54). Familial capital is informed by the work of scholars who have addressed the *communal bonds* within African American communities (Foley, 1997; Morris, 1999), the *funds of knowledge* within Mexican American communities (Moll *et al.*, 1992; Vélez-Ibáñez & Greenberg, 1992; Gonzalez *et al.*, 1995; Olmedo, 1997; Rueda *et al.*, 2004) and *pedagogies of the home* that Students of Color bring with them to the classroom setting (Delgado Bernal, 2002).
4. *Social capital* can be understood as networks of people and community resources. These peer and other social contacts can provide both instrumental and emotional support to navigate through society's institutions (see Gilbert, 1982; Stanton-Salazar, 2001). For example, drawing on social contacts and community resources may help a student identify and attain a college scholarship. These networks may help a student in preparing the scholarship application itself, while also reassuring the student emotionally that she/he is not alone in the process of pursuing higher education. Scholars note that historically, People of Color have

utilized their social capital to attain education, legal justice, employment and health care. In turn, these Communities of Color gave the information and resources they gained through these institutions back to their social networks. *Mutualistas* or mutual aid societies are an example of how historically, immigrants to the US and indeed, African Americans even while enslaved, created and maintained social networks (Gómez-Quiñones, 1973, 1994; Gutman, 1976; Sanchez, 1993; Stevenson, 1996). This tradition of 'lifting as we climb' has remained the motto of the National Association of Colored Women's Clubs since their organization in 1896 (see Gurnier, Fine & Balin, 1997, p. 167). Concha Delgado-Gaitan's (2001) ethnographic research with the Mexican immigrant community of Carpinteria, California further confirms that 'Families transcend the adversity in their daily lives by uniting with supportive social networks' (p. 105).

5. *Navigational capital* refers to skills of maneuvering through social institutions. Historically, this infers the ability to maneuver through institutions not created with Communities of Color in mind. For example, strategies to navigate through racially-hostile university campuses draw on the concept of academic invulnerability, or students' ability to 'sustain high levels of achievement, despite the presence of stressful events and conditions that place them at risk of doing poorly at school and, ultimately, dropping out of school' (Alva, 1991, p. 19; see also Allen & Solórzano, 2000; Solórzano *et al.*, 2000; Auerbach, 2001). Scholars have examined individual, family and community factors that support Mexican American students' academic invulnerability—their successful navigation through the educational system (Arrellano & Padilla, 1996). In addition, resilience has been recognized as 'a set of inner resources, social competencies and cultural strategies that permit individuals to not only survive, recover, or even thrive after stressful events, but also to draw from the experience to enhance subsequent functioning' (Stanton-Salazar & Spina, 2000, p. 229). Indeed, People of Color draw on various social and psychological 'critical navigational skills' (Solórzano & Villalpando, 1998) to maneuver through structures of inequality permeated by racism (see Pierce, 1974, 1989, 1995). Navigational capital thus acknowledges individual agency within institutional constraints, but it also connects to social networks that facilitate community navigation through places and spaces including schools, the job market and the health care and judicial systems (Williams, 1997).
6. *Resistant capital* refers those knowledges and skills fostered through oppositional behavior that challenges inequality (Freire, 1970, 1973; Giroux, 1983; McLaren, 1994; Delgado Bernal, 1997; Solórzano & Delgado Bernal, 2001). This form of cultural wealth is grounded in the legacy of resistance to subordination exhibited by Communities of Color (Deloria, 1969). Furthermore, maintaining and passing on the multiple dimensions of community cultural wealth is also part of the knowledge base of resistant capital. For example, even from within internment camps, Japanese communities resisted racism by maintaining and nurturing various forms of cultural wealth (Wakatsuki Houston & Houston, 1973).[7] Extending on this history, Tracy Robinson and Janie Ward's

(1991) research shows a group of African American mothers who consciously raise their daughters as 'resistors'. Through verbal and nonverbal lessons, these Black mothers teach their daughters to assert themselves as intelligent, beautiful, strong and worthy of respect to resist the barrage of societal messages devaluing Blackness and belittling Black women (Ward, 1996). Similarly, Sofia Villenas and Melissa Moreno (2001) discuss the contradictions Latina mothers face as they try to teach their daughters to *valerse por si misma* (value themselves and be self-reliant) within structures of inequality such as racism, capitalism and patriarchy. In each of these research studies, Parents of Color are consciously instructing their children to engage in behaviours and maintain attitudes that challenge the status quo. These young women are learning to be oppositional with their bodies, minds and spirits in the face of race, gender and class inequality. In analyzing students' historical and contemporary efforts to transform unequal conditions in urban high schools, Daniel Solórzano and Dolores Delgado Bernal (2001) reveal that resistance may include different forms of oppositional behavior, such as self-defeating or conformist strategies that feed back into the system of subordination. However, when informed by a Freirean critical consciousness (1970), or recognition of the structural nature of oppression and the motivation to work toward social and racial justice, resistance takes on a transformative form (see Solórzano & Yosso, 2002b). Therefore, transformative resistant capital includes cultural knowledge of the structures of racism and motivation to transform such oppressive structures (Pizarro, 1998; Villenas & Deyhle, 1999).

Discussion

Recently, *The Journal of African American History* dedicated an entire issue to 'Cultural capital and African American education' (see Franklin, 2002). In this issue, Franklin (2002) defines cultural capital as 'the sense of group consciousness and collective identity' that serves as a resource 'aimed at the advancement of an entire group' (p. 177). Franklin (2002) goes on to explain that various forms of cultural capital 'became a major resource historically for the funding of African American schools and other educational institutions and programs' (pp. 177–178). This research indicates that 'African Americans were willing to contribute their time, energies, and financial and material resources to support these educational institutions because they knew they were important to the advancement of African Americans as a group (Franklin, 2002, pp. 177–178).

Furthermore, in discussing implications of his ethnographic work with two African American school communities in the US urban south and midwest, Jerome Morris (2004) explains, 'Black people shared their cultural capital with one another and developed their social capital (Black social capital) for survival and success in a segregated world bounded by the omnipresent forces of racism and discrimination' (p. 102). This scholarship documenting community mobilization efforts to create access and equity for African Americans in education, bolsters the examples of cultural wealth offered above. Such work also demonstrates that the forms of capital comprising community cultural wealth are engendered from within the context of a legacy of racism and are thus tied to a larger social and racial justice project (Perea *et al.*, 2000). Morris (2004) asserts, 'it is important that social capital theory also consider the agency and sustenance that are characteristic of African American people, culture and institutions—apart from and in response to oppressive forces' (p. 102). Indeed, the main goals of identifying and documenting cultural wealth are to transform education and empower People of Color to utilize assets already abundant in their communities.

As demonstrated through the concept of cultural wealth, CRT research begins with the perspective that Communities of Color are places with multiple strengths. In contrast, deficit scholars bemoan a lack of cultural capital or what Hirsch (1988, 1996) terms 'cultural literacy' in low income Communities of Color. Such research utilizes a deficit analytical lens and places value judgments on communities that often do not have access to White, middle or upper class resources. In contrast, CRT shifts the research lens away from a deficit view of Communities of Color as places full of cultural poverty or disadvantages, and instead focuses on and learns from these communities' cultural assets and wealth (Solórzano & Solórzano, 1995; Valencia & Solórzano, 1997; Villalpando & Solórzano, 2005).

CRT centers the research, pedagogy, and policy lens on Communities of Color and calls into question White middle class communities as the standard by which all others are judged. This shifting of the research lens allows critical race scholars to 'see' multiple forms of cultural wealth within Communities of Color. CRT identifies various indicators of capital that have rarely been acknowledged as cultural and social assets in Communities of Color (i.e., aspirational, social, navigational, linguistic, resistant and familial capital). These forms of capital draw on the knowledges Students of Color bring with them from their homes and communities into the classroom. They are not conceptualized for the purpose of finding new ways to co-opt or exploit the strengths of Communities of Color.[8] Instead, community cultural wealth involves a commitment to conduct research, teach and develop schools that serve a larger purpose of struggling toward social and racial justice.

In the opening epigraph of this essay, Anzaldúa urges the generation of theories based on those whose knowledges are traditionally excluded from and silenced by academic research. She further asserts that beyond creating theories, 'we need to find practical application for those theories. We need to de-academize theory and to connect the community to the academy' (Anzaldúa, 1990, p. xxvi). Anzaldúa (2002) also notes that 'Change requires more than words on a page—it takes perseverance, creative ingenuity and acts of love' (p. 574). CRT offers a response to Anzaldúa's challenge in listening to the experiences of those 'faces at the bottom of society's well' (Bell, 1992, p. v). These experiences expose the racism underlying cultural deficit theorizing and reveal the need to restructure US social institutions around those knowledges, skills, abilities and networks—the community cultural wealth—possessed and utilized by People of Color.

Notes

1. Although not exhaustive, the following resources are some examples of the different frameworks cited: ethnic studies (see *Aztlan: A Journal of Chicano Studies*); feminist studies (see *Frontiers: A Journal of Women's Studies*); cultural nationalist paradigms (see Asante, 1987); critical legal studies (see Kelman, 1989); Marxist and neo-Marxist frameworks (see Bowles & Gintis, 1976; Barrera, 1979); internal colonial models (see Bonilla & Girling, 1973); LatCrit (see Arriola, 1998; Valdes, 1997, 1998); WhiteCrit (see Delgado & Sefancic, 1997); FemCrit (see Wing, 1997); AsianCrit (see Chang, 1993).
2. Solórzano and Yosso (2001) note that while each individual tenet of CRT is not 'new', synthesizing these tenets into a CRT framework in education is relatively recent. For instance, William Tate's 1994 autobiographical article in the journal *Urban Education*—titled 'From inner city to ivory tower: does my voice matter in the academy'—represents (to my knowledge) the first use of CRT principles in education. A year later, in 1995, Gloria Ladson-Billings and William Tate wrote a paper titled, 'Toward a critical race theory of education' in the *Teachers College Record*. Two years later, Daniel Solórzano's 1997 essay on 'Images and words that wound: critical race theory, racial stereotyping and teacher education' in *Teacher Education Quarterly* applied CRT to a specific subfield of teacher education. Also in 1997, William Tate's 'Critical race theory and education: history, theory and implications' in the *Review of Research in Education* furthered our understanding of the history of CRT in education. The field was expanded significantly with the 1998 'Special issue on critical race theory in education' in the *International Journal of Qualitative Studies in Education*. The 1999 edited book on *Race is—race isn't: critical race theory and qualitative studies in education* (Parker *et al.*, 1999) was followed by individual scholars presenting on panels at professional conferences across the country and publishing their work in various journals. In 2002, the journals *Qualitative Inquiry* and *Equity and Excellence in Education* dedicated a special issue to CRT in education. In 2004, the American Education Research Association conference symposium 'And we are still not saved: critical race theory in education ten years later' acknowledged the ten year anniversary of Tate's 1994 article introducing CRT officially to education.
3. As is consistent with the concept of community cultural wealth, this working definition demonstrates an accumulation of collaborative work. Thank you to Daniel G Solórzano who originally conceptualized cultural wealth. He shared with me a model in progress and later a collaboratively written piece (with Octavio Villalpando), and asked me to 'run with it'. Since that time, cultural wealth has taken on multiple dimensions. I also acknowledge those personal and professional experiences, community histories and students' research projects that have informed this work. I look forward to the ways that cultural wealth will take on new dimensions as others also 'run with it'.
4. Thanks to Rebeca Burciaga, whose identification of linguistic and familial capital added important dimensions to cultural wealth.
5. Thanks to UCSB undergraduate students, Pablo Gallegos, Moises Garcia, Noel Gomez and Ray Hernandez, whose research conceptualizing graffiti and hip hop poetry as unacknowledged sources of community cultural wealth expanded my thinking about linguistic capital.
6. Chicana scholars note for example that in Spanish, *educación* holds dual meanings (Delgado-Gaitan, 1992, 1994, 2001; Elenes *et al.*, 2001). A person can be formally educated with multiple advanced degrees, but may still be rude, ignorant, disrespectful or unethical (immoral)—*mal educada*. On the other hand, a person with only a second grade formal education may be *una persona bien educada* or a well-mannered, kind, fair-minded, respectful (moral) individual.
7. The book *Farewell to Manzanar* (Wakatsuki Houston & Houston, 1973) offers a first-hand account of some of the ways Japanese internees held onto hope, fostered caring, coping and responsibility, maintained skills of language, poetry, music, social networks and critical navigational skills, and challenged social and racial inequality.

8. I recognize that the notion of capital may be associated with capitalism, which is a system that is exploitative and has historically been an oppressive force against Communities of Color. The concept of schooling itself can be contradictory, given that schools have historically oppressed Students of Color, while still having the potential to be transformative places of empowerment. Similarly, as viewed through mainstream media, hip-hop's contradictory nature offers an example of how historically some aspects of community cultural wealth are co-opted and utilized for exploitative purposes (see Spike Lee's film *Baboozled*, 2000). Still, hip-hop maintains amazing potential to be a revolutionary art form and transformative cultural expression that can inspire and inform social movement. I believe community cultural wealth and forms of capital nurtured in the histories of People of Color holds the same potential.

References

Allen, W. (1993) A response to a 'white discourse on white racism', *Educational Researcher,* 22, 11–13.

Allen, W. & Solórzano, D. (2001) Affirmative action, educational equity, and campus racial climate: A case study of the university of Michigan law school, *Berkeley La Raza Law Journal,* 12(2), 237–363.

Alva, S. (1991) Academic invulnerability among Mexican American students: the importance of protective resources and appraisals, *Hispanic Journal of Behavioral Sciences,* 13(1), 18–34.

Anzaldúa, G. (1987) *Borderlands/La Frontera: the New Mestiza* (San Francisco, CA, Aunt Lute Book Company).

Anzaldúa, G. (1990) *Haciendo Caras/making face, making soul: creative and critical perspectives by women of color* (San Francisco, CA, Aunt Lute Press).

Anzaldúa, G. (2002) Now let us shift … the path of conocimiento … inner work, public acts, in: G. Anzaldúa & A. Keating (Eds) *This bridge we call home: radical visions for transformation* (New York, Routledge), 540–578.

Arrellano, A. R. & Padilla, A. M. (1996) Academic invulnerability among a select group of Latino university students, *Hispanic Journal of Behavioral Sciences,* 18(4), 485–507.

Arriola, E. (1997) LatCrit theory, international human rights, popular culture and the faces of despair in ins raids, *Inter-American Law Review,* 28(2), 245–262.

Arriola, E. (1998) Difference, solidarity and law: building Latina/o communities through LatCrit theory, *Chicano-Latino Law Review,* 19, 1–612.

Asante, M. K. (1987) *The Afrocentric idea* (Philadelphia, PA, Temple University Press).

Auerbach, S. (2001) *Under co-construction: parent roles in promoting college access for students of color,* unpublished doctoral dissertation, University of California, Los Angeles.

Auerbach, S. (2004) From moral supporters to struggling advocates: reconceptualizing parent involvement through the experience of Latino families, paper presented at annual meeting of the *American Educational Research Association.* San Diego, CA.

Baca Zinn, M. (1989) Family, race and poverty in the eighties, *Signs: Journal of Woman in Culture and Society,* 14, 856–874.

Barnes, R. (1990) Race consciousness: the thematic content of racial distinctiveness in critical race scholarship, *Harvard Law Review,* 103, 1864–1871.

Barrera, M. (1979) *Race and class in the southwest: a theory of inequality* (London, University of Notre Dame Press).

Bell, D. (1986) Application of the 'tipping point' theory to law faculty hiring practices, *Nova Law Journal,* 10, 319–327.

Bell, D. (1987) *And we will not be saved: the elusive quest for racial justice* (New York, Basic Books).

Bell, D. (1992) *Faces at the bottom of the well: the permanence of racism* (New York, Basic Books).

Bell, D. (1995) Who's afraid of critical race theory?, *University of Illinois Law Review,* 1995, 893–910.

Bell, D. (1996) *Gospel choirs: psalms of survival for an alien land called home* (New York, Basic Books).

Bell, D. (1998) *Afrolantica legacies* (Chicago, IL, Third World Press).

Blauner, B. (2001) *Still the big news: racial oppression in America* (Philadelphia, Temple University Press).

Bonilla, F. & Girling, R. (Eds) (1973) *Structures of dependency* (Stanford, CA, Stanford Institute of Politics).

Bonilla-Silva, E. (2001) *White supremacy and racism in the post civil rights era* (Boulder, CO, Lynne Rienner Publishers).

Bourdieu, P. & Passeron, J. (1977) *Reproduction in education, society and culture* (London, Sage).

Bowles, S. & Gintis, H. (1976) *Schooling in capitalistic America: educational reform and the contradictions of economic life* (New York, Basic Books).

Brayboy, B. (2002) Tribal critical race theory in education, paper presentation at annual conference of the *American Educational Research Association,* New Orleans, LA, April.

Brayboy, B. (2001) Toward a tribal critical theory in higher education, paper presentation at *Annual Conference of the Association for the Study of Higher Education,* Richmond, VA.

Caldwell. P. (1995) A hairpiece: perspectives on the intersection of race and gender, in: R. Delgado (Ed.) *Critical race theory: the cutting edge* (Philadelphia, PA, Temple University Press), 267–277.

Calmore, J. (1992) Critical race theory, Archie Shepp and fire music: securing an authentic intellectual life in a multicultural world, *Southern California Law Review,* 65, 2129–2231.

Calmore, J. (1997) Exploring Michael Omi's 'messy' real world of race: an essay for 'naked people longing to swim free', *Law and Inequality,* 15, 25–82.

Carrasco, E. (1996) Collective recognition as a communitarian device: or, of course we want to be role models!, *La Raza Law Journal,* 9, 81–101.

Chang, R. (1993) Toward an Asian American legal scholarship: critical race theory, post-structuralism, and narrative space, *California Law Review,* 81, 1243.

Chang, R. (1998) Who's afraid of Tiger Woods?, *Chicano-Latino Law Review,* 19, 223.

Chon, M. (1995) On the need for Asian American narratives in law: ethnic specimens, native informants, storytelling and silences, *UCLA Asian Pacific American Law Journal,* 3(1), 4–32.

Crenshaw, K. (1989) Demarginalizing the intersection of race and sex: A Black feminist critique of antidiscrimination doctrine, feminist theory and antiracist politics, *University of Chicago Legal Forum,* 1989, 139–167.

Crenshaw, K. (1993) Mapping the margins: intersectionality, identity politics and the violence against Women of Color, *Stanford Law Review,* 43, 1241–1299.

Crenshaw, K., Gotanda, N., Peller, G. & Thomas, K. (Eds) (1995) *Critical race theory: the key writings that formed the movement* (New York, The New Press).

Crenshaw, K. (2002) The first decade: critical reflections, or 'a foot in the closing door', in: F. Valdes, J. McCristal Culp & A. Harris (Eds) *Crossroads, directions and a new critical race theory* (Philadelphia, PA, Temple University Press), 9–31.

Cummins, J. (1986) Bilingual education and anti-racist education, *Interracial Books for Children Bulletin,* 17(3&4), 9–12.

Darder, A. (1991) *Culture and power in the classroom: a critical foundation for bicultural education* (New York, Bergin & Garvey).

Davis, P. (1989) Law as microaggression, *The Yale Law Journal*, 98, 1559–1577.
Delgado, R. (1984) The imperial scholar: reflections on a review of civil rights literature, *University of Pennsylvania Law Review*, 132, 561–578.
Delgado, R. (1988) Critical legal studies and the realities of race: does the fundamental contradiction have a corollary?, *Harvard Civil Rights–Civil Liberties Law Review*, 23, 407–413.
Delgado, R. (1989) Storytelling for oppositionists and others: a plea for narrative, *Michigan Law Review*, 87, 2411–2441.
Delgado, R. (1992) The imperial scholar revisited: how to marginalize outsider writing, ten years later, *University of Pennsylvania Law Review*, 140, 1349–1372.
Delgado, R. (1993) On telling stories in school: a reply to Farber and Sherry, *Vanderbilt Law Review*, 46, 665–676.
Delgado, R. (Ed.) (1995a) *Critical race theory: the cutting edge* (Philadelphia, PA, Temple University Press).
Delgado, R. (1995b) *The Rodrigo chronicles: conversations about America and race* (New York, New York University Press).
Delgado, R. (1996) *The coming race war?: and other apocalyptic tales of American after affirmative action and welfare* (New York, New York University Press).
Delgado, R. (1997) Rodrigo's fifteenth chronicle: racial mixture, Latino-critical scholarship, and the black-white binary, *Texas Law Review*, 75, 1181–1201.
Delgado, R. (1999) *When equality ends: stories about race and resistance* (Boulder, CO, Westview Press).
Delgado, R. (2003) *Justice at war: civil liberties and civil rights during times of crisis* (New York, New York University Press).
Delgado, R. & Stefancic, J. (1992) Images of the outsider in American law and culture: can free expression remedy systematic social ills?, *Cornell Law Review*, 77, 1258–1297.
Delgado, R. & Stefancic, J. (1993) Critical race theory: an annotated bibliography, *Virginia Law Review*, 79, 461–516.
Delgado, R. & Stefancic, J. (1994) Critical race theory: an annotated bibliography 1993, a year of transition, *University of Colorado Law Review*, 66, 159–193.
Delgado, R. & Stefancic, J. (Eds) (1997) *Critical white studies: looking behind the mirror* (Philadelphia, Temple University Press).
Delgado, R. & Stefancic, J. (2001) *Critical race theory: an introduction* (New York, New York University Press).
Delgado Bernal, D. (1997) *Chicana school resistance and grassroots leadership: providing an alternative history of the 1968 East Los Angeles blowouts*, unpublished doctoral dissertation, University of California, Los Angeles.
Delgado Bernal, D. (1998) Using a Chicana feminist epistemology in educational research, *Harvard Educational Review*, 68(4), 555–582.
Delgado Bernal, D. (2001) Living and learning pedagogies of the home: the mestiza consciousness of Chicana students, *International Journal of Qualitative Studies in Education*, 14(5), 623–639.
Delgado Bernal, D. (2002) Critical race theory, LatCrit theory and critical raced-gendered epistemologies: recognizing Students of Color as holders and creators of knowledge, *Qualitative Inquiry*, 8(1), 105–126.
Delgado Bernal, D. & Villalpando, O. (2002) An apartheid of knowledge in academia: the struggle over the 'legitimate' knowledge of Faculty of Color, *Equity and Excellence in Education*, 35(2), 169–180.
Delgado-Gaitan, C. (1992) School matters in the Mexican American home: socializing children to education, *American Educational Research Journal*, 29(3), 495–513.
Delgado-Gaitan, C. (1994) Socializing young children in Mexican-American families: an intergenerational perspective, in: P. Greenfield & R. Cocking (Eds) Cross-cultural roots of minority development (New Jersey, Lawrence Erlbaum Associates), 55–86.
Delgado-Gaitan, C. (2001) *The power of community: mobilizing for family and schooling* (Boulder, CO, Rowman and Littlefield Publishers).

Deloria, V. (1969) *Custer died for your sins: an Indian manifesto* (New York, Avon).

DuBois, W. E. B. (1989) *The soul of black folks* (New York, Bantam). (Originally published in 1903.)

Elenes, C. A., Gonzalez, F., Delgado Bernal, D. & Villenes, S. (2001) Introduction: Chicana/Mexicana feminist pedagogies: Consejos respeto, y educación, *International Journal of Qualitative Studies in Education,* 14(5), 595–602.

Ellison, R. (1990) *Invisible man* (New York, Vintage Books).

Espinoza, L. G. (1990) Masks and other disguises: exposing legal academia, *Harvard Law Review,* 103, 1878–1886.

Espinoza, L. G. (1998) Latino/a identity and multi-identity: community and culture, in: R. Delgado & J. Stefancic (Eds) *The Latino/a condition: a critical reader* (New York, New York University Press), 17–23.

Espinoza, L. & Harris, A. (1998) Embracing the tar-baby: LatCrit theory and the sticky mess of race, *La Raza Law Journal,* 10(1), 499–559.

Essed, P. (1991) *Understanding everyday racism: an interdisciplinary theory* (Newbury Park, Sage Publications).

Faulstich Orellana, M. (2003) *In other words: en otras palabras: learning from bilingual kids' translating/interpreting experiences* (Evanston, IL, School of Education and Social Policy, Northwestern University).

Fay, B. (1987) *Critical social science: liberation and its limits* (Ithaca, NY, Cornell University Press).

Foley, D. E. (1997) Deficit thinking models based on culture: the anthropological protest, in: R. Valencia (Ed.) *The evolution of deficit thinking: educational thought and practice* (London, The Falmer Press), 113–131.

Franklin, V. P. (2002) Introduction: cultural capital and African-American education, *The Journal of African-American History,* 87, 175–181.

Freire, P. (1970) *Education for critical consciousness* (New York, Continuum Publishing Company).

Freire, P. (1973) *Pedagogy of the oppressed* (New York, The Seabury Press).

Gándara, P. (1982) Passing through the eye of the needle: high-achieving Chicanas, *Hispanic Journal of Behavioral Sciences,* 4, 167–179.

Gándara, P. (1995) *Over the ivy walls: the educational mobility of low-income Chicanos* (Albany, State University of New York Press).

Garcia, R. (1995) Critical race theory and proposition 187: the racial politics of immigration law, *Chicano-Latino Law Review,* 17, 118–148.

García, O. & Baker, C. (1995) *Policy and practice in bilingual education: a reader extending the foundations* (Philadelphia, Multilingual Matters).

García, S. B. & Guerra, P. L. (2004) Deconstructing deficit thinking: working with educators to create more equitable learning environments, *Education and Urban Society,* 36(2), 150–168.

Gilbert, M. J. (1982) *Los parientes: social structural factors and kinship relations among second generation Mexican Americans in two southern California communities,* unpublished doctoral dissertation, University of California, Santa Barbara.

Giroux, H. (1983) Theories of reproduction and resistance in the new sociology of education: a critical analysis, *Harvard Educational Review,* 55, 257–293.

Gómez-Quiñones, J. (1973) The first steps: Chicano labor conflict and organizing 1900–1920, *Aztlan,* 3(1), 13–49.

Gómez-Quiñones, J. (1977) *On culture* (New York, UCLA Chicano Studies Center Publications).

Gómez-Quiñones, J. (1994) *Roots of Chicano politics, 1600–1940* (Albuquerque, NM, University of New Mexico Press).

Gonzalez, N. & Moll, L. C. (2002) Cruzando el puente: building bridges to funds of knowledge, *Educational Policy,* 16(4), 623–641.

Gonzalez, N., Moll, L. C., Tenery, M. F., Rivera, A., Rendon, P. Gonzales, R. & Amanti, C. (1995) Funds of knowledge for teaching in Latino households, *Urban Education,* 29(4), 443–470.

Gotanda, N. (1991) A critique of 'our constitution is color-blind', *Stanford Law Review,* 44, 1–68.

Guinier, L., Fine, M. & Balin, J. (1997) *Becoming gentleman: women, law school, and institutional change* (Boston, MA, Beacon Press).

Gutiérrez, K. (2002) Studying cultural practices in urban learning communities, *Human Development,* 45(4), 312–321.

Gutiérrez-Jones, C. (2001) *Critical race narratives: a study of race, rhetoric and injury* (New York, New York University Press).

Gutman, H. (1976) *The Black family in slavery and freedom, 1750–1925* (New York, Pantheon Books).

Harris, A. (1994) Forward: the jurisprudence of reconstruction, *California Law Review,* 82, 741–785.

Hill Collins, P. (1986) Learning from the outsider within: the sociological significance of Black feminist thought, *Social Problems,* 33, S14–S32.

Hill Collins, P. (1998) *Fighting words: Black women and the search for justice* (Minneapolis, MN, University of Minnesota Press).

Hill Collins, P. (2000) *Black feminist thought: knowledge, consciousness and the politics of empowerment* (New York, Routledge).

Hirsch, E. D. Jr. (1988) *Cultural literacy: what every American needs to know* (New York, Vintage Books).

Hirsch, E. D. Jr. (1996) *The schools we need and why we don't have them* (New York, Doubleday).

hooks, b. (1990) *Yearning: race, gender and cultural politics* (Cambridge, MA, South End Press).

hooks, b. (1994) *Teaching to transgress: education as the practice of freedom* (New York, NY, Routledge).

Hurtado, A. (1996) *The color of privilege: three blasphemes on race and feminism* (Ann Arbor, University of Michigan Press).

Ikemoto, L. (1992) Furthering the inquiry: race, class and culture in the forced medical treatment of pregnant women, *Tennessee Law Review,* 59, 487.

Johnson, K. (1999) *How did you get to be Mexican? A White/brown man's search for identity* (Philadelphia, PA, Temple University Press).

Ladson-Billings, G. (1998) Preparing teachers for diverse student populations: a critical race theory perspective, *Review of Research in Education,* 24, 211–247.

Ladson-Billings, G. (2000) Racialized discourses and ethnic epistemologies, in: N. Denzin & Y. Lincoln (Eds) *Handbook of qualitative research* (Thousand Oaks, CA, Sage), 257–277.

Ladson-Billings, G. & Tate, W. (1995) Toward a critical race theory of education, *Teachers College Record,* 97, 47–68.

LatCrit Primer (1999) Fact sheet: LatCrit, presented to the *Fourth Annual LatCrit Conference,* Stanford Sierra Conference Center, Lake Tahoe, Nevada, 29 April–5 May.

Lawrence, C. (1987) The id, the ego, and equal protection: reckoning with unconscious racism, *Stanford Law Review,* 39, 317–388.

Lawrence, C. (1992) The word and the river: pedagogy as scholarship as struggle, *Southern California Law Review,* 65, 2231–2298.

Lawrence, C. & Matsuda, M. (1997) *We won't go back: making the case for affirmative action* (Boston, MA, Houghton Mifflin).

Lawson, R. (1995) Critical race theory as praxis: a view from outside to the outside, *Howard Law Journal,* 38, 353–370.

Lopez, G. (2003) Parental involvement as racialized performance, in: G. Lopez & L. Parker (Eds) *Interrogating racism in qualitative research methodology* (New York, Peter Lang Publishing), 71–95.

Lopez, G. & Parker, L. (Eds) (2003) *Interrogating racism in qualitative research methodology* (New York, Peter Lang Publishing).

Lynn, M. (1999) Toward a critical race pedagogy: a research note, *Urban Education,* 33, 606–626.

Lynn, M. & Adams, M. (Eds) (2002) Special issue of critical race theory in education, *Equity and Excellence in Education,* 35(2), 87–199.

Lynn, M., Yosso, T., Solórzano, D. & Parker, L. (2002) Special issue: critical race and qualitative research, *Qualitative Inquiry,* 8(1), 3–126.

Macedo. D. & Bartolomé, L. (1999) *Dancing with bigotry: beyond the politics of tolerance* (New York, Palgrave).

Marable, M. (1992) *Black America* (Westfield, NJ, Open Media).

Matsuda, M. (1991) Voices of America: accent, antidiscrimination law and a jurisprudence for the last reconstruction, *Yale Law Journal,* 100, 1329–1407.

Matsuda, M., Lawrence, C., Delgado, R. & Crenshaw, K. (1993) *Words that wound: critical race theory, assaultive speech, and the first amendment* (Boulder, CO, Westview Press).

McLaren, P. (1994) *Life in schools: an introduction to critical pedagogy in the foundations of education* (2nd edn) (New York, Longman).

Moll, L. C., Amanti, C., Neff, D. & Gonzalez, N. (1992) Funds of knowledge for teaching: using a qualitative approach to connect homes and classrooms, *Theory into Practice,* 31(2), 132–141.

Montoya, M. (1994) Mascaras, trenzas, y grenas: un/masking the self while un/braiding Latina stories and legal discourse, *Chicano-Latino Law Review,* 15, 1–37.

Montoya, M. (2002) Celebrating racialized legal narratives, in: F. Valdes, J. McCristal Culp & A. Harris (Eds) *Crossroads, directions and a new critical race theory* (Philadephia, PA, Temple University Press), 243–250.

Moraga, C. (1983) La güera, in: C. Moraga & G. Anzaldúa (Eds) *This bridge called my back: writings by radical women of color* (2nd edn) (New York, Kitchen Table), 24–33.

Morris, J. (1999) A pillar of strength: an African-American school's communal bonds with families and community since *Brown, Urban Education,* 33(5), 584–605.

Morris, J. (2004) Can anything good come from Nazareth? Race, class and African-American schooling and community in the urban south and Midwest, *American Educational Research Journal,* 41(1), 69–112.

Olivas, M. (1990) The chronicles, my grandfather's stories and immigration law: the slave traders chronicle as racial history, *Saint Louis University Law Journal,* 34, 425–441.

Oliver, M. & Shapiro, T. (1995) *Black wealth/White wealth: a new perspective on racial inequality* (New York, Routledge).

Olmedo, I. M. (1997) Voices of our past: using oral history to explore funds of knowledge within a Puerto Rican family, *Anthropology and Education Quarterly,* 28(4), 550–573.

Parker, L. Deyhle, D., Villenas, S. & Crossland, K. (1998) Special issue: critical race theory and education, *International Journal of Qualitative Studies in Education,* 11, 1–184.

Parker, L., Deyhle, D. & Villenas, S. (Eds) (1999) *Race is ... race isn't: critical race theory and qualitative studies in education* (Boulder, CO, Westview Press).

Perea, J., Delgado, R., Harris, A. & Wildman, S. (2000) *Race and races: cases and resources for a multiracial America* (St Paul, MN, West Group).

Pierce, C. (1974) Psychiatric problems of the Black minority, in: S. Arieti (Ed.) *American handbook of psychiatry* (New York, Basic Books), 512–523.

Pierce, C. (1989) Unity in diversity: thirty-three years of stress, in: G. Berry & J. Asamen (Eds) *Black students: psychological issues and academic achievement* (Newbury Park, Sage), 296–312.

Pierce, C. (1995) Stress analogs of racism and sexism: terrorism, torture, and disaster, in: C. Willie, P. Rieker, B. Kramer & B. Brown (Eds) *Mental health, racism and sexism* (Pittsburgh, PA, University of Pittsburgh Press), 277–293.

Pizarro, M. (1998) 'Chicano power!' Epistemology and methodology for social justice and empowerment in Chicana/o communities, *International Journal of Qualitative Studies in Education,* 11(1), 57–80.

Reese, L. J. (1992) *Ecocultural factors influencing the academic success of young Latino students,* unpublished doctoral dissertation, University of California, Los Angeles.

Robinson, T. & Ward, J. (1991) 'A belief in self far greater than anyone's belief': cultivating resistance among African-American female adolescents, in: C. Gilligan, A. Rogers & D. Tolman (Eds) *Women, girls and psychotherapy: reframing resistance* (New York, Haworth), 87–103.

Rueda, R., Monzo, L. D. & Higareda, I. (2004) Appropriating the sociocultural resources of Latino paraeducators for effective instruction with Latino students: promises and problems, *Urban Education,* 29(1), 52–90.

Russell, M. (1992) Entering great America: reflections on race and the convergence of progressive legal theory and practice, *Hastings Law Journal,* 43, 749–767.

Saldivar-Hill, S. (2000) *Feminism on the border: Chicana gender politics and literature* (Berkeley, CA, University of California Press).

Scheurich, J. & Young, M. (1997) Coloring epistemologies: are our research epistemologies racially biased?, *Educational Researcher,* 26, 4–16.

Shapiro, T. (2004) *The hidden cost of being African-American: how wealth perpetuates inequality* (New York, Oxford University Press).

Solórzano, D. (1989) Teaching and social change: reflections on a Freirean approach in a college classroom, *Teaching Sociology,* 17, 218–225.

Solórzano, D. (1992) Chicano mobility aspirations: a theoretical and empirical note, *Latino Studies Journal,* 3, 48–66.

Solórzano, D. (1997) Images and words that wound: critical race theory, racial stereotyping and teacher education, *Teacher Education Quarterly,* 24, 5–19.

Solórzano, D. (1998) Critical race theory, racial and gender microaggressions, and the experiences of Chicana and Chicano Scholars, *International Journal of Qualitative Studies in Education,* 11, 121–136.

Solórzano, D., Ceja, M. & Yosso, T. (2000) Critical race theory, racial microaggressions and campus racial climate: the experiences of African-American college students, *Journal of Negro Education,* 69(1/2), 60–73.

Solórzano, D. & Delgado Bernal, D. (2001) Critical race theory, transformational resistance and social justice: Chicana and Chicano students in an urban context, *Urban Education,* 36, 308–342.

Solórzano, D. & Solórzano, R. (1995) The Chicano educational experience: a proposed framework for effective schools in Chicano communities, *Educational Policy,* 9, 293–314.

Solórzano, D. & Villalpando, O. (1998) Critical race theory, marginality, and the experience of minority students in higher education, in: C. Torres & T. Mitchell (Eds) *Emerging issues in the sociology of education: comparative perspectives* (New York, SUNY Press), 211–224.

Solórzano, D. & Yosso, T. (2000) Toward a critical race theory of Chicana and Chicano education, in: C. Tejeda, C. Martinez, Z. Leonardo & P. McLaren (Eds) *Charting new terrains of Chicana(o)/Latina(o) education* (Cresskill, NJ, Hampton Press), 35–65.

Solórzano, D. & Yosso, T. (2001) Critical race and LatCrit theory and method: counterstorytelling Chicana and Chicano graduate school experiences, *International Journal of Qualitative Studies in Education,* 14(4), 471–495.

Solórzano, D. & Yosso, T. (2002a) A critical race counterstory of race, racism and affirmative action, *Equity and Excellence in Eduction,* 35(2), 155–168.

Solórzano, D. & Yosso, T. (2002b) Maintaining social justice hopes within academic realities: a freirean approach to critical race/LatCrit pedagogy, *Denver Law Review,* 78(4), 595–621.

Stanton-Salazar, R. D. (2001) *Manufacturing hope and despair: the school and kin support networks of US–Mexican youth* (New York, Teachers College Press).

Stanton-Salazar, R. & Spina, S. U. (2000) The network orientations of highly resilient urban minority youth: a network-analytic account of minority socialization and its educational implications, *The Urban Review,* 32(3), 227–261.

Stefancic, J. (1998) Latino and Latina critical theory: an annotated bibliography, *La Raza Law Journal,* 10, 423–498.

Stevenson, B. (1996) *Life in Black and White: family and community in the slave south* (New York, Oxford University Press).

Tate, W. (1994) From inner city to ivory tower: does my voice matter in the academy?, *Urban Education,* 29(3), 245–269.

Tate, W. (1997) Critical race theory and education: history, theory and implications, *Review of Research in Education,* 22, 191–243.

Tatum, B. D. (1997) *Why are all the Black kids sitting together in the cafeteria? And other conversations about race* (New York, Basic Books).

Tierney, W. (1993) *Building Communities of difference: higher education in the twenty-first century* (Westport, CT, Bergin & Garvey).

US Bureau of the Census (2000) *2000 census of the population: general population characteristics, United States summary* (Washington, DC, US Government Printing Office).

Valdes, F. (1997) LatCrit theory: naming and launching a new direction of critical legal scholarship, *Harvard Latino Law Review,* 2, 1–501.

Valdes, F. (1998) LatCrit: Latinas/os and the law, *La Raza Law Journal,* 10, 1–600.

Valdes, F., McCristal Culp, J. & Harris, A. (2002) *Crossroads, directions and a new critical race theory* (Philadelphia, PA, Temple University Press), 243–250.

Valencia, R. (1991) *Chicano school failure and success: research and policy agenda for the 1990s* (New York, Falmer Press).

Valencia, R. (2002) *Chicano school failure and success: past, present and future* (New York, Routledge/Falmer).

Valencia, R. & Solórzano, D. (1997) Contemporary deficit thinking, in: R. Valencia (Ed.) *The evolution of deficit thinking in educational thought and practice* (New York, Falmer Press), 160–210.

Valenzuela, A. (1999) *Subtractive schooling: US-Mexican youth and the politics of caring* (New York, SUNY Press).

Vélez-Ibáñez, C. & Greenberg, J. (1992) Formation and transformation of funds of knowledge among U.S.-Mexican households, *Anthropology and Education Quarterly,* 23(4), 313–335.

Villalpando, O. (2003) Self-segregation or self-preservation? A critical race theory and Latina/o critical theory analysis of findings form a longitudinal study of Chicana/o college students, *International Journal of Qualitative Studies in Education,* 16(5), 619–646.

Villalpando, O. & Solórzano, D. (2005) The role of culture in college preparation programs: a review of the literature, in: W. Tierney, Z. Corwin, & J. Kolyar (Eds) *Preparing for college: nine elements of effective outreach* (Albany, NY, SUNY Press), 13–28.

Villenas, S. & Deyhle, D. (1999) Critical race theory and ethnographies challenging the stereotypes: Latino families, schooling, resilience and resistance, *Curriculum Inquiry,* 29(4), 413–445.

Villenas, S. & Moreno, M. (2001) To valerse por si misma between race, capitalism, and patriarchy: Latina mother-daughter pedagogies in north Carolina, *International Journal of Qualitative Studies in Education,* 14(5), 671–688.

Wakatsuki Houston, J. & Houston, J. D. (1973) *Farewell to Manzanar: a true story of Japanese American experience during and after the World War II internment* (Boston, Houghton Mifflin).

Ward, J. (1996) Raising resisters: the role of truth telling in the psychological development of African-American girls, in: B. Leadbetter & N. Way (Eds) *Urban girls: resisting stereotypes, creating identities* (New York, New York University Press), 85–99.

Williams, P. (1991) *The alchemy of race and rights: diary of a law professor* (Cambridge, MA, Harvard University Press).

Williams, P. (1997) Spirit-murdering the messenger: the discourse of fingerprinting as the law's response to racism, in: A. Wing (Ed.) *Critical race feminism: a reader* (New York, New York University Press), 229–236.

Williams, R. (1997) Vampires anonymous and critical race practice, *Michigan Law Review,* 95, 741–765.

Wing, A. (Ed.) (1997) *Critical race feminism: a reader* (New York, New York University Press).

Wing, A. (Ed.) (2000) *Global critical race feminism: an international reader* (New York, New York University Press).

Zavella, P. (1991) Reflections on diversity among Chicanas, *Frontiers: A Journal of Women Studies,* 2(2), 73–85.

Racial microaggressions as a tool for critical race research

Lindsay Pérez Huber and Daniel G. Solorzano

This conceptual article utilizes critical race theory (CRT) to explain how everyday forms of racism – racial microaggressions – emerge in the everyday experiences of People of Color. We provide a framework for understanding and analyzing racial microaggressions that demonstrates how everyday racist events are systemically mediated by institutionalized racism (i.e. structures and processes), and guided by ideologies of white supremacy that justify the superiority of a dominant group (whites) over non-dominant groups (People of Color). To demonstrate the conceptual utility of the framework, we utilize historical and contemporary examples of racial micoraggressions, and offer varied ways to use the framework in critical race research. We argue racial microaggressions can be a powerful 'tool' for identifying, disrupting, and dismantling the racism that marginalizes, subordinates and excludes People of Color in and outside of education.

Recently, the concept of racial microaggressions has received national attention across the US. In spring 2014, Students of Color at colleges and universities throughout the US engaged in social media campaigns to bring attention to these subtle, everyday forms of racism they encounter on their campuses (see St. Olaf microagressions 2014; Vega 2014). In these campaigns, the students challenge claims of a 'post-racial' society where racism is no longer a significant barrier in the lives of Communities of Color (Hodge and Vega 2014). At Harvard University, African American students organized and performed a play called, 'I, too, Am Harvard' that included skits and monologues about their experiences with racial microaggressions as students (see 'I too Am Harvard' 2014; Vega 2014). Even Music Television Network (MTV) has taken an interest in the concept of microaggressions, using the term 'racial bias' to explain the everyday racist slights experienced by People of Color. In 2014, the network launched the 'Look

Different' campaign, with a website that offers viewers a chance to learn about their raced and gendered 'biases' (www.lookdifferent.org).[1]

Despite this very recent national attention, the concept of microaggressions has been utilized in academic research since the late 1960's (Pierce 1969). Dr Chester Pierce, an African American psychiatrist, medical doctor, and scholar first introduced the term microaggressions in 1970. Pierce (1988) argued, '[a]ll blacks must have a firm theoretical grasp of racism in order to dilute its crippling effects' (33). In effect, Pierce has meticulously theorized the concept of racial microaggressions for over 40 years to understand how African Americans experience this form of everyday racism. Building on Pierce's conceptual work, scholarship has examined racial microaggressions in education settings from a critical race theory (CRT) perspective (Allen 2010; Cappiccie et al. 2012; Ek et al. 2010; Gildersleeve, Croom, and Vasquez 2011; Jay 2009; Katsarou 2009; Kohli and Solorzano 2012; Matias 2012; Masko 2005; Mosley 2010; Orozco 2012; Pérez Huber 2011; Rollock 2012; Rolón-Dow 2011; Smith, Yosso, and Solorzano 2006; Smith et al. 2007a, 2007b; Solorzano 1998; Solorzano and Villalpando 1998; Solorzano, Ceja, and Yosso 2000; Urrieta and Villenas 2014; Yosso et al. 2009). This article follows in that theoretical tradition. To that end, racial microaggressions are a form of systemic, everyday racism used to keep those at the racial margins in their place. They are: (1) verbal and non-verbal assaults directed toward People of Color, often carried out in subtle, automatic or unconscious forms; (2) layered assaults, based on race and its intersections with gender, class, sexuality, language, immigration status, phenotype, accent, or surname; and (3) cumulative assaults that take a psychological, physiological, and academic toll on People of Color (Kohli and Solorzano 2012; Pérez Huber and Cueva 2012; Solorzano and Pérez Huber 2012; Pierce 1970, 1995).

We argue that the concept of racial microaggressions is a useful 'tool' for research on race, racism and the everyday experiences of People of Color. It allows us to identify the often subtle acts of racism that can emerge in schools, college campuses, classrooms and in everyday conversations and interactions. In this article, we offer a racial microaggressions framework that demonstrates how everyday racist events are systemically mediated by institutionalized racism (i.e. structures and processes), and guided by ideologies of white supremacy that justify the superiority of a dominant group (whites) over non-dominant groups (People of Color).

The first objective of this article is to provide this framework as a tool to illustrate the inextricable and complex relationship between the everyday microaggressions experienced by People of Color, with institutional racism (i.e. structures and processes), and ideologies of white supremacy that maintain racial subordination. The second objective is to provide examples of how the framework can be used to analyze historical and contemporary forms of racial microaggressions in the lives of People of Color. Through these examples, we illustrate how a racial microaggressions framework can be a robust conceptual tool to understand how People of Color experience racial microaggressions and how those everyday assaults emerge from ideologies of white supremacy. Before undertaking these objectives, we briefly explain the conceptual development of racial microaggressions, originating from the research of Dr Chester Pierce. We then explain how we position our theorizing of a racial microaggressions framework from a CRT perspective, noting how this is different from other approaches used to examine microaggressions. Next, we provide a model that serves as the foundation for the analytic framework developed later in the article. Finally, we use the model to analyze one historical and one contemporary example of racial microaggressions, illustrating its conceptual utility across time.

Dr Chester Pierce and the conceptual development of racial microaggressions

> What is needed for example is a sweeping new theoretical concept. … The poor black may need care based on other models such as the negotiation of 'offensive mechanisms.' (Pierce 1969, 308)

Pierce first described the subtle forms of racism experienced by African Americans as 'offensive mechanisms' in a 1969 chapter titled 'Is Bigotry the Basis of the Medical Problem of the Ghetto?' As a medical doctor and psychiatrist, he explored the means to support the psychiatric needs of African American communities. In this chapter, Pierce suggests that existing theories used to address these needs were inefficient and new frameworks be developed to consider the role of race and racism in the lives of African Americans. As a result, Pierce (1969) develops the concept, offensive mechanisms. He explained:

> To be black in the United States today means to be socially minimized. For each day blacks are victims of white *'offensive mechanisms'* which are designed to reduce, dilute, atomize, and encase the hapless into *his 'place.'* The incessant lesson the black must hear is that he is insignificant and irrelevant. (303)

In the 1970 chapter 'Offensive Mechanisms,' Pierce extends this concept and first introduces the term *microaggression* to explain these 'subtle and stunning' forms of racism. He states:

> Most offensive actions are not gross and crippling. They are subtle and stunning. The enormity of the complications they cause can be appreciated only when one considers that these subtle blows are delivered incessantly. Even though any single negotiation of offense can in justice be considered of itself to be relatively innocuous, the cumulative effect to the victim and to the victimizer is of an unimaginable magnitude. Hence, the therapist is obliged to pose the idea that offensive mechanisms are usually a *micro-aggression.* (265–66, emphasis in original)

Here, we see Pierce begin to extend and transition from the term 'offensive mechanisms' he uses in earlier work, to the concept he names here as, 'micro-aggressions.' Although all his work was on African Americans, it is not until 1980 that Pierce explicitly uses the term 'racial microaggression.' In the chapter, 'Social Trace Contaminants: Subtle Indicators of Racism in TV,' Pierce (1980) tells us that:

> The subtle, stunning, repetitive event that many whites initiate and control in their dealings with blacks can be termed a *racial microaggression*. Any single microaggression from an offender to a defender (or victimizer to victim) in itself is minor and inconsequential. However, the relentless omnipresence of these noxious stimuli is the fabric of black–white relations in America. (251, emphasis added)

Pierce does not use the term again in his writing until 2000 when he and his colleagues explicitly use race and microaggression in an encyclopedia entry on 'Blacks, Stress in' (Profit, Mino, and Pierce 2000). Pierce and his colleagues explain:

> The chief energy demand on blacks is how to recognize, evaluate, anticipate, and dispose of *race-inspired microaggressions*. These are automatic, subtle, stunning, seemingly innocuous messages, often non-verbal, which devaluate the blacks; e.g. a black man and a white man enter an elevator whereupon the single white female passenger clutches her handbag as she moves as close as possible to the white man. Microaggressions, the major and inescapable expression of racism in the United States, take a cumulative toll on black individuals. As such they enter into the formation of black group stress. What may be more important is that these cumulative, minor but incessant put-downs often remain as psychopollutants in the social environment. Their lingering intractability is a major contributor to the continuing traumatic stress suffered by blacks as individuals and as a group. (327–328, emphasis added)

We borrow from and extend this rich conceptual history of racial microaggressions provided by Chester Pierce to develop the framework for understanding and analyzing racial microaggressions. First however, we explain the theoretical perspective we use to advance this conceptual development.

Theorizing racial microaggressions from a CRT perspective

We approach the concept of racial microaggressions from a CRT perspective. CRT is an explanatory framework that accounts for the role of race and racism in education and works toward identifying and challenging racism as a larger goal of identifying and challenging all forms of subordination.[2] Specifically, Solorzano (1998) outlines five tenants of CRT that guide the use of this framework. They include the: (1) centrality and intersectionality of race and racism; (2) challenge to dominant ideologies and deficit perspectives; (3) centrality of experiential knowledge; (4) interdisciplinary analyses; and (5) explicit commitment to social justice. Approaching an examination of microaggressions from a CRT perspective means we engage an interdisciplinary analysis that centers the lived experiences of People of Color to understand how everyday racism, and other forms of oppression, intersect to mediate life experiences and outcomes. Moreover, we engage CRT as a strategic goal of recognizing, analyzing and dismantling racism and other forms of subordination encountered by Communities of Color.

It is not only important to explain our use of CRT, but also how this theoretical approach is different in the study of microaggressions. Currently, Derald Wing Sue et al's work on microaggressions is widely cited in the fields of psychology, education and beyond. In this work, Sue (2010) and his colleagues provide a 'taxonomy' of microaggressions that articulates how microaggressions are delivered (verbal, behavioral, environmental) and the various forms they take (microassault, microinsult, and microinvalidation) (Constantine 2007; Constantine and Sue 2007; Sue 2010; Sue and Constantine 2007; Sue et al. 2007a, 2007b) that has proved very useful in microaggressions research. Sue (2010) argues that white supremacy serves as the foundation for the individual and institutional racism People of Color experience, and thus examines how the unconscious participation in microaggressions is harmful to whites.[3] Theorizing microaggressions from a CRT perspective does not focus the analyses on how whites experience racial microaggressions. Rather, a CRT analysis centers on the lived experiences of People of Color, those targeted by microaggressions. Moreover, we challenge dominant ideologies of meritocracy and colorblindness prevalent in education by acknowledging how white supremacy has historically and continues to mediate the everyday experiences of People of Color. Finally, our approach is interdisciplinary, building from Chester Pierce's work in the health sciences. Moreover, we do this to honor the Scholars of Color who had the courage and took the risks to engage this research, particularly at times when critical perspectives on race were unpopular and delegitimized (Griffith 1998).

Analyzing everyday racism: a racial microaggressions model

Theorizing racial microaggressions from a CRT perspective challenges us to more clearly articulate the structural and systemic forms of racism that operate in everyday racist acts. To meet this challenge, we offer a racial microaggressions model that can help researchers analyze how everyday experiences with racism are more than an individual experience, but part of a larger systemic racism that includes institutional and ideological forms. Figure 1 illustrates this model.

A critical race analysis centers the lived experiences of People of Color. Thus, at the center of the model is the experience with the racial microaggression (in white). The second layer of the model (in black) is institutional

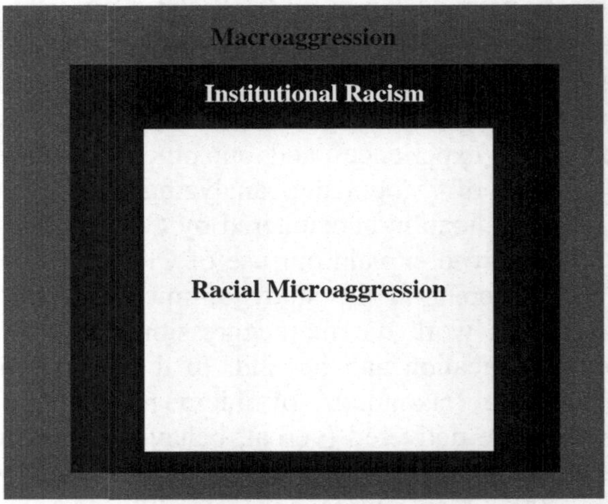

Figure 1. A racial microaggressions model.

racism, which provides the structural articulation of how racism operates institutionally to perpetuate everyday racism. For this reason, the layer of institutional racism in the model surrounds the racial microaggression. The final layer in the model, the macroaggression (in grey), encompasses both institutional racism and the racial microaggression. The macroaggression provides the ideological foundations for the reproduction and perpetuation of institutional and everyday racism – white supremacy. We explain further by providing the following definitions of these components in the model.

Racial microaggression

As mentioned earlier, racial microaggressions are a form of systemic, everyday racism used to keep those at the racial margins in their place. They are: (1) verbal and non-verbal assaults directed toward People of Color, often carried out in subtle, automatic or unconscious forms; (2) layered assaults, based on race and its intersections with gender, class, sexuality, language, immigration status, phenotype, accent, or surname; and (3) cumulative assaults that take a psychological, physiological, and academic toll[4] on People of Color. Microaggressions allow us to 'see' those tangible ways racism emerges in everyday interactions. At the same time, they have a purpose. For instance, whether conscious or not, microaggressions perpetuate a larger system of racism. Microaggressions are the layered, cumulative and often subtle and unconscious forms of racism that target People of Color. They are the everyday reflections of larger racist structures and ideological beliefs that impact People of Color's lives. Thus, the layers illustrated in Figure 1 represents the inextricability of microaggressions with institutional racism and macroaggressions.

Institutional racism

Institutional racism can be understood as *formal or informal structural mechanisms, such as policies and processes that systematically subordinate, marginalize, and exclude non-dominant groups and mediates their experiences with racial microaggressions.* Institutional racism is a key component to understanding the function and permanence of racism in the US.[5] Indeed, systemic racism is imbedded within social institutions that in turn, serve as structural mechanisms that perpetuate racism (Marable 2002). Without a structural understanding of the racism that manifests in the everyday lives of People of Color, it remains an elusive concept that becomes difficult to 'see' in any tangible way. However, when institutional racism is understood as a mechanism that strategically guides policies and processes in education, government, politics and the law, the depth and breadth of institutional racism's significance in the everyday lives of *all* (whites and People of Color alike) emerges. The concept of institutional racism then, articulates the larger structural conditions that exist which allow racial microaggressions to occur.

Manning Marable (2002) uses the term 'structural racism' to explain the imbeddedness of racism within US social institutions. In this work, Marable (2002) states '[I]t is not the objective reality of difference between "races" that produces disparities and social inequality between groups; it is structural racism that reproduces "races"' (28). Here, Marable highlights a critical function of institutional racism and its relationship to what we call macroaggressions. He explains that the 'objective' perceptions – the dominant set of ideologies or beliefs – about racial groups cannot alone produce actual inequalities in the lives of People of Color. It is the structural forms of racism that (re)produce the actual or perceived social arrangements that legitimate the inequitable positions of whites and non-whites in US society. This leads us to define the final layer illustrated in the model – macroaggression.

Macroaggression

The final layer in the model, the macroaggression, encompasses both institutional racism and racial microaggressions. We define a macroaggression as *the set of beliefs and/or ideologies that justify actual or potential social arrangements that legitimate the interests and/or positions of a dominant group over non-dominant groups, that in turn lead to related structures and acts of subordination.* These ideologies provide the 'mental frames' or 'common sense' (Lakoff 2006) understandings and perceptions of dominant and non-dominant groups needed to justify the oppression experienced by the latter. Thus, macroaggressions provide the ideological foundations that justify the actions of racism in the many forms they take, including institutional racism and racial microaggressions. To further clarify the role of the macroaggression in this framework, we use Judge Robert Carter's (1988) reflection on the landmark *Brown v. Board* (1954) Supreme Court decision. He stated:

> … the NAACP lawyers erred. The lawyers did not understand then how effective white power could be in preventing full implementation of the law; nor did it realize at the time that the basic barrier to full equality for blacks was not racial segregation, a symptom, but white supremacy, the disease. (1095)

Carter provides us with a powerful metaphor to better understand racism as a 'symptom' of white supremacy, 'the disease.' Carter's reflection urges that an analysis of white supremacy must be included within an analysis of racism – in our case, a framework of racial microaggressions – to move beyond the acknowledgement of 'symptoms' and understand the 'disease' from where they emerge. The concept of macroaggressions allows for this analysis – to identify the ideologies of white supremacy (the disease) that uphold institutional racism, from where racial microaggressions (symptoms) emerge.

Our conceptualization of racial macroaggressions is different than many other scholars who define racial macroaggressions as the overt, 'large scale' (i.e. state acts) of racism experienced by People of Color (Gildersleeve, Croom, and Vasquez 2011; Smith et al., 2007a). We argue that the terms 'micro' and 'macro' should not define acts of racism as subtle or blatant. In fact, Pierce (1974) makes a similar argument about the limitations of terminology when he stated, '[t]hese problems are only micro in name, since their very number requires a total effort that is incalculable' (520). We concur with Pierce that we are limited by the terms we use to describe the complexities of racism and the harm they can cause. We certainly do not intend to depreciate everyday racism by using the term micro. To the contrary, we would agree with scholars like Dumas (2014) who argue that microaggressions are in fact a form of 'everyday suffering' that have become socially and systemically normalized and effectively minimized. We make a strategic effort to re-appropriate the power of the term microaggression that has endured throughout the decades to capture a historically situated meaning for everyday racism.[6] We offer a racial microaggressions analytic framework as a response to Pierce's (1988) urging that 'All blacks [and other People of Color] must have a firm theoretical grasp of racism in order to dilute its crippling effects' (33). The definitions, frameworks, and examples presented here are necessary conceptual steps toward advancing efforts to dismantle racism and the many forms it takes in the everyday lives of People of Color.

Applying the framework

Now that we have explained the model and defined its components, we apply it to two examples of racial microaggressions, one historical and one contemporary. We do this to demonstrate the conceptual utility of the model. Furthermore, with both historical and contemporary examples, we also demonstrate its utility to analyze microaggressions across time. The first example utilizes a historical artifact, an archival photograph, to illustrate an example of a racial microaggression, institutional racism, and macroaggression in the 1930s Jim Crow state of North Carolina. In the second contemporary example we use the 2013 class-action lawsuit, *Floyd et al. v. City of New York*. This case challenged New York Police Department (NYPD) racial profiling practices and the unconstitutional stop and frisks in predominately African American and Latina/o communities in New York City. Here, we explain how the model can be conceptually expanded when additional facts and data are available about the everyday racist acts, as the *Floyd* case provided. As a result, we build on the racial microaggressions model (Figure 1), providing additional components for a more in-depth analysis. This analysis articulates how People of Color are targeted by and experience racial microaggressions, and how those experiences are connected to institutional racism and ideologies of white supremacy. Thus, we refer to this more complex model as a racial microaggressions analytic framework. First, we begin with the historical example.

Example 1: photograph as historical artifact

Photography, particularly historical photography, provides an insightful venue to America's racist past. Scholars such as Abel (2010) and Smith (2004) recognize the significance of visual photography to capture historically situated meanings of race. We agree such historical images are powerful and is why we chose to use a photograph as our first example of racial microaggressions. Figure 2 is a 1938 photograph cataloged by the US Library of Congress titled, 'A Drinking Fountain on the County Courthouse Lawn' taken in Halifax, North Carolina. Photographers working for the US Farm Security Administration Historical Section were charged with visually documenting 'continuity and change' in America during the 1930s and 1940s, with a particular focus on visual signage (Library of Congress 2013). This photograph is included in a collection titled, 'Photographs of Signs Enforcing Racial Discrimination.'[7]

In the photograph, a young African American boy stands next to a water fountain located on the lawn of a county courthouse. The entrance of the courthouse can be seen in the background to the left. A sign is posted on a tree to the left of the water fountain that reads, 'COLORED.' The boy seems to gaze at the photographer as the photo is taken.

The model in Figure 2 can be used to analyze the young boy's experience with racial microaggressions in this photograph. We argue that the racial microaggression in the photo is the 'colored' water fountain that the boy stands next to. Although the 'COLORED' sign would not be considered

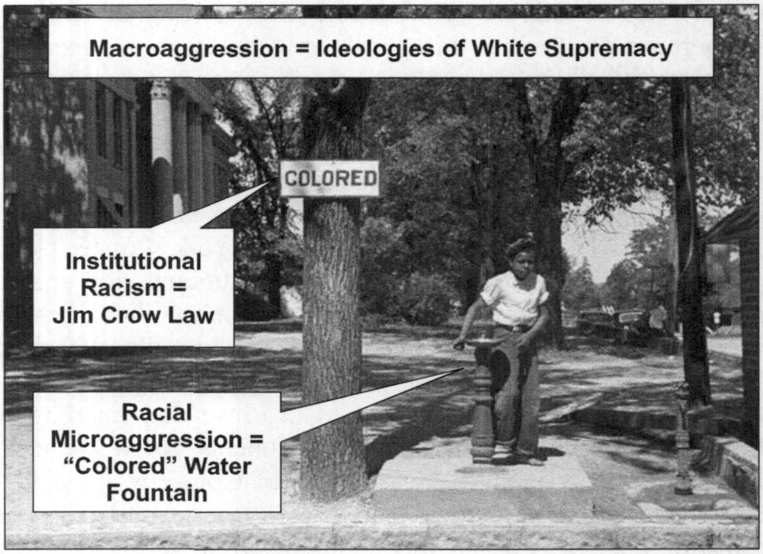

Figure 2. 'A Drinking Fountain on the County Courthouse Lawn,' photograph by J. Vachon, 1938.

subtle today, this was an everyday form of *de jure* racism (Jim Crow) experienced by this young boy at this particular historical moment (1930s), and in this particular geographic location (the Southern United States). Separate public facilities for African Americans in the Southern United States were an everyday experience in 1938.[8] We argue that consistent with our definition of racial microaggressions, the separate water fountain was a form of systemic, everyday racism used to keep those at the racial margins in their place. This was a non-verbal assault directed towards the African American boy. Separate facilities for People of Color in the 1930's 'South' were normative in dominant society, practiced and enforced accordingly in automatic and unconscious ways by many whites, accepted as a 'natural' way of life (Alexander 2012). If we could speak to this young boy as a grown man, he might no doubt, describe the cumulative psychological and physiological toll he had experienced during his life, subjected to this form of everyday racism.

Where a racial microaggression occurs, institutional racism operates to enforce it. The institutional racism we identify in this photo is the Jim Crow *de jure* policy that maintained separate public facilities for whites and People of Color upheld at the time in the South – the Jim Crow 'Colored Only' law. In the photo, we argue that the signage posted on the tree that reads 'COLORED' represents Jim Crow. Jim Crow law is the institutional racism that functioned as a structural mechanism to systemically subordinate, marginalize, and exclude People of Color through policies like separate public facilities. In effect, Jim Crow laws were the forms of institutional racism that enforced and maintained the everyday racial microaggressions we see in this photo.

Although ideologies remain unseen to the eye, there are powerful ideologies at play that justified Jim Crow laws and mediated this young boy's everyday experience with racial microaggressions. Thus, the macroaggression we identify here are ideologies of white supremacy. These ideologies justified the social arrangements maintained by Jim Crow (institutional racism) that systematically subordinated People of Color at the time, and mediated experiences with racial microaggressions. Without the ideological foundations of white supremacy neither institutional racism nor racial microaggressions could be justified or sustained.

With this historical artifact we identified the various ways racism manifests, from the everyday, to the institutional, to the ideological. Furthermore, the racial microaggressions model illustrates how each of these forms of racism are intricately connected in the experience of the young boy in the photograph. Returning to Carter's (1988) metaphor of symptom and disease, the water fountain and signage only allow us to see symptoms, while the macroaggression identifies the ideologies of white supremacy that are present, the disease. In the following section, we expand on this model to provide a more detailed analysis of racial microaggressions that includes how a Person of Color experiences a microaggression, using a class-action lawsuit as a contemporary example, *Floyd et al. v. City of New York* (2013).

Example 2: contemporary legal case

The federal class-action lawsuit *Floyd v. City of New York* (2013) challenged NYPD racial profiling practices and unconstitutional stop and frisks in predominately African American and Latina/o communities in the city. The legal opinion held in *Floyd* provides information about why and how the lawsuit was brought to the court. The opinion provided key evidence presented by the plaintiffs through an independent statistical analysis of data collected over a two-year period on stop and frisks and crime complaint reports conducted by the NYPD (Fagan 2010). In two expert reports presented to the court, plaintiff attorneys provided data on how and why NYPD practiced stop and frisks, the frequency of these practices in particular neighborhoods, and the race, gender and suspected crimes of those stopped. Using the final court opinion (*Floyd v. City of New York* 2013) in *Floyd* and the expert reports (Fagan 2010, 2012), we expand the racial microaggressions model to articulate with greater detail how the plaintiffs experienced these racist acts. We argue that the illumination this conceptual expansion offers provides more than a model, but an analytic framework to examine racial microaggressions. We present and explain a racial microaggressions analytic framework in this example.

In *Floyd*, African American plaintiffs David Floyd, Lalit Clarkson, Deon Dennis, and David Ourlichtand represented 'hundreds of thousands' of New Yorkers stopped by NYPD officers for 'suspicion-less' stop and frisks that disproportionately targeted African Americans and Latinas/os in the city (Fagan 2010). According to an expert report presented in the case, African Americans and Latinas/os constituted 84% of stops from 2010 through 2012 under the city's stop and frisk policy, although these groups comprise only 50% of the city's total population. Further, nearly all of those stopped where released by officers who found no basis for summons or arrest (Fagan 2012). During 2010–2012, there were over 1.6 million stops by police in New York City. Approximately 1.3 million of those stopped were African American and Latina/o, mostly male (Fagan 2012). This would mean that NYPD stopped and frisked more African Americans and Latinas/os than the entire city populations of Buffalo, Rochester, Yonkers, Syracuse, Albany and New Rochelle combined (New York State's six largest cities after New York City). The *New York Times* reported NYPD superior officers provided explicit orders for police to target 'male blacks 14 to 20, 21' years of age under the same policy (New York Times Editorial Board 2013). Using the example of unlawful stop and frisks in *Floyd*, we apply and further develop the racial microaggressions model.

In the opinion of the case, the court recognized that People of Color, and more often African American and Latino males, are targeted by racial profiling practices such as stop and frisk 'on the way to work, in front of their house or just walking down the street, without any cause and primarily because of their race' (Fagan 2012, 3). We argue that the NYPD practice of stop and frisks were the racial microaggressions that targeted the plaintiffs (and the many, many others as reported in the case). However, with the additional information *Floyd* provides about how these racial microaggressions often happened in New York City, we can expand on the racial microaggressions model to include a more detailed analysis of how a Person of Color experiences a racial microaggression. Thus, we will add the following additional components to the model. We present these components first in Figures 3 and 4, then add them to the racial microaggressions model in Figure 5, creating a racial microaggressions analytic framework.

To understand how a Person of Color can experience a racial microaggression, we must first understand how they happen. We begin with Figure 3 that identifies a 'perpetrator,' the individual enacting the microaggression, and the 'primary target' – the individual targeted by it. In the case of *Floyd*, the police officer is the 'perpetrator' and the 'primary target' is David Floyd. However, there can also be 'secondary targets' impacted by the microaggression committed by the perpetrator. The 'secondary targets' may not have been the intended target of the microaggression, but they can also experience its effects.[9] For example, a friend that was walking with Floyd while he was stopped, or a relative who was told of the event and also

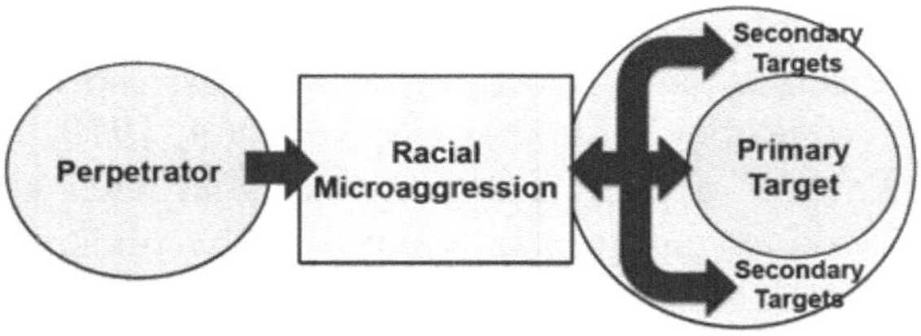

Figure 3. Perpetrator-target model component.

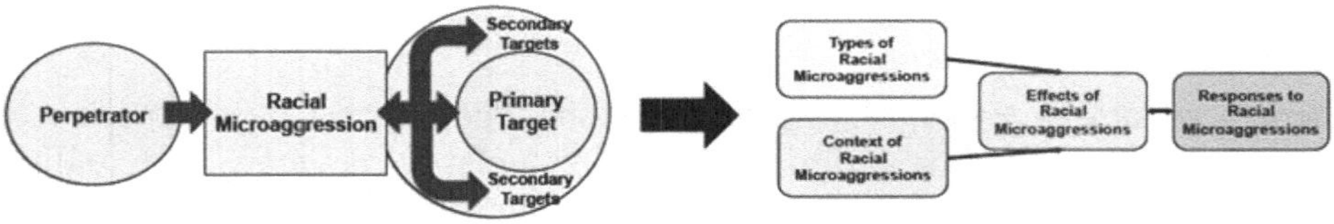

Figure 4. Types, context, effects, responses model component.

experienced emotions of anger, violation, and disappointment. As Critical Race Theorists, we focus on the experiences of the primary and secondary targets, the Person or People of Color that experiences microaggressions. Yet, it is important to understand that the perpetrators of racial microagges-sions often unconsciously engage in microaggressive acts and thus, can commit the act with little thought or attention paid to the interaction. Furthermore, this unconscious intent of perpetrators make confronting microaggressions difficult for People of Color, and is one way racism can be perpetuated while rendered invisible. This is the danger of subtle racism

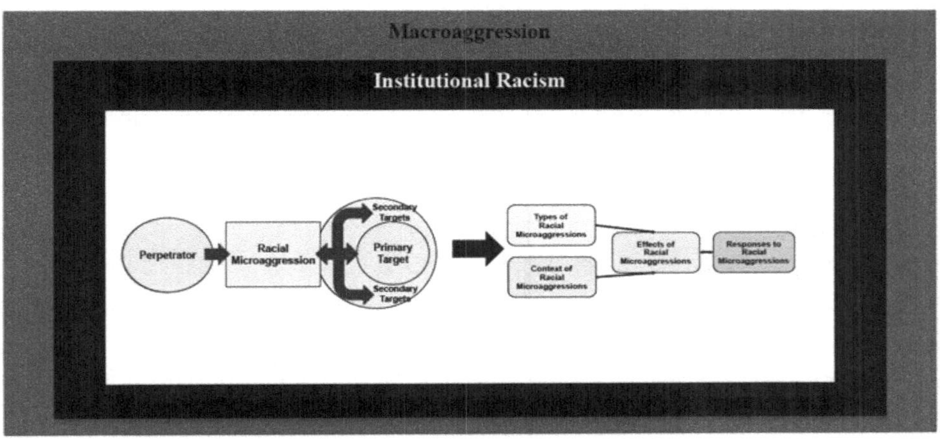

Figure 5. Racial microaggressions analytic framework.

Chester Pierce cautioned – for the People of Color targeted by microaggressions, there can be serious and lasting repercussions, especially when experienced consistently over one's lifetime (Pierce 1969, 1970, 1974).

While Figure 3 would explain how Floyd was targeted by this racial microaggression, we add an additional component to understand how Floyd experienced the microaggression. To understand how one experiences microaggressions, we must understand the type and context of the microaggression, and the effects and responses to them. To illustrate, we add the following component in Figure 4 and explain each of the elements.

Types of microaggressions

There are various types of microaggressions People of Color experience, based on race and/or ethnicity, gender, class, language, sexuality, immigration status, phenotype, accent, surname, and/or culture (Kohli and Solorzano, 2012). From a CRT perspective, we know that racism often occurs at intersections with other forms of oppression. Thus, in analyzing 'types' it is important to acknowledge that a microaggression may be based on multiple characteristics and positionalities that define the identities and experiences of People of Color.[10] In the *Floyd* case, when a police officer engages in practices of stop and frisk, based on raced and gendered stereotypes of perceived criminality, racial and gendered microaggressions are at play.[11]

Context of microaggressions

There is also a context — *where* and *how* the microaggression occurs. In the example of stop and frisk, the *Floyd* case told us that stop and frisks often occurred in the streets. Microaggressions can also occur in schools, classrooms, on the play yard, in laboratories, at meetings, and on college campuses, among others. The context of the microaggression not only refers to the location or space that the microaggression occurred, but also the larger circumstances and conditions present that allowed it to happen. The remaining components of this model account for the ways microaggressions impact People of Color who are targeted by them.

Effects of microaggressions

Through years of research, Chester Pierce (1970, 1974, 1989) found that there were negative psychological and physiological effects of microaggressions. Moreover, Pierce argued that the effects were cumulative, taking a toll on the bodies, minds, and spirits of People of Color over time. For example, those young men targeted by stop and frisk practices may become angry or frustrated, their blood pressure may rise, and heart rates may increase (Clark et al. 1999; Gravlee, Dressler, and Bernard 2005; Smith 2004). Over time, he/she may develop feelings of self-doubt and more serious symptomatic conditions such as high blood pressure, depression, and anxiety (Hill, Kobayashi, and Hughes 2007; Pérez Huber, and Cueva 2012). Mundane extreme environmental stress (MEES) (Carroll 1998), racial battle fatigue (Cueva 2010; Smith 2004; Smith, Allen, and Danley 2007; Smith, Yosso, and Solorzano 2006), and racial trauma (Truong and Museus 2012), are conditions researchers use to describe such race-related health consequences. Some studies have attributed more fatal conditions such as cardiovascular disease and even increased morbidity to race-related stressors such as microaggressions (Adelman 2008; Gee et al. 2009; Geronimus et al. 2006; Pierce 1969).

As a result of the legal charges brought by *Floyd*, a report by the Center for Constitutional Rights (CCR) (2012) compiled 'testimonies' from New Yorkers who had experienced stop and frisk. The report detailed the 'human impact' of the stop and frisks conducted by the NYPD, that found those stopped experienced trauma, humiliation and endured 'fear as a way of life' (7). Furthermore, the report found stop and frisk not only impacted individuals directly targeted by them, but entire communities who reported feeling the presence of NYPD as a 'military-style occupation' due to these everyday acts of racism consistently committed in their communities (19). These findings confirm that and the and the primary and secondary targets, as articulated in our model, can experience the effects of microaggressions. However, just as important is understanding that People of Color are certainly not idle to them. The final element of this analysis addresses the ways People of Color respond to microaggressions.

Responses to microaggressions

Pierce (1995) explained, 'The most baffling task for victims of racism and sexism is to defend against microaggressions. Knowing how and when to defend requires time and energy that oppressors cannot appreciate' (282). Pierce highlights the significance of developing responses to racial microaggressions. Such responses can vary, according to the type and context of the microaggression, as well as the effect it had on the individual. Moreover, one's response can be influenced by the effect, and vice versa. These responses can include engaging in counterspaces, places located within or outside of educational institutions where People of Color develop strategies for healing, empowerment, and building a sense of community (Grier-Reed 2010; Solorzano, Ceja, and Yosso 2000; Solorzano and Villalpando 1998; Yosso et al. 2009).

The Center for Constitutional Rights (2012) reported that even before *Floyd*, New York communities were taking action against stop and frisk and other forms of police misconduct. Community-based organizations were created that conducted 'know your rights' trainings and other public education campaigns, as well as 'copwatch' programs to document police misconduct in their neighborhoods. We would argue these were collective responses to the racial microaggressions perpetrated by police enforcement. Another response was the *Floyd* case itself, where plaintiffs challenged New York City's stop and frisk policy by filing a class-action lawsuit on behalf of the countless People of Color targeted by these racial microaggressions. This response to the microaggressions perpetrated by NYPD proved to be transformational. The outcome of the case acknowledged that NYPD was liable for the unconstitutional patterns and practices of racial profiling and stops by its officers, and prompted a citywide examination of such discriminatory practices.

In Figure 5, we illustrate how these additional components can be added to the racial microggressions model, providing a more complex analytical framework. With the data and information presented in *Floyd*, we were able to identify the perpetrators, and the primary and secondary targets of microaggressions. In addition, we were able to analyze the type, context, effects, and responses plaintiffs had to them.

Now that we have explained how racial microaggressions were experienced in *Floyd*, the model calls for us to identify the institutional racism in the case. The most obvious form of institutional racism is the stop and frisk policy itself, as a formal structural mechanism that systematically subordinated the plaintiffs targeted by racial microaggressions. The more conspicuous form of institutional racism operating within this example is what the court opinion called the 'unwritten' policy of 'targeting the right people for stops' or, the informal structural mechanisms of institutional racism that subjected many members of the African American and Latina/o communities in the city to be held under suspicion of criminality.[12] According to the opinion delivered by US District Court Judge Shira Sheindlin:

> [T]he City adopted a policy of indirect racial profiling by targeting racially defined groups for stops based on local crime suspect data. This has resulted in the disproportionate and discriminatory stopping of [b]lacks and Hispanics. … Both statistical and anecdotal evidence showed that minorities are indeed treated differently than whites … despite the fact that whites are more likely to be found with weapons or contraband. (*Floyd et al. v. City of New York* 2013, 16)

In effect, the *Floyd* ruling acknowledged both formal and informal mechanisms of institutional racism that mediated police stop and frisk practices, or the racial microaggressions. Moreover, it was found that these racist practices disproportionately targeted African Americans and Latinas/os compared to whites, who were more often found 'with weapons and contraband' when stopped. What the *Floyd* ruling did not address, is how the perpetrators of these racial microaggressions developed their racist beliefs and perceptions about African American and Latina/o communities. This is addressed by the final component of the model, the macroaggression.

Identifying the macroaggression in *Floyd* exposes the powerful ideologies at play that articulate racist perspectives of Communities of Color. The *Floyd* case found police officers engaged racial profiling strategies based on racist perceptions of People of Color, and that these practices were formally and informally enforced by the city's written and unwritten stop and frisk policies. What the case does not explain is that without widely-held, normative, racist beliefs about People of Color maintained by many of the police officers that served in the NYPD, these stop and frisk policies and practices could not have emerged in such a pronounced way.

Based on the evidence presented in the *Floyd* case, the opinion revealed that African Americans and Latinas/os were: (1) Stopped more than whites 'even when other relevant variables' were held constant; (2) were more likely than whites to be arrested for the same suspected crimes and; (3) were more likely than whites to be 'subjected to the use of force' even when whites were more likely to require further enforcement action in a stop (*Floyd et al. v. City of New York* 2013, 12). Based on the facts of the case, we would argue that the macroaggression here, are ideologies of white supremacy. Thus, the macroaggression that operates in *Floyd* is in fact, the ideological beliefs in white superiority that led to actions of law enforcement to criminalize Men of Color through such policies[13] (see Alexander 2012).

We acknowledge that for some, being stopped and frisked by police because of your race would not be understood as subtle racism. For example, in a study examining the racist experiences of African American college students, Smith et al. (2007) used the example of racial profiling, or, 'driving-while-black' as a macroaggression experienced by African American males. In the framework we provide in this article, we define racial microaggressions as taking on both covert and overt forms. Thus, in our definition of microaggressions, we state that they are 'often subtle,' but argue they can also be blatant. Thus, using this framework, racial profiling strategies such as 'driving-while-black' would be microaggressions, racial symptoms of a larger disease. That is, the disease of white supremacy, the macroaggression that justifies racial profiling.

Conclusion

In this article, we have provided a brief history of the conceptual development of racial microaggressions, according to Chester Pierce. This history was provided to honor these significant contributions and demonstrate how our work builds on the conceptual foundations created by him. We explained how further theorizing microaggressions from a CRT perspective centers the experiences of People of Color targeted by them and challenges race research to focus on the systemic nature of racism. We then presented a model to understand how racial microaggressions emerge from institutional racism and ideologies of white supremacy. A historical artifact was utilized to apply this model to an experience with racial microaggressions in North Carolina in the 1930s. The model was then applied to a contemporary 'stop and frisk' example with *Floyd et al. v. City of New York* (2013). Due to the additional facts and data provided by the case, we were able to expand the model to articulate a more complex understanding of how People of Color experience racial microaggressions. This conceptual expansion provides a framework to analyze racial microaggressions in Critical Race research. The framework allows for an understanding of racial microaggressions beyond a perpetrator-target interaction and illustrates that these everyday racist acts have a purpose, whether committed consciously or not, to perpetuate and justify a larger system of racial domination.

We acknowledge that there is much more work to be done on racial microaggressions. Here, we have explained the theoretical implications of this conceptual tool to examine every day racism. However, we believe there are also pedagogical implications. Microaggressions can be a powerful tool for People of Color to 'name their pain,' as Paulo Freire (1970) describes, to engage anti-oppressive strategies for liberation. Furthermore, the two examples presented demonstrate the possibility for using historical and contemporary artifacts as pedagogical tools for teaching about racial microaggressions. Finally, an important discussion outside the purview of this article remains. That is, if racial microaggressions emerge from ideologies of white supremacy, and are understood as a form of 'white violence' (Leonardo 2010), how can we explain the race-based forms of discrimination People of Color engage against each other? For example, many NYPD officers in the *Floyd* case were white, but many were also People of Color. What does this mean for the ways we understand racial microaggressions? This is a question we intend to theorize in a future study, as we hope others will do as well. As we have built from the conceptual foundation of Chester Pierce, we hope others find the concepts, models and frameworks provided here useful for their own work in Critical Race Research, and continue to build and move the field forward

Our analysis of the examples in this article demonstrate that every day and systemic racism have certainly not gone away, only changed form throughout the decades. Despite recent Supreme Court decisions that have come down that maintain arguments steeped in color-blindness, we know racism today is alive and well. For example, in May 2014 the US Supreme Court upheld the ban on the use of race in college admissions in Shuette v. BAMN (2014).[14] Justice Sonia Sotomayor stated in her dissent to the decision:

> In my colleagues' view, examining the racial impact of legislation only perpetuates racial discrimination. This refusal to accept the stark reality that race matters is regrettable. The way to stop discrimination on the basis of race is

> to speak openly and candidly on the subject of race, and to apply the Constitution with eyes open to the unfortunate effects of centuries of racial discrimination. As members of the judiciary tasked with intervening to carry out the guarantee of equal protection, we ought not sit back and wish away, rather than confront, the racial inequality that exists in our society. (46)

As Justice Sotomayor stated in her dissent, race is not something that can be 'wished away' by refusing its existence in US society. The recent murder of Michael Brown in Ferguson, Missouri in the summer of 2014 at the hands of white police is a solemn reminder that there is a long road ahead to social justice for Communities of Color.[15] Yet, we are given a sense of hope from the success of *Floyd*. It serves as a reminder that transformation and justice is possible if we continue the work to name, resist, and challenge everyday racism.

Notes

1. MTV has partnered with the Ohio State University's Kirwan Institute for the Study of Race and Ethnicity and a coalition of other organizations to develop the 'Look Different' campaign. This multi-year project was launched in 2014 and seeks to assist youth in identifying their raced and gendered biases. It also provides a process of 'debiasing' through participating in a 'racial bias cleanse' (see http://kirwaninstitute.osu.edu/kirwan-institute-partners-with-mtv-on-multi-year-campaign-to-help-youth-combat-hidden-biases-inequality/). As the analysis reflects in this article, we would argue that the deconstruction of racism is not possible through the simple recognition of racial bias, as racism is a symptom of white supremacy. Therefore, the deconstruction of racism must include a detachment from white supremacist ideologies.
2. Here, education is broadly defined as a process that occurs within and outside of formal schooling institutions. In effect, we recognize that racial microaggressions occur within these varied contexts, as evident in the examples we present later in this article.
3. Sue (2010) theorizes racial microaggressions within the context of the counseling psychology field, and specifically to provide counseling practicioners with strategies address the unconscious racism inform their practice with clients of color. In this context, the focus on the perpetrator is important and much-needed. Here, we acknowledge these contributions, while differentiating a theory of racial microaggressions from a CRT perspective.
4. We use the term 'toll' in the same way as Chester Pierce (1974, 1989), to describe the cumulative effects of racial microaggressions over time.
5. Derrick Bell (1992) uses the concept of 'racial realism' to describe the permanence of racism in the US. In his work, he cautions us in focusing intently on efforts that merely change racism's form. Rather, he argued, we must develop and implement 'strategies that can bring fulfillment and even triumph' (374). Institutional racism articulates a systematic positioning of race and racism in the US that leads to racial realism. Racial microaggressions then, become a tool, or 'strategy' in understanding how everyday racism occurs in order to confront and dismantle structures of oppression.
6. Through this re-appropriation of terminology, we engage a discursive shift of power that allows us to (re)create and (re)envision the meaning of microaggression. Historically, People of Color have engaged similar strategies with

terminology, particularly for terms to describe racial/ethnic identity (i.e. black, Chicana, Chicano).

7. Full title of collection is, 'Photographs of Signs Enforcing Racial Discrimination: Documentation of Farm Security Administration – Office of War Information Photographers' (see http://www.loc.gov/rr/print/list/085_disk.html).
8. One could also argue that *dejure* and *defacto* racism also occurred in other parts of the US.
9. Shelley Harrell's (2000) research on race-related 'stressors' offers insight into the discussion of primary and secondary targets of microaggressions with what she terms 'vicarious' racist experiences. She asserts that, 'racism exerts its influence not only through direct personal experience, but also vicariously, through observation and report. The inclusion of vicarious experiences is critical in understanding the nature of racism's effect on individuals' (45). Harrell offers insight on how secondary targets of racial microaggressions vicariously experience the racism of the primary target, even when this racism was not directed to them.
10. For other types of microaggressions, see Solorzano (1998) on gender microaggressions and Pérez Huber (2011) on racist nativist microaggressions. See also Sue (2010) on sexual-orientation microaggressions.
11. We would argue racial profiling practices like stop and frisk would be both racial and gender microaggressions, as research has shown racial profiling strategies disproportionately impact Men of Color (Glover 2009; Johnson 2003; Marable 2002; Smith, Allen, and Danley 2007).
12. Could this be an example of what Michelle Alexander (2012) refers to as the 'New Jim Crow.'
13. While we argue for this different conceptual understanding of macroaggressions, it is not our intention to claim there is only one way to conceptualize macro or microaggressions. We do not attempt to articulate universal definitions, but alternative perspectives we believe useful for examining the everyday forms of racism in the lives of People of Color.
14. In *Schuette v. BAMN* (2014), the US Supreme Court ruled to uphold Michigan's Proposal 2, passed in 2006, to ban the use of race (among other characteristics) in state college and university admissions. Justice Scalia delivered his concurring opinion that cited the dissent of Justice Harlan in *Plessy v. Ferguson* (1896) that the constitution is 'color-blind and neither knows nor tolerates classes among citizens' and that in passing Proposal 2, 'the people of Michigan wish the same for their governing charter' (17). See concurring opinion retrieved from Supreme Court of the United States at http://www.supremecourt.gov/opinions/13pdf/12-682_8759.pdf. In 2013, a similar argument is made in *Shelby County v. Holder* where the Supreme Court ruled to overturn a key section of the Voting Rights Act that required states with a history of discriminating against racial minority voters (mostly in the South) to get federal permission to change voting requirements.
15. Michael Brown was an unarmed 18-year-old African American teenager who was shot and killed by a white police officer while walking in his neighborhood of Ferguson, Missouri. The murder led to weeks-long demonstrations and riots against policy violence in this city and cities across the country. The Los Angeles Times comments that Brown's murder has become on 'international incident' that casts a grim spotlight on race relations in the US (Makinen 2014).

References

Abel, E. 2010. *Signs of the Times: The Visual Politics of Jim Crow*. Berkeley, CA: University of California Press.

Adelman, L. 2008. "Unnatural Causes: Is Inequality Making Us Sick?" [Television Series]. San Francisco, CA: Public Broadcasting Service (PBS).

Alexander, M. 2012. *The New Jim Crow: Mass Incarceration in the Age of Colorblindness*. New York: The New Press.

Allen, Q. 2010. "Racial Microaggressions: The Schooling Experiences of Black Middle-class Males in Arizona's Secondary Schools." *Journal of African merican Males in Education* 1 (2): 125–143.

Bell, D. 1992. *Faces at the Bottom of the Well: The Permanence of Racism*. New York: Basic Books.

Cappiccie, A., J. Chadha, M. B. Lin, and F. Snyder. 2012. "Using Critical Race Theory to Analyze How Disney Constructs Diversity: A Construct for the Baccalaureate Human Behavior in the Social Environment Curriculum." *Journal of Teaching in Social Work* 32 (1): 46–61.

Carroll, G. 1998. *Environmental Stress and African Americans: The Other Side of the Moon*. Westport, CT: Praeger.

Carter, R. 1988. "The NAACP's Legal Strategy against Segregated Education, 1925–1950." *Michigan Law Review* 86: 1083–1095.

Center for Constitutional Rights. 2012. "Stop and Frisk, the Human Impact: The Stories behind the Numbers, the Impact on Our Communities." http://stopandfrisk.org/the-human-impact-report/

Clark, R., N. Anderson, V. Clark, and D. Williams. 1999. "Racism as a Stressor for African Americans: A Biopsychosocial Model." *American Psychologist* 54 (10): 805–816.

Constantine, M. 2007. "Racial Microaggressions against African American Clients in Cross-racial Counseling Relationships." *Journal of Counseling Psychology* 54 (1): 1–16.

Constantine, M. G., and D. W. Sue. 2007. "Perceptions of Racial Microaggressions among Black Supervisees in Cross-racial Dyads." *Journal of Counseling Psychology* 54 (2): 142–153.

Cueva, B. 2010. "A Testimonial of Resistance, Survival, and Hope: Breaking the Silences of Racial Battle Fatigue in Academia." *Social Sciences and Comparative Education Newsletter* 2 (2): 3–5.

Dumas, M. 2014. "Losing an Arm: Schooling as a Site of Black Suffering." *Race, Ethnicity and Education* 17 (1): 1–29.

Ek, L. D., P. D. Q. Cerecer, I. Alanís, and M. A. Rodríguez. 2010. "'I Don't Belong Here':Chicanas/Latinas at a Hispanic Serving Institution Creating Community through Muxerista Mentoring." *Equity & Excellence in Education* 43 (4): 539–553.

Fagan, J. 2010. *Second Supplementary Report in Floyd et al. v. City of New York et al.* New York: United States District Court, Southern District of New York. Accessed September 2, 2013. http://ccrjustice.org/files/FaganSecondSupplementalReport.pdf.

Fagan, J. 2012. *Executive Summary, Stop and Frisk: Updated Data Confirms Earlier Findings Ofrights Violations*. New York: Center for Constitutional Rights. http://www.ccrjustice.org/files/Fagan-2012-summary-FINAL.pdf.

Floyd v. City of New York. 2013. No. 08 Civ. 01034 (SAS) 2013 U.S. Dist. LEXIS 132881 (S.D.N.Y Aug. 12).

Freire, P. 1970. *Pedagogy of the Oppressed*. New York: Continuum.

Gee, G., A. Ro, S. Shariff-Marco, and D. Chae. 2009. "Racial Discrimination and Health among Asian Americans: Evidence, Assessment, and Directions for Future Research." *Epidemiologic Reviews* 31 (1): 130–151.

Geronimus, A., M. Hicken, D. Keene, and J. Bound. 2006. "'Weathering' and Age Patterns of Allostatic Load Scores among Blacks and Whites in the United States." *American Journal of Public Health* 96 (5): 826–833.

Gildersleeve, R., N. Croom, and P. Vasquez. 2011. "'Am I Going Crazy?!': A Critical Race Analysis of Doctoral Education." *Equity & Excellence in Education* 44 (1): 93–114.

Glover, K. S. 2009. *Racial Profiling: Research, Racism, and Resistance*. Lanham, MD: Rowman & Littlefield.

Gravlee, C., W. Dressler, and H. Bernard. 2005. "Skin Color, Social Classification, and Blood Pressure in Southeastern Puerto Rico." *American Journal of Public Health* 95 (12): 2191–2197.

Grier-Reed, T. 2010. "The African American Student Network: Creating Sanctuaries and Counterspaces for Coping with Racial Microaggressions in Higher Education Settings." *Journal of Humanistic Counseling, Education, and Development* 49 (2): 181–188.

Griffith, E. E. H. 1998. *Race and Excellence: My Dialogue with Chester Pierce*. Iowa City: University Of Iowa Press.

Harrell, S. 2000. "A Multidimensional Conceptualization of Racism-related Stress: Implications for the Well-being of People of Color." *American Journal of Orthopsychiatry* 70 (1): 42–57.

Hill, L., I. Kobayashi, and J. Hughes. 2007. "Perceived Racism and Ambulatory Blood Pressure in African American College Students." *Journal of Black Psychology* 33 (4): 404–421.

Hodge, C., and T. Vega. 2014, March 21. "Microaggressions: Comments That Sting." [Video file]. http://www.nytimes.com/video/us/100000002769668/microaggressions-comments-that-sting.html

"I, too, am Harvard". 2014. [web log]. http://itooamharvard.tumblr.com/

Jay, M. 2009. "Race-ing through the School Day: African American Educators' Experiences with Race and Racism in Schools." *International Journal of Qualitative Studies in Education* 22 (6): 671–685.

Johnson, K. R. 2003. "Case for African American and Latina/O Cooperation in Challenging Racial Profiling in Law Enforcement." *Florida Law Review* 55: 341–363.

Katsarou, E. 2009. "Reading African-American Literature to Understand the World: Critical Race Praxis in Teacher Preparation." *Race, Ethnicity, and Education* 12 (2): 253–266.

Kohli, R., and D. Solórzano. 2012. "Teachers, Please Learn Our Names!: Racial Microaggressions and the K-12 Classroom." *Race Ethnicity and Education* 1–22.

Lakoff, G. 2006. *Thinking Points: Communicating Our American Values and Vision*. New York: Farrar, Straus and Giroux.

Leonardo, Z. 2010. "Pedagogy of Fear: Toward a Fanonian Theory of 'Safety' in Race Dialogue." *Race, Ethnicity and Education* 13 (2): 139–157.

Library of Congress. 2013. Photograph by Vachon, J. (c. 1938). *A Drinking Fountain on the County Courthouse Lawn*. [Photograph.]. Washington, DC: Library of Congress. http://www.loc.gov/rr/print/list/085_disc.html

Makinen, J. 2014, Aug. 18. "Michael Brown Shooting in Ferguson Becomes in International Incident." *Los Angeles Times*. http://www.latimes.com/world/asia/la-fg-ferguson-michael-brown-shooting-world-reaction-20140818-story.html#page=1

Marable, M. 2002. *The Great Wells of Democracy: The Meaning of Race in American Life*. New York: BasicCivitas.

Masko, A. L. 2005. "'I Think About it All the Time': A 12-Year-Old Girl's Internal Crisis with Racism and the Effects on Her Mental Health." *Urban Education* 37 (4): 329–350.

Matias, C. E. 2012. "Who You Callin' White?! a Critical Counter-story on Colouring White Identity." *Race Ethnicity and Education* 1–25.

Mosley, M. 2010. "'That Really Hit Me Hard': Moving beyond Passive Anti-racism to Engage Withcritical Race Literacy Pedagogy." *Race Ethnicity and Education* 13 (4): 449–471.

New York Times Editorial Board. 2013, March, 23. "Walking While Black in New York." *New York Times* A16.

Orozco, R. 2012. "Framing Hostilities: Analysis of Mission Statements from Segregated Chicana/O Schools." *Journal of Latinos and Education* 11 (2): 80–93.

Pérez Huber, L. 2011. "Discourses of Racist Nativism in California Public Education: English Dominance as Racist Nativist Microaggressions." *Educational Studies* 47 (4): 379–401.

Pérez Huber, L., and B. Cueva. 2012. "Chicana/Latina Testimonios on Effects and Responses to Microaggressions." *Equity & Excellence in Education* 45 (3): 392–410.

Pierce, C. 1969. "Is Bigotry the Basis of the Medical Problem of the Ghetto?" In *Medicine in the Ghetto*, edited by J. Norman, 301–314. New York: Meredith Corporation.

Pierce, C. 1970. "Offensive Mechanisms." In *The Black Seventies*, edited by F. Barbour, 265–282. Boston, MA: Porter Sargent.

Pierce, C. 1974. "Psychiatric Problems of the Black Minority." In *American Handbook of Psychiatry*, edited by S. Arieti, 512–523. New York: Basic Books.

Pierce, C. 1980. "Social Trace Contaminants: Subtle Indicators of Racism in TV." In *Television and Social Behavior: Beyond Violence and Children*, edited by S. Withey and R. Abeles, 249–257. Hillsdale, NJ: Lawrence Erlbaum.

Pierce, C. 1988. "Stress in the Workplace." In *Black Families in Crisis: The Middle Class*, edited by A. Coner-Edwards and J. Spurlock, 27–34. New York: Brunner/Mazel.

Pierce, C. 1989. "Unity in Diversity: Thirty-three Years of Stress." In *Black Students: Psychological Issues and Academic Achievement*, edited by G. Berry and J. Asamen, 296–312. Newbury Park: Sage.

Pierce, C. 1995. "Stress Analogs of Racism and Sexism: Terrorism, Torture, and Disaster." In *Mental Health, Racism, and Sexism*, edited by C. Willie, P. Rieker, B. Kramer, and B. Brown, 277–293. Pittsburgh, PA: University of Pittsburgh Press.

Plessy v. Ferguson. 1896. 163 U.S. 537.

Profit, W., I. Mino, and C. Pierce. 2000. "Blacks, Stress in." In *Encyclopedia of Stress*. Vol. 1 (A-D), edited by G. Fink, 324–330. San Diego, CA: Academic Press.

Rollock, N. 2012. "Unspoken Rules of Engagement: Navigating Racial Microaggressions in Theacademic Terrain." *International Journal of Qualitative Studies in Education* 25 (5): 517–532.

Rolón-Dow, R. 2011. "Race(Ing) Stories: Digital Storytelling as a Tool for Critical Race Scholarship." *Race Ethnicity and Education* 14 (2): 159–173.

Schuette v. BAMN, No. 12-682 slip op. (S. Ct. Apr. 22, 2014).

Smith, W. 2004. "Black Faculty Coping with Racial Battle Fatigue: The Campus Racial Climate in a Post-civil Rights Era." In *A Long Way to Go: Conversations about Race by African American Faculty and Graduate Students*, edited by D. Cleveland, 171–190. New York: Peter Lang.

Smith, W., W. Allen, and L. Danley. 2007a. "'Assume the Position ... You Fit the Description.' Psychosocial Experiences and Racial Battle Fatigue among African American Male College Students." *American Behavioral Scientist* 51 (4): 551–578.

Smith, W., T. J. Yosso, and D. G. Solórzano. 2007b. "Racial Primes and Black Misandry on Historically White Campuses: Toward Critical Race Accountability in Educational Administration." *Educational Administration Quarterly* 43 (5): 559–585.

Smith, W., T. Yosso, and D. Solorzano. 2006. "Challenging Racial Battle Fatigue on Historically White Campuses: A Critical Examination of Race-related Stress." In *Faculty of Color Teaching in Predominantly White Colleges and Universities*, edited by C. A. Stanley, 299–328. Bolton, MA: Anker.

Solorzano, D. 1998. "Critical Race Theory, Race and Gender Microaggressions, and the Experiences of Chicana and Chicano Scholars." *Qualitative Studies in Education* 11 (1): 121–136.

Solorzano, D., M. Ceja, and T. Yosso. 2000. "Critical Race Theory, Racial Microaggressions, and Campus Racial Climate: The Experiences of African American College Students." *The Journal of Negro Education* 69 (1/2): 60–73.

Solorzano, D., and L. Pérez Huber. 2012. "Microaggressions, Racial." In *Encyclopedia of Diversity in Education*, edited by J. Banks, 1489–1492. Thousand Oaks, CA: Sage Publications.

Solorzano, D., and Villalpando, O. 1998. "Critical Race Theory, Marginality and the Experience of Students of Color in Higher Education." In *Sociology of Education: Emerging Perspectives*, 181–210. Albany: State University of New York Press.

St. Olaf microagressions. 2014. [web log]. http://stolafmicroaggressions.tumblr.com/

Sue, D. W. 2010. *Microaggressions in Everyday Life: Race, Gender, and Sexual Orientation*. Hoboken, NJ: John Wiley & Sons.

Sue, D., J. Bucceri, A. Lin, K. Nadal, and G. Torino. 2007a. "Racial Microaggressions and the Asian American Experience." *Cultural Diversity and Ethnic Minority Psychology* 13 (1): 72–81.

Sue, D. W., C. Capodilupo, G. Torino, J. Bucceri, A. Holder, K. Nadal, and M. Esquilin. 2007b. "Racial Microaggressions in Everyday Life: Implications for Clinical Practice." *American Psychologist* 62 (4): 271–286.

Sue, D. W., and M. G. Constantine. 2007. "Racial Microaggressions as Instigators of Difficultdialogues on Race: Implications for Student Affairs Educators and Students." *College Student Affairs Journal* 26 (2): 136–143.

Truong, K., and S. Museus. 2012. "Responding to Racism and Racial Trauma in Doctoral Study: An Inventory for Coping and Mediating Relationships." *Harvard Educational Review* 82 (2): 26–254.

Urrieta, L., and S. Villenas. 2014. "The Legacy of Derrick Bell and Latina/O Education: A Critical Race Testimonio." *Race, Ethnicity and Education* 16 (4): 514–535.

Vega, T. 2014, March 21. "Student See Many Slights as 'Racial Microaggressions'." *New York Times*. http://www.nytimes.com/2014/03/22/us/as-diversity-increases-slights-get-subtler-but-still-sting.html?_r=0

Yosso, T., W. Smith, M. Ceja, and D. Solorzano. 2009. "Critical Race Theory Racial Microaggressions and Campus Racial Climate for Latina/O Undergraduates." *Harvard Educational Review* 79 (4): 659–690.

Against the politics of desperation: educational justice, critical race theory, and Chicago school reform

David Stovall

As a center for education 'reform' in the United States, Chicago sheds light on state apparatuses seeking to end public education and replace it with market-driven ventures, largely by way of public–private partnerships. Critical to this process is the idea of 'choice' which has come to operate as a political device providing the illusion that students, parents, and families have options leading to educational improvement. In this article, Stovall pays specific attention to what he calls the *politics of desperation*, suggesting that entities such as central school offices and educational management organizations are using popular rhetoric coupled with marketing tools to solicit buy-in on their specific brand of educational improvement. He argues that this strategy targets groups facing uncertainty in education and housing, and who therefore attempt to navigate choices they have little say in defining. Instead of said improvements, Stovall contends we are witnessing a 'more-of-the-same' game, including dispossession and continued disenfranchisement of working-class communities of color. At the same time, he highlights the absolute necessity of resistance. Borrowing from Duncan-Andrade's notion of *critical hope*, he suggests we must be painfully honest about current educational conditions, while also building grassroots networks that challenge these realities. Stovall identifies strategies and resources mobilized by Chicago residents through direct-action organizing, coalition building, and school–community partnerships to challenge neoliberal reform.

Introduction

This article is an analytical and theoretical essay on the realities faced by low-income/working-class communities of color in K-12 urban schools in the United States. Chicago, as a center for education 'reform' in the United States, sheds light on state apparatuses seeking to end public education and replace it with neoliberal market-driven ventures, largely by way of public–private partnerships. Critical to this process is the idea of 'choice' which has come to operate as a political device providing the illusion that students, parents, and families are offered options that lead to educational improvement. For the purpose of this account, I will pay specific attention to what I am calling the *politics of desperation*, suggesting that entities like central school offices, educational management organizations (EMOs), and other state agencies are using a combination of popular rhetoric coupled with marketing tools to solicit buy-in on their specific brand of educational improvement; in particular, this strategy targets racially and economically marginalized groups facing uncertainty in education and housing, and who therefore attempt to navigate a set of choices that they have had little say in defining. Instead of said improvements, what we are witnessing is a 'more-of-the-same' game. Instead of the ability of these new instruments of reform to contribute to wholesale academic improvement, students and families in cities like Chicago are witnessing an entirely different dynamic. In the new data-driven mode of educational reform, there is an undercurrent that deserves attention and that is heavily rooted in dispossession and continued disenfranchisement of particular populations.

Simultaneously, this article is not intended to contribute to a sense of hopelessness. Instead, my concern is to provide a critical analysis for the purpose of highlighting the absolute necessity of resistance. Borrowing from Duncan-Andrade's (2009) notion of *critical hope*, I am of the understanding that hope must be supported by connection to the material conditions of the people we are accountable to and engaged with through active struggle. Critical hope also requires that we must be painfully honest about the realities of current educational conditions in urban areas, while at the same time building networks that challenge these conditions. As an emerging global city, Chicago has set forth policies that unfortunately are becoming blueprints for cities in the United States and across the globe. Nevertheless, this reality does not have to be a foregone conclusion. Instead, these realities deserve specific study to develop the necessary tools for resistance.

In order to frame the aforementioned issues in the context of Chicago and potential ramifications for urban centers, this article is divided into three sections. The first section places Chicago in context, explaining the current realities facing low-income families of color and trends in educational reform over the last decade. Additionally, this section is dedicated to providing examples of said reforms and what they have meant to numerous groups throughout the city. The second section combines Critical Race Theory (CRT) and the concept of the politics of desperation to explain the sentiments at play when families are presented with educational 'options' that are often direct attempts to maintain the existing allocation of resources to a select group of residents in the city. The concluding section highlights various forms of resistance and the necessity of such struggles at a time when the aforementioned reforms are positioned as the only response to addressing educational concerns in historically marginalized and under-resourced communities.

Into the realities of Chicago: Renaissance 2010 and educational reform for the few

Documented extensively in the works of Lipman (2003, 2004, 2011), Saltman (2007, 2010), and Fabricant and Fine (2012), Chicago has been a hotbed for educational reforms. I am reluctant to use the word 'reform' because the changes have been touted as positive changes, but they have largely resulted in the further marginalization of low-income and working-class communities of color. Instead of considering the current policies as justice-minded reforms, a more accurate description of these policies and their implementation is neoliberal policy reform. Largely rooted in the belief that free-market economies provide solutions to the vast majority of social concerns, neoliberal reform centers on the rights of the individual. The market is understood as self-correcting, resulting in the rationale for privatization of public goods for the purposes of cost-effectiveness, maximizing of profits, and better choices for those traditionally excluded from market transactions. For low-income families of color, this often results in a rhetorical charge that the market can solve the vast majority of political, economic, and social issues that confront them. Because the resources on offer in the marketplace are falsely positioned as available to all, low-income and working-class families of color are often blamed for not accessing said resources.

This manifestation has been most evident in Chicago over the last two decades. Based on the 1995 educational policy shift resulting in mayoral control of Chicago Public Schools (CPS), the mayor currently has sole authority in appointing the school board, which is responsible for final approval of school-related issues (e.g., financial matters, curricular shifts, contract procurement, approval of new schools, etc.). In addition to the mayor's ability to appoint members of the school board, he or she has the ability to overturn any decision made by the board. Facilitated by the 22-year mayoral tenure of Richard M. Daley, Chicago has laid a blueprint for numerous cities in the United States, where advocates of educational markets desire to centralize control of the school system in the hands of like-minded state actors. During this time, the number of educators on the school board has decreased significantly. Currently, the board membership largely consists of people from business, legal, and philanthropic sectors. This fosters a reciprocal relationship between the board and the mayor's office, as board members are usually individuals or employees of entities that have contributed significantly to the mayor's reelection campaign.

In addition to mayoral control and likewise rooted in neoliberal ideology, there has been a convergence of housing and education policies. In Chicago's attempt to market itself as a global city (attracting international investment from tourism and business ventures), housing has been paired with education as a key component in the city's development. Dating back to 1971, Mayor Richard J. Daley (father of Richard M.) spearheaded a policy and planning initiative known as the Chicago 21 Plan, targeting 21 geographic and political districts for redevelopment. Considered as part of the last wave of urban renewal strategies, the Chicago 21 Plan should be understood as the blueprint for neoliberal reform in the city.

Fast-forward approximately 40 years to the present, and actions by the mayor and other state actors to secure corporate contributions through free-market strategies have become the norm locally, nationally, and internationally. Parts of the Chicago model of reform have been duplicated in cities like New York, Los Angeles, and Houston. Officials from all three cities have come to Chicago to study mayoral control (of the school board) and how to connect education, housing, and business with the intent to foster long-term development. Internationally, Chicago has been cited for its improvements in these sectors. As a central hub for global finance, advancements in information technology, and management of systems of production, Chicago has fashioned itself as a viable competitor for investment from transnational global firms in business, industry, and entertainment (Smith & Stovall, 2008).

All of this has implications for education. Through a collaborative of business interests known as the Commercial Club of Chicago, its Civic Committee developed a 2003 report known as 'Left behind'. Included in this report was the argument that students in the United States are falling behind internationally in reading, math, and science. Their suggested solution was to retool the public education landscape by infusing 'innovation' from the business sector. These innovations would be for the purposes of strengthening the US workforce and returning the US economy to supremacy in the global marketplace. The people best suited to foster change in this direction were those who possessed an intimate knowledge of free-market strategies to boost competition among education providers (Civic Committee, 2003). Key to this strategy is the idea that competition ultimately will boost academic performance. Under free-market capitalism, the belief is that if one school is performing well, it will push others to improve or else be closed due to decreasing enrollment as families 'choose' better education providers. Contrary to this understanding is the fact that each school serves a different set of students requiring a unique set of resources germane to that particular population. Neoliberal competition-based models ignore this fact and assume that schools are best imagined/developed as sites of efficiency and replication. This also fosters patterns of exclusion as 'winners' (those who do well on standardized tests) are championed, while losers (those who don't) are subject to further marginalization or dismissal.

Nevertheless, the city moved forward with policy recommendations suggested in the aforementioned report and rolled out a plan in 2004, called Renaissance 2010. Indeed, the suggestions of the Civic Committee were promoted to the public. By 2010, CPS proposed to target up to 70 'chronically underperforming' schools for 'transformation' into 100 schools with the designation of charter, contract, or performance school. Whereas charters are granted by the state, contract schools distinguish individuals or groups that have secured contracts with the city to create schools. While contract schools are a close cousin to charter schools with regard to funding formulas, the distinct difference lies in the direct partnership with the city rather than the state. Currently, the largest contract institution in Chicago is the Academy of Urban School Leadership (AUSL). Schools in the performance category were yet another manifestation, aimed at giving principals and teachers some level of autonomy regarding curriculum and schedule. Simultaneously, the internal understanding was to lessen the city's financial commitment to education through the use of partners that could in turn use their contributions to education as tax subsidies (through the federal tax code's provision for charitable donations). Such transformations were posited to community residents as CPS moving to provide 'choice' and 'options' in the so-called education marketplace (Chicago Public Schools, 2012).

The first site where this experiment would take place was in a group of neighborhoods known as the mid-South region. Consisting of the neighborhoods of Kenwood, Oakland, Grand Boulevard, and Douglass, 20 of the 22 schools in the four-neighborhood area were targeted for closure or restructuring in the aforementioned forms. Fortunately, due to the collective efforts of community organizations and a team of collaborating researchers, the first effort to implement the experiment was curtailed. Thanks to grassroots efforts, it was discovered that many of the schools targeted for reconfiguration were performing at or exceeding the standards set forward by the state. One specific community organization, the Kenwood Oakland Community Organization (KOCO), staged a sleep-in at the central office building of CPS. Coupled with the work of a local activist-scholar, Pauline Lipman, these efforts garnered attention and resulted in the curtailing of the original rollout plan targeting 20 schools. Instead, CPS targeted 10 schools, reconfiguring the majority as charter and contract schools.

As mentioned earlier, critical to the process of market-based education reform is its intimate relationship to the housing market. Because housing stock is key in attracting business interests to the city, education becomes an important conduit in solidifying long-term investment in schools (Arrastia, 2007; Lipman, 2003, 2011, 2012; Smith & Stovall, 2008). With the main determinant of a family's home purchase being the schools in the prospective neighborhood, the mid-South region became a hotbed for gentrification, most notably through the mass destruction of public housing through the Chicago Housing Authority's (CHA's) Plan for Transformation (Lipman, 2011). Touted as a $1.6 billion plan, its aim is to redevelop areas once occupied by high-rise public housing as mixed-income communities. As housing stock in the redeveloped areas will be distributed in thirds among low-income, moderate-income, and upper-income groups, questions arise about the dubious qualifications have been placed on the low-income group (Olszewski & Sadovi, 2003). To receive any of the homes in the new developments, public housing families have to go through a battery of screenings for health (specifically for substance abuse), employment (applicants must now work at least 30 hours per week unless they are not able or are in a training/educational program), and criminal activity (a person cannot rent an apartment if anyone in the household has a felony conviction) (Olivio, 2004). In the Plan for Transformation, schools are framed as an important component, and the change in housing has been projected to mean an increase in families of moderate and affluent incomes. Because this requires strategic planning on the part of CPS, the convergence of Renaissance 2010 and the Plan for Transformation are critical to bringing the larger neoliberal plan into fruition. Despite the provisions for low-income families in the new mixed-income communities, the aforementioned health, employment, and criminal compliances help to carefully sanitize the community marketed to newcomers. Schools, as the final frontier, provide the necessary push for buyers to take the step in securing life in the city.

Fortunately for the families that remain in some of the targeted areas, a collective of community organizations has been able to develop strategies to contest the efforts of CPS. Local Chicago organizations like the KOCO, Blocks Together, Brighton Park Neighborhood Council (BPNC), Albany Park Neighborhood Council, Logan Square Neighborhood Association (LSNA), Organization of the Northeast (ONE), Grand Boulevard Federation, Southwest Organizing Project (SWOP), and ENLACE Chicago have organized separately and collectively to address school closings, teacher removal, and restorative justice. Central to these organizations is their focus on community education and achieving results directly connected to their organizing efforts. A specific example of collective strategizing would be the multi-organizational coalition Voices of Youth in Chicago Education (VOYCE). Collectively, they have won victories in eliminating 10-day suspensions in CPS, established pilot student surveys for teacher evaluation, and developed peer juries in local schools.

Revisiting Renaissance 2010 and the Plan for Transformation

The residual effects of the convergence of Renaissance 2010 and the Plan for Transformation have been devastating for a growing number of African-American and Latino/a communities in Chicago. According to the 2010 US Census, Chicago lost 200,000 residents from 2000 to 2010 (Glanton, Mullen, & Olivio, 2011). The Plan for Transformation began in 1999, while Renaissance 2010 was unveiled and first implemented in 2004. As the two policies converged during a six-year period, Chicago witnessed 178,000 African-American residents depart from the city. Additionally, since the initial rollout of Renaissance 2010, 101 schools have been permanently closed, phased out (when students are no longer admitted), or labeled as turnaround (when the existing staff is fired and an EMO is hired to re-staff the school, usually with a new curricular focus). Ninety-nine of the 101 schools in these categories were predominantly African-American or Latino/a (Lipman, Smith, Gutstein, & Dallacqua, 2012). Coupled with the destruction of over 80% of public housing stock (whose population was 95% African-American), many schools became depopulated, while others were converted to 'receiver schools'. Such institutions would conduct an intake of students from the depopulated or closed schools. Massive overcrowding in historically underfunded and underresourced African-American and Latino/a schools on the South and West sides of the city resulted from this strategy, while populations in affluent regions of the city actually grew (Lipman et al., 2012).

As neoliberal educational reform, Renaissance 2010 has since morphed into numerous entities, securing private monies through organizations such as the Renaissance Schools Fund (a private philanthropic entity), the Chicago Public Education Fund (a philanthropic entity specifically for securing resources for charter and turnaround schools), and the Office of New Schools (an internal office to CPS). Coupled with new policy initiatives from the federal government (e.g., Race to the Top, No Child Left Behind re-authorization, etc.), this particular brand of school reform has been touted as a replicable model for nearly two decades. In addition to CPS having five CEOs over the last 12 years, the rotating door of administration has created a central office structure with minimal transparency for communities that are demanding fair and equitable education for students of color in low-income and working-class areas of the city. Despite some slowing in the housing market due to the international economic downturn of 2008, the housing market in Chicago is trending upward despite periods of volatility. With Chicago's considerable loss of its African-American population over the last decade combined with the mass destruction of public housing, the current school restructuring plan has been able to move forward without significant stoppage. As I discuss in the final section, however, communities have been able to mobilize to challenge the trends exacerbated by Renaissance 2010.

While some would cite the convergence of Renaissance 2010 and the Plan for Transformation as conspiratorial, I offer to take it a step further in that there is no longer a clandestine conversation surrounding policy aims. Instead, we should understand these policy machinations as public, where state actors and private parties are implementing strategies to permanently remove particular residents from urban areas. The expressed public purpose of these policies is to attract a majority White affluent gentry from suburban areas and international destinations. Coupled with the neoliberal push for privatization of the public sector, schools become the conduit for an illusion of progress.

CRT, interest convergence, and the politics of desperation: realities and contradictions

First utilized in legal scholarship, CRT has relevance to this discussion, especially to understanding the nuances and intersections of race, class, and gender in urban educational policy (Crenshaw, Gotanda, Peller, & Thomas, 1995; Ladson-Billings, 1997). Indeed, CRT provides a framework to analyze the ever-shifting phenomenon of race, class, and gender in housing and education. As a result of the endemic nature of racism in US society, laws aimed at treating people of color and whites 'alike' only promise to curtail extreme cases of injustice. In this instance in Chicago, because the vast majority of the affected populations are either African-Americans or Latino/as from low-income communities, we are propelled to seek a deeper understanding of white supremacy not only as a single act wrongly committed by a perpetrator but also as a structural manifestation of the continued subjugation of people of color. Instead of suffering victimhood, however, communities negatively affected by the aforementioned policies have developed a language by which to name, address, and actively resist the current trend of neoliberal reform in education.

CRT is traditionally rooted in *counterstories* or accounts based on the experiential knowledge of the racially oppressed (Solórzano & Yosso, 2009). Ultimately, the intent is for those who share counterstories to begin to interrogate the underpinnings of policies that are purported as beneficial to the academic achievement of urban youth of color from low-income and working-class communities, particularly when those policies have the opposite effect. In excavating the counterstory in the convergence of Renaissance 2010 and the Plan for Transformation, CRT can be utilized to reveal the realities of such projects.

In addition to counterstories, I also find utility in a construct popularized by critical race legal theorist Derrick Bell known as interest convergence. Stemming from Bell's legal scholarship, the principal idea is that White-dominated mainstream society will promote racial justice only to the extent that it advantages White mainstream society (Bell, 1980). Considering the realities presented through the policy convergence of Renaissance

2010 and the Plan for Transformation, the dynamic set in motion is best understood as a form of 'consolation without consultation'. In Chicago, for African-American and Latino/a residents from low-income and working-class communities who are able to remain in the city, there is a consolation prize offered to them in the form of Renaissance 2010 education options. As I discuss later, there is also a bevy of traditional neighborhood public schools that have been repurposed in title to make them attractive to students, parents, and families.

Complicating the issue is the fact that a portion of the population that is gentrifying the aforementioned neighborhoods is not White, but middle-class and affluent African-American and Latino/a residents. On the surface, the new CPS options are positioned as a move toward social (racial), economic, and educational justice with the retooling of schools for African-American and Latino/a students. In reality, many of these consolation prizes are offered to communities without their consultation. Charter, contract, and performance schools are presented as improvements over educational conditions in the past. Without assessing the needs of the community in question, however, schools developed under Renaissance 2010 have delivered more of the same to residents on the far West and South sides of the city (Brown & Gutstein, 2009).

More specifically, changing the school curriculum and then restricting access to newly redeveloped schools makes 'good sense' as far as interest convergence goes: it is in the best interests of white policy makers to shift the curricular focus of schools in ways that make them attractive to traditionally marginalized communities, while at the same time rendering them less accessible to the least desired segments of the population by way of academic admissions requirements, lottery systems (to regulate the number of 'undesirables'), and inaccessible housing. Where mixed-income developments become the logical solution to the problem of blighted public housing, Renaissance 2010 becomes the solution to a 'failing' school system.

Toward a politics of desperation

In the aftermath of Renaissance 2010 and the Plan for Transformation, it becomes important to focus on the population of African-American and Latino/a residents that was able to remain in the city. While the vast majority of these residents remain in areas that have little proximity to the rail systems and the central business district and have a history of community disinvestment by the city, there are a number of African-American and Latino/a residents who were able to keep their homes or apartments. Similar to the group of African-American residents cited in Pedroni's work in Milwaukee, Wisconsin, this group of families is either living in the areas that are experiencing gentrification or are in close proximity to them (Pedroni, 2007). In many instances, this population is combined with a group of more affluent, middle-class African-Americans and Latino/as who may have moved away from the neighborhood and are returning as part of the new regimen of gentrifying residents. In this instance, members of both groups understand the history of CPS and its inability to collectively serve the broadest range of students. As a byproduct of Renaissance 2010, schools that once were neighborhood public schools have become magnet schools, language academies, math and science academies, military academies, or visual and performing arts centers.

The 'academy' title seems appealing to incoming and remaining residents, but it is part of a larger strategy that provides 'incentive for professional and middle-class families to live in the city' (Lipman, 2003, p. 56). The key to the argument for building new public schools and redeveloping public housing was that current residents would benefit. However, such redevelopment can also help to attract middle-income families who might otherwise move to the suburbs or are likely to once their children reach school age. Strategies to redevelop poorly performing 'inner-city' schools and the poor neighborhoods where they are usually located have real potential to do more harm than good for the families the policy is supposed to benefit.

For both sets of residents, their experiences as either former CPS students or through observations of family members attending CPS equip them with a working knowledge of the district and its history. Because many families have experienced or are fearful of exposing their child to the worst that CPS has to offer, some families embrace a *politics of desperation*. In this instance, the politics of desperation should be understood as *the complex assemblage of thoughts and actions that guide educational decisions in periods of housing and schooling uncertainty, especially when available choices have not been defined by affected communities*. For many of these families, if their child does not gain admission to a selective enrollment school, the vast majority of the remaining public school options come in the form of charter, contract, or a renamed neighborhood school with a supposedly new curricular focus.

With the aforementioned in mind, I would like readers to consider the following counterstory: of the 95% African-American residents in Chicago public housing before the Plan for Transformation was implemented, 40% were senior citizens living on a fixed income. Many of the senior citizens living on fixed incomes are women of color (specifically grandmothers) who often have the responsibility of childrearing in their respective families. With them rests the responsibilities for registering children for school, staying current with immunizations, and remaining abreast of any shifts in current educational policy that may affect their grandchildren's educational experiences.

Instead of acknowledging these facts, public officials noted that the majority of units in the proposed Plan for Transformation will not be public housing for low-income families – usually not more than one-third of the total. Because they will not have access to newly developed housing, it is likely that such families will not have a place to live within the confines of the city. Moreover, children under a grandparent's care are not allowed to live in public housing specifically designated for senior citizens; families such as these often have to apply for what is known as project-based subsidized housing vouchers (commonly known as Section 8 housing). If afforded a Section 8 voucher, the family may be allowed to secure housing in the area. Yet, this is rarely the case – Section 8 vouchers are not generally granted in the city of Chicago and waiting lists can have backlogs of up to 2 years. Under these conditions, schools become an important and often exclusive venue for the remaining population. While receiver schools are concentrated in particular areas where low-income families remain, charter schools, usually run by EMOs, recruit the children of the upper-income residents. Despite the fact that charter schools locally in Chicago and nationally have not proven to outperform traditional public schools (Fabricant & Fine, 2012), the presentation of such 'choices' makes for a spectacle that is often attractive to parents and families whose children are fortunate enough to be admitted.

It becomes important to note that the politics of desperation are based on an understanding of the peculiar realities around educational options in the city. When charter or contract schools hold open houses and community presentations, parents and potential students understandably are drawn to the immaculate presentation of the physical plant. The newly scrubbed floors, new lockers, and professional presentation of the school by a young and energetic new staff are key factors in engendering a sense of desire and belonging. For many families, in fact, *anything* is better than what they have traditionally had at their disposal.

Simultaneously, once parents enter these schools, the situation changes completely. One particular EMO, the Noble Street Network of charter schools, reported collecting $386,745 in fines over the last 3 years from students for disciplinary infractions (Parents United for Responsible Education, 2012). Even as it touts itself as serving African-American and Latino/a students from low-income and working-class communities, students are encumbered and not allowed to advance to the next grade if fines are not collected.

Other charter networks give families contracts upon a student's acceptance to the school. Some of these contracts contain a nondisciplinary dismissal clause, stating that if a student receives two failing grades in consecutive grading periods, they will be expelled from the school. Many school reform organizations consider this as representative of a 'tough love, no-excuses' shift toward parental accountability, but there is another rationale that should be considered. Many EMOs retain these policies because students with a failing grade for consecutive grading periods decrease the achievement data reported to the district. Charter schools have promoted themselves as the alternative to traditional neighborhood schools due to their success in test score gains and college acceptance. At the same time, little attention is paid to the students who were removed from the school to protect test score performance and other forms of achievement data reported to the district. In all of these instances, appealing to a family's desperation for quality education has the potential to create long-term deleterious effects if these issues are not brought into the larger discussion of education reform.

Conclusion: all is not lost – critical hope, critical race praxis, and authentic community engagement

My hope is that the previous discussion did not paint a gloom-and-doom scenario. Although the road forward may appear daunting, there are efforts across the United States and internationally that are fueling resistance to neoliberal education reform. Such efforts illuminate the type of critical hope that Duncan-Andrade (2009) speaks about – a hope rooted in the material realities of those who are working to collectively address and transform their conditions. Eric Yamamoto (1997), in his challenge to legal scholars, pushes us to spend less time with abstract theorizing and more time with on-the-ground issues concerning historically marginalized communities of color. Known as Critical Race Praxis, there is a growing number of scholars who are willing to engage affected communities in praxis toward transformative education and equity.

Recently, in Chicago, the organization Stand for Children introduced legislation that would limit the power of teachers to organize to address school conditions; this organization receives funding from major corporations such as Adidas, the Nike School Innovation Fund, and Intel. The legislation requires a 75% approval vote of union membership to authorize a strike. Due to the organizing efforts of the Chicago Teachers Union (CTU), its delegation of community partners, and its own Caucus of Rank-and-File Educators (CORE), they were able to get 90% of their membership to authorize a strike. This has never happened in the history of large-scale organized labor in Chicago. The key to their success was CTU's ability to abandon tactics common to labor organizing. Instead, the CTU through CORE reached out to community partners to develop a strategy that centered the needs of students and parents as key in developing effective education reform. They have been tirelessly active in supporting community efforts to halt school closings and turnarounds as well (CORE, 2012).

At the time of writing, a teachers' strike led by the CTU has just concluded. Critical to the success of the strike was CORE's aforementioned organizing strategy within the CTU that garnered support from parents, students, and other large-scale labor unions in the city (Fraternal Order of Police, International Firefighters Union, etc.). While all of the demands were not met (e.g., smaller class size and wraparound support services for students and teachers), significant gains were achieved (specifically protection for laid-off teachers due to school closings, re-infusion of art, music and physical education into the curriculum, seniority rights, rejection of test-based merit pay). For 9 days, CPS was entirely shut down, representing a needed alternative to the neoliberal deluge currently ravaging public school systems. Nationally and internationally, the ability of a union to organize 90% of their 30,000-plus members is indicative of a moment where the rank and file citizenry have mobilized to make demands on the neoliberal state (Lipman, 2012).

Predating the recent strike, a team of education researchers began a collective in 2010 to actively challenge popular rhetoric around school reform. Known as Chicagoland Researchers and Advocates for Transformative Education (CReATE), they have begun to develop a number of research reports that are directly distributed to community organizations. Additionally, they have been in collaboration with community organizations to host public forums for families who have been affected by neoliberal education reform (CReATE, 2012).

Receiving minimal media coverage in the United States, teachers in the Canadian province of Quebec have joined forces with students and families to protest neoliberal education reform and the overreliance on high-stakes standardized tests. Culminating in a series of work stoppages, communities have begun to harness their power in resisting state-sanctioned reforms. Their effort has served as an inspiration to groups in cities that are often fighting a sense of hopelessness in the battle for quality education, including Chicago.

As the efforts move forward, the fight must be named and engaged. The recent attack on the Raza Studies program in Tucson, Arizona, is of particular importance; this program was built on the voices, cultures, and histories of Latino/as. Since this is a student-centered effort by teachers and community members to develop authentic education for students in the Tucson Unified School District, the state's efforts to thwart this initiative should be condemned. Any effort to support a transformative education for historically underserved students should be championed, especially when it is developed by and for the community – unlike the education reforms in Chicago. Finally, the struggles of our comrades in Tucson should serve as further inspiration to fight systems of power despite the appearance of insurmountable odds. If our bodies are not able to get there, our hearts, minds, and souls are connected by the work we do on the ground in other parts of the world.

References

Arrastia, L. (2007). Capital's daisy chain: Exposing Chicago's corporate coalition. *Journal of Critical Education Policy Studies*, *5*, Retrieved from http://www.jceps.com/

Bell, D. (1980). *Brown v. Board of Education* and the interest convergence dilemma. *Harvard Law Review*, *93*, 518–533.

Brown, L., & Gutstein, E. (2009). *The charter difference: A comparison of Chicago charter and neighborhood high schools*. Chicago, IL: Collaborative for Equity and Justice in Education.

Caucus of Rank-and-File Educators. (2012). *Homepage*. Retrieved from www.coreteachers.org

Chicago Public Schools. (2012). *New schools and programs*. Retrieved from www.cps.edu/NewSchools/Pages/ONS.aspx

Chicagoland Researchers and Advocates for Transformative Education. (2012). *Blog*. Retrieved from http://createchicago.blogspot.com/

Civic Committee of the Commercial Club of Chicago. (2003). *Left behind: Student achievement in Chicago's public schools*. Chicago, IL: Commercial Club of Chicago.

Crenshaw, K., Gotanda, N., Peller, G., & Thomas, K. (Eds.). (1995). *Critical race theory: The key writings that formed the movement*. New York, NY: The New Press.

Duncan-Andrade, J.M.R. (2009). Note to educators: Hope required when growing roses in concrete. *Harvard Educational Review*, *79*(2), 1–13.

Fabricant, M., & Fine, M. (2012). *Charter schools and the corporate makeover of public education: What's at stake?* New York, NY: Teachers College Press.

Glanton, D., Mullen, W., & Olivio, A. (2011, February 18). Neighborhood population drain: Census shows central Chicago grew while outlying areas lost. *Chicago Tribune*, pp. B10–11.

Ladson-Billings, G. (1997). Just what is critical race theory and what's it doing in a 'nice' field like education. *International Journal of Qualitative Studies in Education*, *11*, 7–24.

Lipman, P. (2003). Chicago school policy: Regulating Black and Latino youth in the global city. *Race, Ethnicity, and Education*, *6*, 331–355.

Lipman, P. (2004). *High stakes education: Inequality, globalization, and urban school reform*. New York, NY: Routledge.

Lipman, P. (2011). *The new political economy of urban education: Neoliberalism, race, and the right to the city*. New York, NY: Routledge.

Lipman, P. (2012, September 22). What we won in Chicago. *Truthout*. Retrieved from www.truthout.org

Lipman, P., Smith, J., Gutstein, E., & Dallacqua, L. (2012). *Examining CPS' plan to close, turnaround, or phase out 17 schools*. Chicago, IL: Collaborative for Equity and Justice in Education.

Olivio, A. (2004, September 22). New CHA housing is tied to jobs: Adults must work 30 hours a week. *The Chicago Tribune*, pp. C12–13.

Olszewski, L., & Sadovi, C. (2003, December 19). Rebirth of schools set for south side CHA and a list of institutions have big plans. *The Chicago Tribune*, pp. C5–6.

Parents United for Responsible Education. (2012). *Fact sheet: Noble street profiting from predatory discipline code*. Retrieved from http://pureparents.org/wp-content/uploads/2012/02/NobleFactSheet-2-13-12.pdf

Pedroni, T. (2007). *Market movements: African-American involvement in school voucher reform*. New York, NY: Routledge.

Saltman, K.J. (2007). *Capitalizing on disaster: Taking and breaking public schools*. Boulder, CO: Paradigm.

Saltman, K.J. (2010). *The gift of education: Public education and venture philanthropy*. New York, NY: Palgrave Macmillan.

Smith, J., & Stovall, D. (2008). Coming home to new homes and new schools: Critical race theory and the new politics of containment. *Journal of Education Policy*, *23*, 135–152.

Solórzano, D.G., & Yosso, T.J. (2009). Critical race methodology: Counter-storytelling as an analytical framework for educational research. In E. Taylor, D. Gillborn, & G. Ladson-Billings (Eds.), *Foundations of critical race theory in education* (pp. 131–147). New York, NY: Routledge.

Yamamoto, E. (1997). Critical race praxis: Race theory and political lawyering practice in post-civil rights America. *Michigan Law Review*, *95*, 821–900.

You can't erase race! Using CRT to explain the presence of race and racism in majority white suburban schools

Thandeka K. Chapman

Employing a critical race analysis of contemporary suburban schooling in the US, the author challenges the ideology of colorblind racial contexts. The concepts of color-blindness, interest-convergence, racial realism, and white privilege are used to explain how federal mandates and common school policies and practices, such as tracking, traditional curricula, teacher classroom practices, and student surveillance, sustain a racially hostile environment for students of color in majority white suburban schools. Critical multicultural education is offered as a means to openly address issue of race and racism in the curriculum, school policies, and teacher practices.

Introduction

The post-racial era, crafted through discourses of American education by the first election of President Barack Obama, has made it increasingly difficult to discuss the ways in which race and racism continue to create and sustain barriers that limit the social and economic gains of people of color in the United States (Crenshaw, 2011). This post-racial moment is predominantly defined by the concept of colorblindness that is cultivated in public spaces. 'Colorblindness has helped to construe race as an "impolite" or even morally suspect subject "politically correct" whites should avoid' (Tarca, 2005, p. 107). The irony of colorblind policies is the *color-conscious* racism that serves as its foundation. A critical race analysis of schools and schooling counters common sense instantiations of colorblind contexts with examples of how race and racism continue as pervasive barriers to equitable schooling for students of color. Employing a critical race analysis of contemporary schooling in the US, I challenge the ideology of colorblind racial contexts in three ways: first, I interrogate the historical underpinnings of race that continue to impact schools; second, I explore the role(s) of race in current education policies; and third, I present empirical evidence demonstrating how race and racism are manifested in majority White suburban school settings.

To accomplish these three goals, I begin the next section with an articulation of the current research on students of color in majority white suburban schools. The following section is an overview of critical race theory and the tenets of the theory used in the paper. Because of its significant impact on schools, the concept of colorblindness is given a more extensive explanation. Next, I illustrate how desegregation reforms, No Child Left Behind, and existing curricula stand as historical and contemporary policies with racialized instantiations of practice that impact today's schools. I then present data from a study about the experiences of students of color in predominately white suburban schools to discuss how supposedly colorblind school contexts further marginalize students of color. I explore how school practices reinstate race and racism and widen the equity gap between white students who are *privileged by* and students of color who are *oppressed by* white supremacist articulations of schooling (Tarca, 2005; Urrieta, 2006). Lastly, I suggest that schools need to commit to a focus on critical multicultural education for social justice to assist educators in predominately white suburban schools to challenge racist practices, which are supported through a colorblind ideology, and create more equitable schooling experiences for students of color (Grant & Sleeter, 1989/1997; Kincheloe, 1993).

Current research on students of color in majority white suburban schools

As racial demographics continue to shift, many scholars are researching the experiences of students of color in majority white high schools (Carter, 2007, 2008; Chapman, 2007; Diamond, 2006; Diamond, Lewis, & Gordon, 2007; Huidor & Cooper, 2010; O'Connor, Mueller, Lewis, Rivas-Drake, & Rosenberg, 2011). O'Connor et al. interviewed 44 black students, and conducted in-depth research of eight high-achievers, to document the schooling experiences of high-achieving African-American students in racially stratified accelerated courses in predominately white schools. The researchers found that students maintained strong connections with their African-American peers, who were in less rigorous classes, as a means to buffer them from acts of racism. A support system was unavailable to black students in the upper-level Advanced Placement (AP) and advanced courses, causing them to seek alliances with other racial groups such as Asian Americans. O'Connor et al. state that the students' resistance to stereotypes, and their negotiation of the school contexts, interacted with the contexts of the school as an unwelcoming space. The researchers also noted that some students were able to trespass racial boundaries in classes by proving themselves as worthy academic partners. However, many of the high-achieving black students in the study espoused a negative view of black low achievers, and they connected these perceptions with negative stereotypes of race.

Diamond et al. (2007) found comparable results pertaining to issues of racial isolation and negative peer pressure in upper-level courses for black students. Among the black students in regular classes, there was a stronger support system. Diamond et al. also noted that the stress and racism of upper level classes caused black students to doubt their academic abilities. They interviewed 70 black and white high school students with a range of grade point averages. The researchers found that the majority of black students felt that being black would limit their life chances for success, while the white students did not believe that race was a factor in their success. However, the black students' belief in racially stratified success did not impact their academic achievement and desire to be successful. In fact, black students at every level of tracking hoped to attend college.

In her study of high-achieving black students at a majority white suburban elite school, Carter (2007, 2008) noted that black students created homogenous racial enclaves to affirm racial identity and shield them from racism in the school. Carter conducted a series of three interviews with nine African-American 10–12th grade students who accessed the school through a race-based desegregation busing program. Although the students recognized the structural and social inequities embedded in their schools, Carter (2008) found that the students' perceptions of race and racism in school varied across individuals. She also documented how African-American students reinforced their black identities through their forms of dress and informal language styles when socializing in certain areas of the school where black students congregated (2007). The students further supported each other through a formal association, the Black Leadership Advisory Council, which gave them the opportunity to meet and voice their frustrations. Carter asserts that formal and informal spaces for black students help them to maintain positive resistance to racism and a positive sense of self and academic achievement.

Huidor and Cooper (2010) explore how students of color choose to participate or abstain from educational activities based on their levels of comfort and ability to negotiate the different circumstances. In their study of 20 students of color who were bused to a predominately white school, the researchers documented the students' perceptions of their school experiences as significantly more rigorous and engaging than the school experiences in their neighborhood schools. The students recognized the racial segregation in both academic and social components of the school, and mediated these issues by forming close bonds with their same race peers.

Henfield, Moore, and Wood's (2008) themes resonate with Huidor and Cooper (2010) and the previously cited research. Henfield et al. conducted a mixed-methods study of gifted high school students of color to explore how racial identity interacted with their academic identity. As with the previously mentioned researchers, they found that black students maintain strong racial identities despite racism and isolation. Black students also were extremely cognizant of racist practices at the school and classroom levels. Interestingly, the gifted students combated issues of 'acting white' and 'nerd' by joining extracurricular activities where they interacted with black students who were outside of the gifted program.

Although the study in this paper shares many of the conclusions of the previous studies, this paper veers from the trajectory of research to focus on how the institutional climate contradicts the colorblind discourse articulated in white high schools. Similar to critical research on the contexts of integrated schools with histories of desegregation (Chapman, 2007; Diamond, 2006), the author interrogates the structural factors that create racially imbalanced settings and deny students full access to the curriculum. Diamond states, 'One cannot separate the educational experiences, attitudes, and achievement of students from the broader patterns of racial inequality that exist in communities, schools, and classrooms. To do so, distorts the understanding of race and educational achievement' (2006, p. 501). The voices of students of color highlight the hypocrisy of colorblind discourses, and legitimate their 'racially based feelings and viewpoints' (Bonilla-Silva, 2009, p. 11), by articulating the very real ways the students are racialized. The shift from focusing on identity formation to institutional instantiations of racism and oppression is an attempt to move the discourse from a focus on the racial group's reaction to racism to the systems and actions that cause the conflict.

Critical race theory

Critical Race Theory (CRT) is used to interpret the students' perceptions of their experiences in majority white suburban schools. As a theoretical lens, it provides a historical filter for explicating and analyzing past and present contexts that create specific learning environments. Scholars (Ladson-Billings & Tate, 1995; Lynn, 2004; Solorzano & Yosso, 2001) have asserted that one of the goals of CRT in education research is to examine issues of race, class, and gender in educational settings with regard to their historical and local contexts. These applications of CRT address issues in teacher education, educational research paradigms, and the historical and present effects of court-ordered desegregation.

CRT connects the suburban districts' histories of racial oppression to the ongoing unequal system propagated by current reforms. Specifically, interest-convergence, color-blind ideologies, the enduring presence of racism, and white privilege are conceptual tools of CRT that frame the analysis in the paper. CRT is an appropriate theoretical lens for connecting students' everyday experiences of racism with institutional policies and social norms that create and sustain barriers to students' current and future academic success. 'Critical race theory has the benefit of hindsight in drawing on previous critiques of educational inequality to expose and challenge macro and micro forms of racism disguised as traditional school curriculum' (Yosso, 2002, p. 95).

Colorblind racism

Nieto, Bode, Kang, and Raible state that the colorblind discourse is 'tacitly accepted by many educators and evident in classroom practices, including both curriculum and pedagogy …' (2008, p. 181). Colorblindness 'is a set of understandings—buttressed by law and the courts, and reinforcing racial patterns of white dominance—that define how people comprehend, rationalize, and act on race' (Lopez, 2006, p. 62). The discourse of color blindness allows school adults to disregard the racial identities of students by solely viewing them as individuals who are divorced from the social, economic, and cultural factors that shape their past and present experiences. By denying the 'historical and current contexts of white domination' (Urrieta, 2006, p. 456), colorblind discourses position the perceptions of students of color as irrational and baseless (Lopez, 2003).

Much of the discussion focused on colorblindness in education centers around the classroom environment. In the classroom context, this usually is identified by the teacher's avoidance of topics about race and the exposition of an equal=fair=equity pedagogical stance that influences individual relationships and behavioral consequences. Colorblindness is a false premise because the conscious avoidance of the topic of race, and the unconscious actions based on race, contradicts the notion of racial blindness. However, the context for colorblindness is larger than the individual teacher and impacts the greater school context. The insidious nature of colorblindness designs barriers to student learning and growth, which speaks more to the institutionalization of racism. Bonilla-Silva (2009) explains,

> Much as Jim Crow racism served as the glue for defending a brutal and overt system of racial oppression in the pre-Civil Rights era, color-blind racism serves today as the ideological armor for a covert and institutionalized system in the post-Civil Rights era. And the beauty of this new ideology is that it aids in the maintenance of white privilege without fanfare, without naming those who it subjects and those who it rewards (2009, p. 2).

In white majority high schools, the connections between colorblindness and white privilege, and the maintenance of white supremacy, pose significant challenges for students of color to overcome. Therefore, Bonilla-Silva asserts, a stronger term, such as 'colorblind racism', more aptly captures the damaging effects of colorblindness on students of color and the privileging effects for white students in majority white public schools.

Educational spaces are saturated with 'colorblind racism'. Although the ways in which colorblind racism is enacted vary across different contexts, the outcomes are the same. It constricts the learning and development of students of color and maintains white privilege by further marginalizing students of color in academic settings. In majority white suburban schools, colorblind racism's most blatant expressions can be viewed through the relationships between adults and students of color; more subtle enactments of colorblind racism are documented by curricular and behavior policies. Ironically, the racialized histories and current policy mandates of public schooling, which impact these enclaves of white privilege, highlight racial inequities at the same moment there is a public call to minimize these conversations.

Racial realism and school desegregation: The ghost of past racism

Historically, the legacy of desegregation litigation continues to significantly impact the schooling experiences of all students in US schools. The children in today's schools are the grandchildren and great-grandchildren of *Brown v. Board of Education*, and the descendants of the policy mandates such as cross-town busing, open enrollment, inter-district enrollment, charter schools, voucher schools, comprehensive reform orders, tax levies, and multicultural education, all of which stem from decades of litigation to secure equitable schooling for non-white children. The schooling experiences of children in the US, particularly for urban and suburban children, are the manifestations of political and social acts by stakeholders who have continually pushed for/opposed greater access to an equitable education based on issues of race and racism. Lopez remarks that 'the past is never really past, especially not when one talks about race and the law in the United States' (2006, p. 62). Research has shown that race, consciously or dysconsciously negated, impacts the schooling experiences of students of color (King, 1991; Lewis, 2003; Pollock, 2005). Therefore, notions of a post-race society, situated in contexts constructed and fortified by issues of race and racial privilege, are untenable.

Interest-convergence and present articulations of race in NCLB

Given the intractable nature of racism, Bell (2004) argues that African-Americans only progress in their battles with civil liberties when whites are allowed to benefit as well. Interest-convergence is one lens for explaining how and why urban districts made certain decisions around the implementation of *Brown*. The interpretations or avoidance of *Brown* benefited whites by creating alternate hierarchies of schooling to maintain racially stratified education opportunities. The schools in this study are from a unique subset of inter-district busing programs that were created in the 1960s and 1970s due to court pressures to desegregate schools (Wells et al., 2009). The 1974 *Milliken v. Bradley* had major implications for desegregation across districts if suburban districts were found complicit of de jure segregation. The decision prevented districts from crossing district boundaries to alleviate racial segregation *if* the suburban district had no past culpability for segregation, therefore maintaining segregation in suburban districts. Fearing court-interventions or adhering to court orders, several districts created inter-district busing programs before and after *Milliken* to alleviate segregation in inner-city schools. In some cases, this interest-convergence allowed the suburban districts to avoid more comprehensive desegregation while a small number of urban students escaped their racially segregated schools. In this city, the suburban schools were found complicit in maintaining segregation and forced to fashion a policy to alleviate inner-city segregation (Wells et al., 2009). Since the initial court order in this district, other suburban schools have voluntarily joined the program. The districts in this study continue to maintain these busing programs for various reasons. Some districts welcome the diversity as a means to better reflect society and give white children the opportunity to interact with students outside their race, while other districts value the student monies that accompany inter-district students.

Additionally, due to the housing market and small amount of rental property listings, many of these suburban enclaves are experiencing an increase in families of color moving into the districts (Orfield, 2002). ‘Communities experiencing increasing diversity and tension between racial and ethnic groups are on the front lines of the struggle against racism in public institutions of education’ (Tarca, 2005, p. 100). Many suburban districts in the area are struggling to respond to families of color who are voting tax-payers in the community. While the number of families moving into these communities remains small, they are making their concerns heard.

A second example of interest-convergence is a result of a No Child Left Behind mandate for schools and districts to disclose student achievement scores using racial demographic data. Before this measure, the majority of white districts with significant achievement gaps between white students and students of color were not concerned with racial disparities. Since these schools, in general, are more highly resourced and rigorous than their urban counterparts, students of color are seen as privileged to acquire the few allotted spots given to them from inter-city busing programs. However, NCLB policy articulations have highlighted current inequities in the schooling experiences of racial minority students in predominately white schools. High-achieving schools with racially mixed populations have a significant gap between the achievement of their students of color and their white students. School/district reputations and funding are now vulnerable to sanctions based on the district’s ability to meet the academic needs of all children. This is different from previous years where high-achieving schools, which claimed to be integrated and thriving educational spaces for all children, used aggregated data to obfuscate their achievement gaps. These potential sanctions make administrators take a new interest in the achievement patterns of their racial minority students. Thus, federal mandates foster interest convergence by compelling predominately white districts to better support the education of racial minorities in order to maintain their privileged and elite school status.

White privilege and traditional curriculum

The concept of curriculum as ‘intellectual property’ (Ladson-Billings & Tate, 1995) is used to explicate reinstantiations of white privilege and supremacy in suburban schools. Curriculum as intellectual property or ‘curriculum property’ is the means by which the materials, programs, rules, structures, and pedagogies of the school reinstantiate white privilege. The reinstantiation of white privilege is apparent through the absence of racially diverse content and critical stances used to examine power and privilege, regulations targeting racial minority groups, hierarchies of extra-curricular activities in which students of color dominate the lower echelons, and tracking. The school curriculum, in its broadest sense, becomes the tool for further marginalization and maintenance of the status quo, rather than a tool of empowerment and social change. In her examination of school contexts in a dual language program, Palmer (2010) affirms that, ‘District and school policies coupled with teachers’ unexamined biases continue to systematically undermine black students’ access to the highest quality programs’ (p. 110). Thus, an examination of colorblind school contexts uncovers the ways in which schools remain complicit in racially stratified educational practices.

A look at majority white schools

When exploring racial stratifications, Teranishi (2002) argues that students' experiences with racism must be understood through their distinct racial contexts. He explains,

> These contexts are predicated by a number of factors such as a school's historical legacy of inclusion or exclusion of various racial/ethnic groups, its structural diversity in terms of the numerical representation of various racial/ethnic groups, the social climate (defined as the racial perceptions and attitudes that different groups have of one another), as well as behavioral climate dimensions characterized by intergroup relations at school (p. 145).

In public schools, the situated nature of race and racism is indelibly bound to the contexts of the schools (Huidor & Cooper, 2010). In predominately white contexts, colorblind discourses become more prominent because issues of equity and equality are framed through the policies and practices that attempt to treat all students the same. White administrators and teachers, who are the majority of adults in suburban schools, create and maintain a facade of colorblind equity by invoking colorblind policies, such as zero tolerance behavior consequences and inflexible tutorial times that students of color who are bused to school cannot attend.

Background to the study

The study was commissioned by a community organization that consists of parents of color from suburban districts, university faculty from multiple universities in the surrounding metropolitan area, and high-ranking school district officials. This organization was created to address the racial achievement gap between students of color and white students in suburban districts. The purpose of the study was a qualitative exploration of the schooling experiences of students of color in predominately white high schools, with the goal to change various aspects of the school curriculum to increase students' academic achievement. The specific objectives of the larger study were:

- to identify successful and unsuccessful relationships, events, and policies in the schools;
- to identify resources and experiences that support students' academic, social, and emotional growth; and
- to identify policies, events, and school practices that support or create barriers to student learning.

The study took place in four predominantly white suburbs that share borders with a Midwest metropolitan area. These suburban high schools participate in two 30-year-old inter-district busing programs that allow students of color from the urban district to attend suburban schools. White suburban students are allowed to attend urban schools as well, but few suburban families utilize this option. Researchers conducted 22 focus group interviews with 97 high school students of color, from six schools in four districts. The participants' ages ranged from 14 to 19 years. Two thirds of the participants were girls. Students from all racial categories, except white, were solicited for interviews. The racial breakdown of the students included African-American (74), Latino/a (5), and Asian American (4), bi-racial (10), Native American (2), multi-racial (2) students. The students interviewed hailed from across the urban center with a few living in the suburban cities. Depending on the suburban district, these students of color experience various levels of school segregation through tracking and low enrollment of students of color.

Data were collected through single session, 1.5-hours long, audio-taped, focus group interviews with 5–7 high school students and one member of the research team during the school day at each high school site. The focus groups functioned as Freirean 'study circles' with the 'goal for the educator or facilitator within these study circles is to engage with people in their lived realities, producing and transforming them' (Kambrelis & Dimitriadis, 2005, p. 890). The semi-structured interviews focused on three categories: general questions about their high school, adult relationships, and academics. These three areas are aligned with scholarship documenting school capacities that foster student success (Fredricks & Eccles, 2006; Johnson, Crosnoe, & Elder, 2001; Shernoff & Schmidt, 2008) and the *Indiana University Survey of High School Student Engagement* previously given to eighth grade students in the same districts.

Data analysis

The research team consisted of two African-American women, one Latina, one Korean man, and one Hmong woman. The primary researcher, and author of the article, is an African-American woman who is an associate professor at an urban university. The four remaining researchers, each with past lives as educators in K-12 schools, were doctoral students at varying levels of program completion who received instruction in qualitative methods and conducted qualitative pilot studies as part of their doctoral course work. Three research team members are bilingual: two speak Spanish and English, one speaks Hmong and English, and one member purposefully code-switches between academic English and African-American Vernacular English.

Data analysis was conducted using contact summary sheets during data collection to capture the researchers' summaries of the main points of emphasis from the group, significant issues, and recurring themes from previous interviews (Miles & Huberman, 1994). A systematic process articulated by LeCompte (2000) was adapted for a research team analysis. The team: (1) read and marked the interviews with marginal remarks; (2) made external notes on areas of frequency, omission, and declaration; (3) used their individual notes to make initial taxonomies as a team; (4) created a visual matrix of these initial taxonomies; (5) used the matrix to identify sub-categories and patterns as a team; and (6) assembled structures as a team. Concerns for data trustworthiness are addressed through the use of a collective team process in which all five members of the research used identical interview protocols for data collection, conducted the steps to analyze the data, and challenged each other's assumptions and characterizations of the data through the collective analysis process.

The following themes represent multiple concepts of CRT. The concepts of colorblindness, interest-convergence, racial realism, and white privilege are used to explain how common school policies and practices, such as tracking, traditional curricula, teacher classroom practices, and student surveillance, create a racially hostile environment for students of color in majority white suburban schools. These normative school practices inhibit students of color from fully engaging in the school and, therefore, from securing equitable schooling experiences.

Academic tracking

The physical composition of the school challenges notions of colorblind school contexts and reinforces the difference between integrated spaces and desegregated spaces. In these suburban schools, the majority of the students of color remain in the lower tracks of classes. High-achieving students of color noted that they were frequently the only black or brown bodies in their advanced placement or advanced subject classrooms. In speaking with high-achieving students of color, most of them could count the number of students of color in their classes.

> **Student:** In AP Spanish there is only one other black person in there. The rest of mine—no. They are all white.
> **Student:** In my AP classes I have more Asian people.
> **Student:** AP English there is one [Asian].
> **Student:** My regular English classes, I have me, my brother, and two other black people. The others are white. Or my Latin class, there are four black people and the majority are white.
> **Student:** Mostly all my classes are predominantly white. I only have one class with one black person in my entire schedule.
> **Student:** For my first time in high school, I had a class with two other black kids and that was the most I ever had.

Conversely, students, who were in lower tracked courses, could not give the number of students because there were too many to quickly count.

> **Researcher:** So most [students of color] are in regular classes?
> **Student:** Yeah
> **Researcher:** … Are they [students of color] in lower levels?
> **Student 1:** Yes, math especially.
> **Student 2:** Yes, I am in the lower level in every course.
> **Researcher:** What is the representation in those courses?
> **Student 1:** A lot.
> **Researcher:** More than in regular?
> **Student 3:** I have formal geometry, and there is only one white kid in there.

In the case of white majority schools, higher tracks of curriculum serve as the property of white students in which few students of color are able to access the rigorous curricular experiences that lead to greater college access (Ladson-Billings & Brown, 2008; Ladson-Billings & Tate, 1995). These stratifications maintain a desegregated context rather than an integrated one, and reinforce the white supremacist ideology of students of color as intellectually inferior. When asked how students chose their courses, many of them explain that counselors and teachers play major roles in placing them into their current classes. Because most of the students of color have matriculated in these districts since kindergarten, their track positions cannot be dismissed as students of color transferring to suburban high schools from lower status urban middle schools. Instead, the placement of students of color in lower tracks reflects 40-year conversations about how students are tracked into classes based on race and socioeconomic status at an early age and unable to cross into upper tracks later in their schooling careers (Rist, 1970; Oakes, 1985).

The visible racialization of curricular tracking also poses an example of interest convergence. Because even the lower track classes at suburban high schools are considered better than the regular school curricula found in the attached urban district, students of color believe, and the research supports (Goldsmith, 2011), that they receive stronger academic preparation in the suburban schools. In this study and the study of students of color bused into white schools (Huidor & Cooper, 2010), the students felt their suburban schools were more rigorous, safe, and offered more extra-curricular activities than their neighborhood schools. Students in the study explained,

Student: I wouldn't say it is an honor but people say it is a good school. So I feel kind of proud that I go to this school rather than [Urban School 1] or [Urban School 2], [urban district] schools.
Student: Yeah. I think that if you get a 2.5 here that is like 3.5 at [Urban School 1] or [urban school 3] or something.
Student: I feel like our school is a lot tougher than most schools. Whenever I talk to my cousins who go to [urban district] schools, they are—oh yeah—it is real easy here. We never get homework. Like here they kind of get on us. We have a sufficient amount of homework that we have to get done.
Student: This school has a good curriculum school, like to get into better colleges. We are kind of like up here to a point, academically. We are higher than a whole lot of other schools in [metropolitan city].

White students maintain the property of curriculum by being over-represented in higher track classes, while students of color regard their lower track education as valuable. Indeed, even in the Huidor and Cooper (2010) study, the students still thought their education was more rigorous than their neighborhood schools, despite not being enrolled in AP courses. From the perspective of most students of color, the goal is to get into a college – any college. For students in the majority of the high schools in the urban center, meeting the goal of going to college is a great challenge. Even from the lower tracks at the suburban school, students of color are able to meet this goal. However, they are unable to attend the high-ranked colleges and universities where many of their white counterparts apply. Tracking these highly motivated students into lower tracks affects the future possibilities of students of color by limiting their college choices, making them less competitive for jobs, and restricting their exposure to new forms of cultural capital that are present in elite environments (Ladson-Billings & Brown, 2008). Therefore, the economic and social possibilities for these students remain stratified by race.

In addition, broadly defined aspects of the curriculum reflect problematic issues of race. The majority of students segregate themselves by race in the cafeteria and extra-curricular activities. Students of color are over-represented in particular sports activities such as basketball and football and under-represented in other sports, clubs, and leadership activities.

Student 1: Do you guys see a breakup of clubs in who the people in those clubs are, like key club? It is white kids. Multicultural club [is] minority kids. Basketball is all black, like the stereotypical.
Student 2: Most of the people on the soccer team are white. Most of the girls are the rich white girls are on the tennis teams.

Segregation in these social settings is another example of the presence of race in supposedly colorblind settings. When the interactions between students of color and affluent white students are limited to academic settings, students have fewer opportunities to engage in informal interactions where cultural capital and social capital are exchanged. In addition, the stratification of extra-curricular activities by race generates a hierarchy of school activities. Homogenous white activities become more valued, and homogenous black and brown activities become less valued. Once again, curriculum serves as property when academic clubs and student leadership opportunities become the purview of white students who use these activities to support their college applications.

Students as racial authority

When defining curriculum as property as a form of access, Ladson-Billings and Brown (2008) state, 'However, even when students have access to the same curriculum, we know that they have it differentially and that the curriculum can serve to reinforce racial ideology' (p. 155). When issues of race and poverty are introduced in the classroom, students of color experience the curriculum in these high schools differently from their white peers. Rather than feeling empowered by conversations on race and society, students of color feel further marginalized in their classrooms. As a single racial minority in the classroom, students of color become the sole proprietors of knowledge about race and poverty from the perspective of all non-white groups at any point in history.

Student: They have discussions where I will feel a little awkward because we are talking about something like that [race], and because I am the only black person in the class. But I feel like they are all looking at me like, 'is it okay talking about this?'
Student: Like in class, it is not like a burden, but when you are talking about something black like all eyes will swivel to you, like you are the Negro-damus [opinion] or something like that. It is kind of annoying at the same time. Well, I am the only the black person in this class. But just because we are talking about slavery, it doesn't mean you have swivel your eyes over here.
Student: When people ask me about Chinese or China … it is like we are reading something about the Chinese and [students ask me] like—Does this happen? I say, 'I am Korean'. Some people kind of assume that if you are Asian, you know the whole Asian culture. Like general stereotyping. Not a lot of people know [the difference].
Student: It is kind of awkward sometimes, like in history class, talking about slavery and Black people. It is kind of weird. It is kind of awkward to hear it because I am the only Black person in class and people will look at me.
Student: We were talking about the Civil War and I was the only black person in class. So everyone expects me to know everything about the Civil War. And like, we were reading, and this stocky man said the N word, and everyone said, 'What do you think?' It was like, if we were reading something, I am not going to get all mad.
Student: Like sometimes, like in English class, we will read stuff. That's all we read are books about black people being slaves. And so when my teacher asks me a question pertaining to race, I am just going to say, 'I don't think that is necessary'. Every time we read a book about a black slave, you want to ask me a question about how would it make me feel. How do you think it will make me feel? How would you feel if you were a slave? I would feel the same way, so why would you ask me that question?

Students feel uncomfortable and defensive when issues of race and racism are part of the formal curriculum. When these issues are highlighted in classes, the teacher makes the student the center of attention for all the wrong reasons. Curriculum stands as property in this context, and as a symbol of white privilege, because white students are not asked to speak for their race or made to feel uncomfortable when their group is the focus of the text. When reading Shakespeare, the white students are not asked, 'What is it like to be a suicidal teenager whose boyfriend is a murderer?' In many ways, these events have implications for the pedagogical practices of teachers in these settings. But more significantly, the events demonstrate the color-consciousness of students and teachers in racially diverse environments.

Double standards

During the interviews, students overwhelmingly remark on the unequal behavior standards in their schools. Students describe incidents in which black girls and Latinas were sent home for violating dress codes regarding leggings and 'short shorts', while white girls were not reprimanded. The students were primarily frustrated about the unfair treatment they received in individual classrooms that resulted in students being sent to the office. Once in the office, the teacher's story goes unchallenged, and unquestioned, and discipline is doled out to the student. Students also remark that students of color are disciplined more severely than their white peers. The following quotes explain a few of these numerous incidents.

> **Student:** It is like they were playing a game on a computer one day. He got done with his work so he went to play on the computer. The white kid two feet down from him was playing on the computer, but the teacher called him out and like he got in trouble. He said, 'Well, he is playing too. And she is like, 'well, I am talking to you'. It is like, why don't you talk to him too? Some teachers do that and it makes you think like [they] are racist. 'Well I am not racist' [student mimicking teachers]. Well okay, that is what it seems like. You are pointing me out, but you are not pointing out some of the other ones.
>
> **Student:** It is a known fact [unequal treatment]. I have turned in stuff late the same day as somebody else did, and we are both late, and I get a lower grade. And [the white] one doesn't even get marked down late. They [teachers] say, 'Oh, it is the quality of it'. So I had the same person write my stuff, but just in a different tone, and the same thing has happened [the paper is still marked down]. So it's just like, I mean I am in a lose-lose situation.
>
> **Student:** Also just say there is like a double standard. It seems like if a black [kid] it is doing something [talking] ... But like white kids are sitting there talking and the black person gets pointed out. Like why are you yelling at him? You know? It is a double standard.
>
> **Student:** When it comes down to it, teachers are like always calling me out. Sometimes I have to use the bathroom in band a lot and he [the teacher] will let a whole bunch of students go. It is like they are all Caucasian. I always feel like that. Teachers always let them go to the bathroom, but when you ask, 'Oh, you need to hold it'. Like, 'Oh, no, you can't go'. Or they always yell at you when everyone is doing something bad, they just yell at you first.

These incidents speak to the over-surveillance of students of color in majority white schools. Students admit their imperfections, and that they may have been doing something wrong; but because the adults in the school are concentrating more on their behavior, the students of color are more likely to be reprimanded. Thus, the system of colorblindness is perpetuated because the student cannot claim innocence and avoid persecution; they can only point out that white students were also complicit in the negative behavior as part of their defense.

Race as an unsafe space

Students implicitly understand that they are not supposed to discuss race or use it as a form to differentiate themselves from the other students. One student said it best when he said, 'They want you to conform, or don't want you to go and create your own [student] government. They would prefer that you participate in their [student] government. They don't want you to identify yourself kind of'. When students ask adults to address issues of racism in the school, they were ignored or marked as trouble-makers. When students of color defend themselves from verbal attacks, either verbally or physically, they are disproportionately punished for their actions. Although several of the schools have ethnic clubs, the students struggle to maintain them because they cannot find teachers who are willing to advise the clubs or secure spaces for their meetings. The students understand that these clubs are unwelcome additions to the school.

However, the schools' attempts to obscure race do not dissolve the students' performances of race. Students feel the need to perform at higher academic levels than their white peers to combat stereotypes that label them as academically inferior to white students.

Student: I would say that us being minorities here in—We have to be careful because you have to be aware of the way, we kind of are put on a pedestal.
Student: You are a black female and no one is going to take pity on you. No one is going to feel sorry for you. You have to work twice as hard as a white female and that is the way it is. Every time a grade comes in a C, maybe a D, she [pointing to friend] don't like. She is working twice as hard.
Student: Talking as a black male, I would say that you would always have to fight the stereotype. If you make one small mistake, they are going to hold it against you.
Student: Because of [race] you are always fighting against [racism] beside what you are regularly fighting against. And for me personally, I always say, I don't want to be a statistic, someone who has dropped out of school, who has not gotten into college.

The burden of performing race causes the students to want to disappear racially in order to smoothly matriculate through school, not because of low racial identity (Diamond, 2006). However, they realize this is not a rational expectation. Instead, students tried to minimize their presence as much as possible by remaining quiet and unobtrusive, not drawing attention to themselves, and getting good grades. One student rationalizes her behavior:

Student: I know I am black, but if I am going to get through a day, a school year, I kind of have to put that aside, and kind of become colorless, just to get through it.

Unlike previous research that would imply that the student is rejecting a positive black identity (Ogbu, 2003), this student attempts to become invisible in opposition to choosing to become white. Carter (2008) explains, 'It is a resistance for survival in that these black students' psyches are constantly under attack in a learning environment in which their racial group membership is often associated with anti-intellectualism and/or intellectual inferiority' (p. 478). The racialized contexts of the school push the student, and others like her, to bracket their race in order to focus on learning.

Critical multiculturalism

Critical multiculturalism is one strategy for addressing the schooling inequities experienced by students of color in majority white schools. McLaren (1994) suggests that critical multicultural teachers unpack the complexities of meaning and identity constructions and confront the larger societal challenges surrounding social justice. McLaren states 'Critical multiculturalism interrogates the construction of difference and identity in relation to a radical politics' (1994, p. 53). Critical multiculturalism advocates systemic change and contests the ideology of cultural deficiency that serves as a commonsense narrative in majority white schools.

Other scholars support the push to use multicultural education as a change agent (Banks, 2007; Grant & Sleeter, 1989/1997; Nieto & Bode, 2008). Grant and Sleeter suggest that multicultural education, as social reconstruction, offers schools the opportunity to build learning environments and programs that re-envision current traditional policies and practices that marginalize students of color and prevent white students and white adults from empathetically engaging with issues of race, culture, and other differences. Banks (2007) offers a transformative model of multicultural education that challenges all stakeholders to make schools reflect a more socially just and critical multicultural society. Similarly, Nieto (2000) calls for multicultural education for social justice to target systemic inequities through a comprehensive approach to school reform.

> … Multicultural education permeates the curriculum and instructional strategies used in schools, as well as in the interactions among teachers, students and parents, and the very way that schools conceptualize the nature of teaching and learning. Because it uses critical pedagogy as its underlying philosophy and focuses on knowledge, reflection, and action (praxis) as the basis for social change, multicultural education furthers the democratic principles of social justice. (Nieto, 2000, p. 305)

With a combined history of over 120 years of experience in the field of multicultural education, these scholars implore districts to restructure schools and support teachers to engage with race and other social markers in ways that strengthen, not debilitate, students' academic achievement and personal growth.

Rather than attempting to obscure the racial realities of majority white high school settings, administrators, teachers, and staff must understand how race is consistently and newly constructed in schooling environments.

> School leaders must be prepared to work with individuals who are culturally different and help create learning environments that foster respect, tolerance, and intercultural understanding. They must also have an awareness of the effect of racism and how it intersects with other areas of difference such as gender, sexual orientation, disability, and class oppression. (Lopez, 2003, p. 71)

These constructions of race must be interrogated to acknowledge how institutional policies and practices reinstantiate white supremacy and support inequitable systems. Moreover, Carter (2008) noted that 'schools and educators need to be counter-hegemonic in their practices, challenging traditional dominant discourses and paradigms about what it means to be successful and who is successful' (2008, p. 494).

Only when systemic changes, which include conversations on race and racism, are implemented will schools become more equitable environments for students of color (Banks, 1995). 'To break the interlocking patterns of racial hierarchy, there is no other way but to focus on, talk about, and put into effect constructive policies explicitly engaged with race' (Lopez, 2006, p. 62). But creating policy is an insufficient means of dealing with colorblind racism when the actors, administrators and teachers, implement policy through deficit paradigms of racial groups. As seen in the examples from the study, white privilege is maintained through the structures of the school, the over-surveillance of students of color, and the discussions allowed in the classroom (Yosso, 2002). Critical multicultural education is a solution to minimizing the gap between institutional policy and its practical implementations. The goal of multicultural education is to serve all children; therefore, it can only be achieved when schools embrace all-inclusive school reforms that reflect the racial milieu of public school classrooms.

Conclusions

Students of color remain deeply impacted by racist schooling practices that they are not allowed to name in their schools. Diamond states,

> However, integrated schools (to the extent that they have existed) have failed to create equal opportunity for all students, in part, because racial inequality in the society as a whole or within the schools, in numerous cases, has not been directly confronted (2006, p. 502).

The colorblind discourses in white suburban schools prevent students of color from having meaningful exchanges with adults and maintain the curriculum's role of intellectual property for white students. Lopez explains what happens when colorblindness is allowed free reign in society,

> As a result, the collective frustrations of people of color and/or Black nationalist groups are simply seen as irrational … This slippage only maintains racism firmly in place by ignoring or downplaying the role of White racism in the larger social order (2003, p. 69).

Students of color are viewed as 'irrational' when they name racism in their schools. 'The trap of colorblindness neither initiates conversations about the influence of race nor empowers those experiencing discrimination to argue their case' (Tarca, 2005, p. 114). Moreover, they are further cast as outsiders and trouble-makers, making it more difficult for them to successfully matriculate through schools.

The irony of the colorblind discourse is evident. Schools in the US cannot erase race. The enforcement of colorblindness serves to exacerbate, not alleviate, issues of race and racism for students of color in predominately white schools. This exploration of colorblind ideology/color-conscious practices in schools serves as an alternate explanation to 'blaming the victim' (Bonilla-Silva, 2009) for under-achievement, racial isolation, and academic disinterest in majority white high schools; and it places the burden of school reform on policy makers and educators to 'dismantle and reconstruct systemic approaches currently in place within the educational system' (Saddler, 2005, p. 53).

References

Banks, J. A. (1995). Multicultural education: Historical development, dimensions, and practice. In C. M. Banks (Ed.), *Handbook of research on multicultural education* (pp. 3–24). New York, NY: MacMillan.

Banks, J. A. (2007). *Educating citizens in a multicultural society.* New York, NY: Teachers College Press.

Bell, D. A. (2004). *Silent covenants: Brown v. board of education and the unfulfilled hopes for racial reform.* Oxford, New York, NY: Oxford University Press.

Bonilla-Silva, E. (2009). *Racism without racists. Colorblind racism and the persistence of racial inequality in America* (3rd ed.). New York, NY: Roman & Littlefield.

Carter, D. J. (2007). Why the Black kids sit together at the stairs: The role of identity-affirming counter-spaces in a predominantly White high school. *Journal of Negro Education*, *76*(4), 542–554. Retrieved from http://search.ebscohost.com/login.aspx?direct=true&db=eft&AN=508007943&site=ehost-live

Carter, D. J. (2008). Achievement as resistance: The development of a critical race achievement ideology among Black achievers. *Harvard Educational Review*, *78*(3), 466–497. Retrieved from http://search.ebscohost.com/login.aspx?direct=true&db=eft&AN=508008080&site=ehost-live

Chapman, T. K. (2007). The power of contexts: Teaching and learning in recently desegregated schools. *Anthropology & Education Quarterly*, *38*(3), 297–315. doi:10.1525/aeq.2007.38.3.297

Crenshaw, K. W. (2011). Twenty years of critical race theory: Looking back to move forward. *Connecticut Law Review*, *43*(5), 1253–1351. Retrieved from http://archive.connecticutlawreview.org/documents/Crenshaw.pdf

Diamond, J. B. (2006). Still separate and unequal: Examining race, opportunity, and school achievement in 'Integrated' suburbs. *Journal of Negro Education*, *75*(3), 495–505. Retrieved from http://search.ebscohost.com/login.aspx?direct=true&db=eft&AN=507901896&site=ehost-live

Diamond, J. B., Lewis, A. E., & Gordon, L. (2007). Race and school achievement in a desegregated suburb: Reconsidering the oppositional culture explanation. *International Journal of Qualitative Studies in Education*, *20*(6), 655–679. doi:10.1080/09518390701630791

Fredricks, J. A., & Eccles, J. S. (2006). Is extracurricular participation associated with beneficial outcomes? Concurrent and longitudinal relations. *Developmental Psychology*, *42*(4), 698–713. doi:10.1037/0012-1649.42.4.698

Goldsmith, P. R. (2011). Coleman revisited: School segregation, peers, and frog ponds. *American Educational Research Journal*, *48*(3), 508–535. doi:10.3102/0002831210392019

Grant, C. A., & Sleeter, C. E. (1989/1997). *Turning on learning: Five approaches for multicultural teaching plans for race, class, gender, and disability*. Columbus: Merrill.

Henfield, M. S., Moore, J. L., & Wood, C. (2008). Inside and outside gifted education programming: Hidden challenges for African American students. *Exceptional Children*, *74*(4), 433–450. Retrieved from http://search.ebscohost.com/login.aspx?direct=true&db=eft&AN=508079747&site=ehost-live

Huidor, O., & Cooper, R. (2009). Examining the socio-cultural dimension of schooling in a racially integrated school. *Education and Urban Society*, *42*(2), 143–167. doi:10.1177/0013124509350047

Johnson, M. K., Crosnoe, R., & Elder, Jr., G. H. (2001). Students' attachment and academic engagement: The role of race and ethnicity. *Sociology of Education*, *74*(4), 318–340. doi:10.2307/2673138

Kambrelis, G., & Dimitriadis, G. (2005). Focus groups: Strategic articulations of pedagogy, politics, and inquiry. In N. Denzin & Y. Lincoln (Eds.), *The Sage handbook of qualitative research* (3rd ed., pp. 887–907). Los Angeles, CA: Sage.

Kincheloe, J. (1993). Representations of identity and difference in education. In L. A. Castenell Jr., & W. F. Pinar (Eds.), *Understanding curriculum as racial text* (pp. 249–262). New York, NY: State University of New York Press.

King, J. E. (1991). Dysconscious racism: Ideology, identity, and the miseducation of teachers. *The Journal of Negro Education*, *60*(2), 133–146. doi:10.2307/2295605

Ladson-Billings, G., & Brown, K. (2008). Curriculum and cultural diversity. In F. M. Connelly, F. H. Ming, & J. Phillion (Eds.), *The SAGE handbook of curriculum and instruction* (pp. 153–175). Los Angeles, CA: Sage.

Ladson-Billings, G., & Tate, W. F. (1995). Toward a critical race theory of education. *Teachers College Record*, *97*(1), 47–68. Retrieved from http://search.ebscohost.com/login.aspx?direct=true&db=eft&AN=508572449&site=ehost-live

LeCompte, M. D. (2000). Analyzing qualitative data. *Theory into Practice*, *39*(3), 146–154. doi:10.1207/s15430421tip3903_5

Lewis, A. E. (2003). *Race in the schoolyard: Negotiating the color line in classrooms and communities*. New Brunswick, NJ: Rutgers University Press.

Lopez, G. R. (2003). The (racially neutral) politics of education: A critical race theory perspective. *Educational Administration Quarterly*, *39*(1), 68–94. doi:10.1177/0013161X02239761

Lopez, I. H. (2006). Colorblind to the reality of race in America. *The Chronicle Review*, *53*(11), B6.

Lynn, M. (2004). Inserting the race into critical pedagogy: An analysis of race-based epistemologies. *Educational Philosophy & Theory*, *36*(2), 153–165. doi:10.1111/j.1469-5812.2004.00058.x

McLaren, P. (1994). White terror and oppositional agency: Towards a critical multiculturalism. In D. T. Goldberg (Ed.), *Multiculturalism: A critical reader* (pp. 33–70). Malden, MA: Blackwell.

Miles, M., & Huberman, A. M. (1994). *Qualitative analysis: An expanded source book* (2nd ed.). Thousand Oaks, CA: Sage.

Milliken v. Bradley. 418 US 717 (1974).

Nieto, S. (2000). *Affirming diversity: The sociopolitical context of multicultural education* (3rd ed.). New York, NY: Allyn & Bacon.

Nieto, S., & Bode, P. (2008). *Affirming diversity: The socio-political context of multicultural education* (4th ed.). New York, NY: Addison Wesley Longman.

Nieto, S., Bode, P., Kang, E., & Raible, J. (2008). Identity, community, and diversity: Retheorizing multicultural curriculum for the postmodern era. In F. M. Connelly, M. F. He, & J. Phillion (Eds.), *Handbook of curriculum and instruction* (pp. 176–197). Los Angeles, CA: Sage.

Oakes, J. (1985). *Keeping track: How schools structure inequality*. Princeton, NJ: Yale Press.

O'Connor, C., Mueller, J., Lewis, R., Rivas-Drake, D., & Rosenberg, S. (2011). 'Being' black and strategizing for excellence in a racially stratified academic hierarchy. *American Educational Research Journal*, *48*(6), 1232–1257. doi:10.3102/0002831211410303

Ogbu, J. U. (2003). *Black American students in an affluent suburb: A study of academic disengagement*. Mahway, NJ: Lawrence Erlbaum.

Orfield, M. (2002). *American metro politics: The new suburban reality.* Washington, DC: Brookings Institute.

Palmer, D. (2010). Race, power, and equity in a multiethnic urban elementary school with a dual-language 'Strand' program. *Anthropology & Education Quarterly, 41*(1), 94–114. doi:10.1111/j.1548-1492.2010.01069

Pollock, M. (2005). *Colormute: Race talk dilemmas in an American school.* Princeton, NJ: Princeton University Press.

Rist, R. (1970). Student social class and teacher expectations: The self-fulfilling prophecy in ghetto education. *Harvard Educational Review, 40*(3), 411–451. Retrieved from http://search.ebscohost.com/login.aspx?direct=true&db=eft&AN=507726591&site=ehost-live

Saddler, C. A. (2005). The impact of Brown on African American students: A critical race theoretical perspective. *Educational Studies: American Educational Studies Association, 37*(1), 41–55. doi:10.1207/s15326993es3701_5

Shernoff, D. J., & Schmidt, J. A. (2008). Further evidence of an engagement-achievement paradox among US high school students. *Journal of Youth and Adolescence, 37*(5), 564–580. doi:10.1007/s10964-007-9241-z

Solorzano, D., & Yosso, T. (2001). From racial stereotyping and deficit discourse toward a Critical Race Theory. *Multicultural Education, 9*(1), 2–8. Retrieved from http://search.ebscohost.com/login.aspx?direct=true&db=eft&AN=507717093&site=ehost-live

Tarca, K. (2005). Colorblind in control: The risks of resisting difference amid demographic change. *Educational Studies: Journal of the American Educational Studies Association, 38*(2), 99–120. doi:10.1207/s15326993es3802_3

Teranishi, R. T. (2002). Asian Pacific Americans and critical race theory: An examination of school racial climate. *Equity & Excellence in Education, 35*(2), 144–154. doi:10.1080/713845281

Urrieta, L. (2006). Community identity discourse and the Heritage Academy: Colorblind educational policy and White supremacy. *International Journal of Qualitative Studies in Education (QSE), 19*(4), 455–476. doi:10.1080/09518390600773197

Wells, A. S., Baldridge, B. J., Duran, J., Grzesikowski, C., Lofton, R., Roda, A., Warner, M., & White, T. (2009). *Boundary crossing for diversity: Equity and achievement. Inter-district school desegregation and educational opportunity.* Cambridge, MA: Charles Hamilton Houston Institute for Race and Justice. Harvard University.

Yosso, T. J. (2002). Toward a critical race curriculum. *Equity & Excellence in Education, 35*(2), 93–107. doi:10.1080/713845283

Pedagogy of fear: toward a Fanonian theory of 'safety' in race dialogue

Zeus Leonardo and Ronald K. Porter

In education, it is common to put the condition of 'safety' around public race dialogue. The authors argue that this procedural rule maintains white comfort zones and becomes a symbolic form of violence experienced by people of color. In other words, they ask, 'Safety for whom?' A subtle but fundamental violence is enacted in safe discourses on race, which must be challenged through a pedagogy of disruption, itself a form of violence but a humanizing, rather than repressive, version. For this, the authors turn to Frantz Fanon's theory of violence, most clearly outlined in *The wretched of the earth*. First, the article outlines the basic assumptions of Fanon's theory of revolutionary, as opposed to repressive, violence. Second, we analyze the surrounding myths that an actual safe space exists for people of color when it concerns public race dialogue. Third, we critique the intellectualization of racism as part of the concrete violence lived by people of color in the academy, which whites continually reduce to an idea. We pedagogically reframe the racial predicament by promoting a 'risk' discourse about race, which does not assume safety but contradiction and tension. This does not suggest that people of color are somehow correct by virtue of their social location. In addition, it does not equate with creating a hostile situation but acknowledges that *violence is already there*. Finally, we consider the practical import of intellectual solidarity, where understanding racism becomes the higher good rather than whether or not one leaves the dialogue looking more or less racist than before.

> [D]ecolonization is always a violent event. (Fanon 2004, 1)

Part of color-blindness is to demand that race dialogue takes place in a 'safe' environment. This is tantamount to premising racial pedagogy on assumptions about comfort, which quickly degrade anti-racist teaching into image and personal management (Thompson 2003). In other words, the higher goal of understanding and fighting racism is exchanged for creating a safe space where whites can avoid publicly 'looking racist', which then overwhelms their reasons for participating in racial dialogue. This approach ironically still leaves intact what bell hooks (1992) has called the 'terrorizing force of white supremacy', even within the context of safety (174). As opposed to this, critical race pedagogy is inherently risky, uncomfortable, and fundamentally unsafe (Lynn 1999), particularly for whites. This does not *equate* with creating a hostile situation but acknowledges that pedagogies that tackle racial power will be most uncomfortable for those who benefit from that power. It also acknowledges that mainstream race dialogue in education perpetuates what the poet Aimé Césaire (2000) would call a 'pseudo-humanism' (37) that establishes white humanity at the expense of people of color, reminding us that 'the only way the European could make himself man was by fabricating slaves and monsters' (Sartre 2004, lviii). In other words, it reaffirms an already hostile and unsafe environment for many students of color whose perspectives and experiences are consistently minimized. It may be a euphemized form of violence, a discursive 'cool violence' compared to the 'hot violence' of economic exploitation (McLaren, Leonardo, and Allen 1999), but linguistic racism is no less a violation (Derrida 1985), maintains links between material distributions of power and a politics of recognition (Fraser 1997), and lowers standards of humanity. It reaffirms Žižek's (2008) insight that violence is part of the fabric of the daily functioning of social life where systemic and symbolic violence passes as natural (see Bourdieu and Passeron 1990; Bourdieu 1977). We suggest that a humanizing form of violence, a non-repressive expression of power, returns people to their rightful place, just as the violence of decolonization can potentially cancel the molesting power of colonialism.[1]

Safety discourses on race are a veiled form of violence and it will require a humanizing form of violence to expose contradictions in the discourse of 'safety'. As a result, a new system of violence is introduced. We want to make it clear that we are not working from the hegemonic and literal appearance of violence and ask the reader to suspend naturalized images of violence as only bloodshed, physical, or repressive. A humanizing form of violence is a pedagogy and politics of disruption that shifts the regime of knowledge about what is ultimately possible as well as desirable as a racial arrangement. It is not violent in the usual and commonsensical sense of promoting war, injury, or coercion. Insofar as the theory of violence we put forth is positioned against racial domination, it is violently anti-violence. To the extent that racial violence is structured in discourse, we argue that dislodging it will require a violent undertaking in order to set pedagogy on a humanizing trajectory. For this we turn to Frantz Fanon's insights – particularly the chapter concerning violence in *The wretched of the earth*. Fanon's work instructs us to consider the dialectics of violence: *education as violent and violence as educative*.

In public settings, people of color find themselves between the Scylla of becoming visible and the Charybdis of remaining silent. If minorities follow an analytics of color, they run the risk of incurring white symbolic racism at best or literal violence at worst. Although some may argue that people of color maintain their dignity and counteract the culture of silence when they come to voice, participating in public race dialogue makes them vulnerable to assaults on many fronts. On one level their actions illuminate what Fanon characterized as the tenuous relationship between humanity and reason. According to Gordon (1995), 'If even reason or the understanding is infected with racism, where unreason stands on the opposite pole as a Manichaean abyss of blackness, then a black man who reasons finds himself in the absurdity of the very construction of himself as a black man *who reasons…*' (8). On another level, by sharing their real perspectives on race, minorities become overt targets of personal and academic threats. It becomes a catch-22 for them. Either they must observe the safety of whites and be denied a space that promotes people of color's growth and development or insist on a space of integrity and put themselves further at risk not only of violence, but also risk being conceived of as illogical or irrational. Thus, white privilege is at the center of most race dialogues, even those that aim to critique and undo racial advantage.

Authentic participation for whites also has its contradictions but it is not marked by oppression. For people of color, race dialogue is more than ironic.

A certain kind of violence that shifts the standards of humanity for people of color and whites is necessary if race dialogue is more than an exercise in safety but a search for liberatory possibilities. It is violent for whites and forces them to account for race in a condition of risk, not safety. *If it is a safe condition, then it is the safety of being able to take risks, of putting oneself at risk, a condition many people of color already navigate*, something Du Bois (1989) once described as 'double consciousness'. It is also violent to people of color as it removes a previously violent regime from being ensconced and grafted onto their bodies. We return to the neutral definition of violence, which is not inherently negative or positive but judged for its consequences. At times, this requires performing violence against a primary violence, thereby making a truly peaceful coexistence possible: *peace as a form of violence*. Avoiding this violent shift allows an existing violence to continue, instituting a permanent state of discursive and ideological warfare. The educative possibilities of violence are found precisely in this consideration.

Fanon was ultimately ambiguous about the role of violence in social change. When Fanon (2004) writes that decolonization 'can only succeed by resorting to every means, including, of course, violence', (3) we take him to mean violence in multiple ways, literal and physical violence only being one of them. For example, he declares:

> In the colonial context the colonist only quits undermining the colonized once the latter have proclaimed loud and clear that white values reign supreme. In the period of decolonization the colonized masses thumb their noses at these very values, shower them with insults and vomit them up. (8)

Colonialism's violence is pervasive and Fanon suggests that an equally complete reversal, from physical to psychical violence, will be required to oppose it: 'Violence among the colonized will spread in proportion to the violence exerted by the colonial regime' (Fanon 2004, 46–7). Ejecting colonialism at the level of values and subjectivity is as much a part of decolonization as material redistribution. As Wallerstein (2009) notes, 'Without violence the wretched of the earth can accomplish nothing. But violence, however therapeutic and however effective, solves nothing' (125). Although we clearly are appropriating Fanon's insights for a context that differs from revolutionary Algeria and colonial Africa, we find his work useful for tackling modern problems with public race dialogues in education. Whether as a form of social analysis or support for policy, Fanon's theory of violence is replete with insights on the racial contradictions of our time. First, we outline below the basic assumptions of Fanon's theory of revolutionary, as opposed to repressive, violence. Second, we analyze the surrounding myths that an actual safe space exists for people of color when it concerns public race dialogue. Third, we critique the intellectualization of racism as part of the concrete violence lived by people of color in the academy, which whites continually reduce to an idea. Here we pedagogically reframe the racial predicament by promoting a 'risk' discourse about race, which does not assume safety but contradiction and tension. This does not suggest that people of color are somehow correct by virtue of their social location. Finally, we consider the practical import of intellectual solidarity, where understanding racism becomes the higher good rather than whether or not one leaves the dialogue looking more or less racist than before.

Toward a Fanonian theory of race and violence

Two dominant discourses exist within debates concerning critical studies of race and education, one focusing on critical race theory (Gillborn 2008; Yosso 2006; Dixson and Rousseau 2005; Parker and Stovall 2005; Brayboy 2005; Bernal and Villalpando 2005; Ladson-Billings 2004; Taylor 1998; Solorzano 1998; Tate 1997; Ladson-Billings and Tate 1995) and the other a resurgent interest in the work of W.E.B. Du Bois (Alridge 1999, 2008; Provenzo 2002: Leonardo 2002). We support this development (Leonardo 2009). However, scant literature exists relating the work of Frantz Fanon to the study of education. This intervention is necessary considering the arguable relationship between education and colonialism, nationally and abroad (Macedo 2000; Ladson-Billings 1998; Altbach and Kelly 1978; Memmi 1965), as well as the recent turn to the decolonial imaginary in social theory (Maldonado-Torres 2006; Grosfoguel 2007; Wynter 1995) and the reassertion of a continuing coloniality in social life even after the fall of official administrative colonialism (Quijano 2000; Maldonado-Torres 2007). Gordon, Sharpley-Whiting, and White (1996) have argued that inquiries into Fanonian thought consist of five progressive stages, which include reactions to his work, biographies, analyses of his contribution to political theory, his role in the development of postcolonial theory, and finally his possible contribution to the generation of original work across the human sciences. We seek to extend this fifth stage in Fanonian thought by applying his theory to the study of education.

Fanon wrote at a time when the grim scenario of colonialism decreased through a moment of possibility when the process of decolonization could have led to the self-determined futures of the former colonies. Fanon (2004) recognized this critical moment and addressed the possibilities inherent in this political situation in his book, *The wretched of the earth* (see also, Fanon 1965, 1967a, 1967b). While Fanon's focus may have been more internationalist in scope, the thin line that he posited to exist between the possibility of liberation and the risk of intensifying repressive violence, is significant for current discussions that seek to dismantle racism within the United States. We suggest that Fanon's theorization of the process of decolonization, both in terms of the violence necessary for its existence and the violent activity required for its undoing, is applicable to a criticism of safe space dialogue concerning race. There is much to learn from Fanon's argument that 'decolonization is always a violent event', be it at the level of the nation or the individual, because it requires 'the substitution of one "species" of mankind by another' (1). What follows is an exploration that seeks to clarify Fanon's position regarding the violence of colonialism as applied to the study of race and education.

The colonial situation of the 1950s and 1960s that Frantz Fanon writes of in *The wretched of the earth* presents us with an incredibly violent situation. According to Fanon, colonialism is a system that works, primarily by force, to permeate the entire lifeworld of the colonized. Those at the very bottom of the colonial hierarchy experience the brunt of physical violence. Yet, a form of educative-psychic violence in the form of racial discourses is also developed by the colonizer in order to keep the very consciousness of the colonized under control. For instance, the colonizer creates a narrative which posits that he is the creator of history, thus justifying conquest as well as racial and cultural supremacy. The colonizer 'makes history and he knows it', according to Fanon, and 'because he refers constantly to the history of his metropolis, he plainly indicates that [at the site of colonization] he is the extension of this metropolis' (15). This form of psychic violence leads to abjection and feelings of inferiority on the part of the colonized (see also Fuss 1994). The colonized thus learn to stay in their place, and participate in a complex process of consent where they enact violence upon each other, are constantly anxious due to the violence they experience, and establish myths and religious systems that relegate their fate to the will of the gods (16–19). Sartre (2004) writes, 'The status of "native" is a neurosis introduced and maintained by the colonist in the colonized *with their consent*' (liv). Through this combination of physical and psychic violence, Fanon argues that the colonizer 'brings violence into the homes and minds of the colonized subject' (4). Fanon was clear that education – far from being neutral or enlightening in and of itself – is at the core of colonial domination. He emphasizes:

> In capitalist societies, education, whether secular or religious, the teaching of moral reflexes handed down from father to son, the exemplary integrity of workers decorated after fifty years of loyal and faithful service, the fostering of love for harmony and wisdom, those aesthetic forms of respect for the status quo, *instill in the exploited a mood of submission and inhibition which considerably eases the task of the agents of law and order*. (3–4; italics added)

A hegemonic system of violence – one that necessitates a relationship of both active force and consent – functions so that the colonized either are forced into or acquiesce to their declared inferiority (Gramsci 1971; Hall 1996). This unraveling of physical and psychic violence would occur through the liberating violence of the colonized. In this sense, both domination and liberation are, in part, an educative question.[2]

For Fanon, violence is a necessary part of the process of decolonization due to the inherent brutality of the colonial situation. He argues firmly that the violence of colonialism can only be undone through the '*cleansing force*' of violence (51). However, we must be clear what Fanon means when he uses the term 'violence' as well as his criticism of 'nonviolence'. According to common sense, violence is defined as involving the exertion of force in order to injure, abuse, or destroy another human being. This kind of violence shifts downward our standards of humanity, a regime under which no human thrives. This is violence in both its negative and uncivilized senses, or the active and willful destruction of property and life, as opposed to a Fanonian conception of violence that is liberatory insofar as it frees humans from an oppressive regime by shifting upward the standards of humanity. The problem with the hegemonic definition of violence is that it acts as a regulatory power and renders violence as unacceptable on both sides of the colonial situation (Foucault 1990). As Angela Davis (1998) pointed out:

> The conservative, who does not dispute the validity of revolutions deeply buried in history, invokes visions of impending anarchy in order to legitimate his demand for absolute obedience. Law and order, with the major emphasis on order, is his watchword. The liberal articulates his sensitivity to certain of society's intolerable details, but will almost never prescribe methods of resistance that exceed the limits of legality – redress through electoral channels is the liberal's panacea. (39)

This limited understanding of violence is dangerous because it stifles any type of dialogue seeking to unpack the complexity of violence and its multifarious use in social movements. However, non-violent tactics that have been praised include electoral politics, protests, the legal system, or dialogue where everyone is made to feel safe and included in the public sphere. The ultimate exemplars of the beneficial qualities of non-violence can be found in the personages of Mohandas Karamchand Gandhi and Martin Luther King Jr. We will have more to say about Gandhi and King below. For now, we want to propose that both Fanon (internationally) and King (United States specifically) give us new understandings of the pitfalls and possibilities of violence, thereby transcending its traditional definition as simply repressive. Like King Jr., Fanon spoke of dreams (2004, 15) but Fanon's projections were the natives' liberation predicated on violence.

It is clear that Fanon was not advocating for the non-violent overthrow of colonial systems. In fact, in his theorization of violence, Fanon was only concerned with political strategy when he focused his attention on the shift that occurs after the moment of decolonization, which involves the construction of the new nation. Fanon was not interested in glorifying violence for the purposes of starting mass upheavals; in fact, he was critical of nationalist movements of this strain. He was skeptical of simplistic nationalist movements, those that were not 'explained, enriched, and deepened … into a social and political consciousness, into humanism'. Such movements, according to Fanon, would only lead 'to a dead end' (2004, 144). Nevertheless, he did accept the fact that violence is a necessary element of decolonization, political struggle, and human liberation (1).[3] Thus, he stated, 'Colonialism is not a machine capable of thinking, a body endowed with reason. It is naked violence and only gives in when confronted with greater violence' (23). This passage is key. Fanon was well aware of the liberatory possibilities of violence, its potential to lead to both a plurality of action and the creation of a new politics. His thoughts on the liberatory properties of violence are worth quoting:

> At the individual level, violence is a cleansing force. It rids the colonized of their inferiority complex, of their passive and despairing attitude. It emboldens them, and restores their self-confidence … Enlightened by violence, the people's consciousness rebels against any pacification. (51–2)

Thus, Fanon leaves us with a dialectical definition of violence, one that accounts for its potential for brutality, but also its power to destroy, create, and unify. Naturalizing violence as only repressive comes with two consequences. One, it constructs legitimate violence as the sole possession of the oppressor enforced on the oppressed. It does not conceive of the oppressed, such as racial minorities, as capable of violence as a revolutionary right. Two, it fails to consider violence in the multitude, or the possibility that it may be used to humanize an oppressive relationship.

Fanon was critical of doctrines of passive non-violence because they created a situation of compromise wherein creative forms of tension and struggle were avoided and left untapped. He argued:

> In its raw state this nonviolence conveys to the colonized intellectual and business elite that their interests are identical to those of the colonialist bourgeoisie and it is therefore indispensable, a matter of urgency, to reach an agreement for the common good. Nonviolence is an attempt to settle the colonial problem around the negotiating table before the irreparable is done, before any bloodshed or regrettable act is committed. (2004, 23)

Here we note that there are more similarities between Fanon's theory of violence and Martin Luther King's doctrine of non-violence than meets the eye. King adopted a non-violent platform, but this did not involve coming to the negotiating table to seek a compromise. To the contrary, the tactics of agitation deployed during the 1960s'

Civil Rights movement were intended to establish a necessary *crisis* and willingly performed violence against both whites and a system of white domination. Dr. King (1996) asserted, 'Nonviolent direct action seeks to create … a crisis and foster such a tension that a community which has constantly refused to negotiate is forced to confront the issue. It seeks so to dramatize the issue that it can no longer be ignored' (741–2). As Lewis Gordon (2008) emphasized, 'Martin Luther King, Jr. is today recognized as an apostle of nonviolence. But when he was waging his nonviolent protest, it was perceived by most white Americans and the U.S. government as *violent*. That is because Dr. King was, in Fanon's formulation, *actional*'. In order to be perceived as being legitimately nonviolent in the eyes of white American society, 'King would have had to cease fighting against U.S. apartheid' (2008). Thus, King's tactic of non-violence was, in content but not in form, an act of violence aimed at liberating both the oppressed and the oppressor. In a quote that is remarkably similar to Fanon's theorization of the creative potential of violence, King (1999) stated:

> The nonviolent approach does not immediately change the heart of the oppressor. It first does something to the hearts and souls of those committed to it. It gives them new self-respect; it calls up resources of strength and courage that they did not know they had. Finally it reaches the opponent and so stirs his conscience that reconciliation becomes a reality. (347)

The empty category of violence can now be further theorized, one filled with a political project. When Mahatma Gandhi and Martin Luther King, Jr. proposed non-violent protest as a favored strategy against empire, they understood very well that *this non-violent expression was a form of violence to whites*.

As a counter-hegemonic challenge to white supremacy, Gandhi and King's methodology of the oppressed (Sandoval 2000) – indeed their violence – was an attempt to shift upward the standards of humanity, which whites would interpret as an assault on their way of life. Dr. King (1996) continued:

> Just as Socrates felt that it was necessary to create a tension in the mind so that individuals could rise from the bondage of myths and half-truths to the unfettered realm of creative analysis and objective appraisal, so must we see the need for nonviolent gadflies to create the kind of tension in society that will help men rise from the dark depths of prejudice and racism to the majestic heights of understanding and brotherhood. (742)

In the US case, whites obliged the world with hegemonic and literal expressions of violence captured by the media and circulated across the globe. Focusing entirely on a definition of violence that is dependent on its appearance – we know it when we see it – would miss the pedagogical lesson of King's gamble and the depth of Fanon's theory of violence. Although the civil rights protests were protected by the constitution, and although they were mostly peaceful, they were clearly violent to white sensibilities, and whites exposed their rage when they returned the violence *with interest* by escalating the tensions. White violence was captured by the media for all the world to see, striking at the legitimacy of US benevolence toward its racial minorities (Bobo and Smith 1998). In a literal sense, white violence was just that: repressive. But theoretically, it was not violent in the sense of altering relations for it maintained the current and false standards of humanity. It was a violence so hegemonic that it became naturalized, one that maintained the world as it was. It became violence as a way of life, a necrophilic one at that. White violence is indicative of a certain death drive whereas the liberating violence of the oppressed possesses a humanizing, life-affirming moment. With Fanon (2004), we ask 'But how do we get from the atmosphere of violence to setting violence in motion?' (31).

Just as not all expressions of protest achieve the theoretical status of resistance, not all expressions of rage achieve the theoretical status of violence insofar as they fail to introduce change into a social system. For example, the armed protest of the Minutemen at the border of the state of Arizona and Mexico does not merit the title of resistance by virtue of the fact that they appear to be resisting when in fact they are assisting the immigration history between the United States and Mexico, which is violent to Mexicans (see Leonardo 2003). In contrast, not all apparently non-violent aspirations are easily assimilable into the convenient category of peaceful protest. In the United States in particular, it took the non-violent violence of the Civil Rights movement to introduce a *different system of violence* into civil society. As Fanon insists, challenging repressive systems of power requires going beyond a 'rational confrontation of viewpoints' (2004, 6). We suggest that there are pedagogical lessons contained in this history. Violence is always present in a social system because the struggle over power structures participation within the system. This is not necessarily deplorable but constitutes the field of discourses that struggle for our subjectivity (Weedon 1997). The issue hinges on a couple of questions. What political project is attached to this or that system of violence? What consequences and relations are produced? What are the standards of humanity in the system? Unless these questions are posed, we cannot arrive at the *practical function of violence*.

Following Foucault (1980), King's 'peaceful' protest was not an act by the powerless but a resistance that summoned every morsel of power against a repressive State. In other words, it was an expression of power that took the form of resistance, unlike whites' reactions, which were deployments of power for the sake of maintaining it. This is an important distinction. Using conventional modes of force against a State that monopolizes its legitimate use, as Weber (1978) reminds us, would likely not have succeeded for it would have been overwhelmed by the military, absent of a coup. As Perry Anderson's (1976) near book-length article on Gramsci makes plain, in modern societies the State becomes an 'outer ditch' filled by a complex system of civil institutions. This fact necessitates an equally complex understanding of civil society, which a 'war of maneuver' against an all-encompassing State fails to illuminate. Instead, a 'war of position' must expose fissures in civil society, exploiting its cultural institutions, such as the media and educational system. We may compare King's peaceful protest with the dismantling of apartheid in South Africa. One may be tempted to suggest that the South African revolution was peaceful, without much bloodshed and ending with the Truth and Reconciliation Commission. Of course as Fanon might argue, the South African case was violent to the core, particularly to whites, whose entitlements were revoked. The same can be said about the achievements of the Civil Rights movement, which was a massive assault on an entire social system. Likewise, a critical education is radically violent if it expects to shift the racial dialogue. It is a humanizing form of violence that puts people back in their rightful place and restores their dignity, both the oppressor and the oppressed (Freire 1993).

A humanizing violence is both necessary and liberatory because the actual system and theoretical backbone of colonialism and systems of domination create unethical situations wherein individuals are relegated to subject positions that make them something below, or other than, human. In Charles Mills' (1997) understanding, people of color become subpersons within the assumptions of such a system. What it means to be human or what it means to be an actional individual in Fanon's sense, is defined via the discourse of the colonizer as the embodiment of the western-white-heterosexual-propertied male (Wynter 2001). Fanon was correct to warn us that non-violence as compromise, electoral politics, political concessions, and appeal to legality only forestalls the overthrow of a *regime of thought* that continues to demarcate between the human and the subperson. If dialogue seeks to undo racism, then we must ask if notions of safe dialogue legitimate an oppressive system or if they engage in a process that is creative enough to produce a new social consciousness, a new human subject 'with a new language and a new humanity' (Fanon 2004, 2). According to Fanon's 'stretched' materialist dialectic, in order to speak to the issue of colonial classes (see De Lissovoy 2008), liberatory violence is the only way to overcome the system while actively reclaiming one's humanity.

The myth of safety in race dialogue for people of color

One of the main premises of safe-space discourse is that it provides a format for people of color and whites to come together and discuss issues of race in a matter that is not dangerous as well as inclusive. Thus, the conventional guidelines used to establish a safe space – such as being mindful of how and when one is speaking, confidentiality, challenge by choice, and speaking from experience – are used to create an environment where fundamental issues can be broached and no one will be offended. Taken unproblematically, this trend is reasonable. However, the ironic twist is that many individuals from marginalized groups become both offended and agitated when engaging in apparently safe spaces.[4] In their naiveté, many white students and educators fail to appreciate the fact – a lived experience – that race dialogue is almost never safe for people of color in mixed-racial company. But before we romanticize its opposite, or same-race dialogues, the idea that homogeneous spaces are automatically safe for people of color is a mystification for they result precisely from a violent condition: racial segregation. That said, something has gone incredibly wrong when students of color feel immobilized and marginalized within spaces and dialogues that are supposed to undo racism. This situation should give us doubt regarding whether or not safe-space dialogue really allows for the creativity necessary to promote a humanizing discussion on race, or if it functions, in Fanon's words, as a negotiating table that seeks peaceful compromise without engaging in the violence necessary to both explore and undo racism.

We want to suggest that the reason why safe-space discussions partly break down in practice, if not at least in theory, is that they assume that, by virtue of formal and procedural guidelines, safety has been designated for both white people and people of color. However, the term 'safety' acts as a misnomer because it often means that white individuals can be made to feel safe. Thus, a space of safety is circumvented, and instead a space of oppressive color-blindness is established. It is a managed health-care version of anti-racism, an insurance against 'looking racist'. Fanon provides a useful counter to the inherent color-blindness of current racial pedagogy. Fanon's arguments in both *Black skin, white masks* and *The wretched of the earth*, show sympathies with what intellectuals now call a post-racial analysis (see Leonardo in press). Fanon (1967a) warned against the inherent narcissism of white racial superiority found in arguments for separatism, what Appiah (1990) terms 'extrinsic racism', which is the inferiorization of an outer group in terms of their moral worth.

Fanon stated, 'I believe that the fact of the juxtaposition of the white and black races has created a massive psychoexistential complex. I hope by analyzing it to destroy it' (12). In destroying the neuroses of blackness, Fanonian violence approaches post-race implications to the extent that the genesis of blackness is a source external to it: that is, whiteness (see Nayak 2006). By hoping to destroy it, Fanon suggests ending race as a neurotic relation. However, to be clear, Fanonian post-race differs from color-blindness because it seeks to destroy race and racism via a practice of full engagement as opposed to a practice of avoidance. Fanon's methodology was phenomenological because he sought to undo racism by engaging the phenomenon itself, of going through race in order to undo it. Thus, a Fanonian post-racial gesture to pedagogy is both different and more beneficial than the color-blind stance taken up in safe-space dialogue, which is hardly blind to color. Perhaps the problem with safe space is that it willingly tries to side step the issues, as well as the educative aspects of anger and frustration, necessary for a beneficial and truly liberatory dialogue on race to take place.

A Fanonian approach leads us back into considerations of violence in race-based dialogue. The question we must ask is how do we go about understanding liberatory discussions on race as necessitating violence? We are not speaking of violence in the sense of a willful act to injure or abuse, but a violence that humanizes, or shifts the standards of humanity by providing space for the free expression of people's thoughts and emotions that are not regulated by the discourse of safety. Our main criticism of safe space is that it is laced with a narcissism that designates safety for individuals in already dominant positions of power, which is not safe at all but perpetuates a systematic relation of violence. Fanon advised against a politics of narcissism, and instead advocated a materialist politics of recognition whereby an individual allows himself to be mediated by the other, or Fanon's appropriation of Hegel's (1977) idealism of the other. Unfortunately, this does not happen because white narcissism is at the very center of safe space. Through the avoidance of conflict and the emphasis on personal and image management, it maintains the self-image and understanding of whiteness and reveals a refusal to change through the other. To be fair, Fanon also took to task people of color's own narcissism, particularly as it concerns the limitations of identity politics and nationalism, what Appiah (1990) calls 'intrinsic racism', or the assumption of a family resemblance within a group necessary in the short term and usually for protection against the assaults of an outer group.[5] African nationalism during decolonization is an example of the second class, whereas Nazism represents the first class; both are problematic, but they differ in purpose and outcome. White indulgence is a gross attempt to understand the self through the self rather than through the other: narcissism par excellence. In fact, Fanon warns us that the 'other' in the self/other dichotomy in racial dialogue may not even exist. According to Gordon (2008):

> In the contemporary academy, much discussion of race and racism is replete with criticism of otherness. Fanon, however, argues that racism proper eliminates such a relationship. Instead of self and other, there are self, others, and non-self, non-others. In other words, there is the category of people who are neither self nor others. *They are no-one.* The dialectics of recognition is disrupted, and the struggle of such people becomes one of achieving such a dialectics. Put differently, they are not fighting against being others. They are fighting to become others and, in so doing, entering ethical relationships. This argument results in a peculiar critique of liberal political theory. Such theory presupposes ethical foundations of political life. *What Fanon has shown is that political work needs to be done to make ethical life possible. That is because racism and colonialism derail ethical life.* (italics added)

A pedagogical approach that avoids safety in the interest of image and personal management makes such an ethical relationship possible.

If we are truly interested in racial pedagogy, then we must become comfortable with the idea that for marginalized and oppressed minorities, *there is no safe space*. As implied above, mainstream race dialogue in education is arguably already hostile and unsafe for many students of color whose perspectives and experiences are consistently minimized. *Violence is already there*. In other words, like Fanon's understanding of colonialism, safe space enacts violence. Those who are interested in engaging in racial pedagogy must be prepared to (1) undo the violence that is inherent to safe-space dialogue, and (2) enact a form of liberatory violence within race discussions to allow for a creativity that shifts the standards of humanity. In other words, anger, hostility, frustration, and pain are characteristics that are not to be avoided under the banner of safety, which only produces Freire's (1993) 'culture of silence'. They are attributes that are to be recognized on the part of both whites and people of color in order to engage in a process that is creative enough to establish new forms of social existence, where both parties are transformed. This is not a form of violence that is life threatening and narcissistic, but one that is life affirming through its ability to promote mutual recognition.

Pedagogy of fear and the intellectualization of race

Teaching race literacy is necessary but difficult. In addition, authentic race dialogue is elusive because over and beyond its emotional register for many educators and students, race dialogue runs into the formidable force of ideology. *In mixed racial company, race dialogue is almost never for the benefit of people of color and race-conscious whites*. In fact, as Nishitani Osamu (2006) observes, race dialogue in mixed-race company works to maintain the Western distinction between 'anthropos' (the inhuman) and 'humanitas' (the human). Osamu points out, '"anthropos" cannot escape the status of being the object of anthropological knowledge, while "humanitas" is never defined from without but rather expresses itself as the subject of all knowledge' (260). Put another way, race dialogue often maintains the status of whiteness as being both natural and unchanging in the white imaginary. In other words, whiteness remains ubiquitous even if it is not named, and noticing whiteness is itself regarded as a form of transgression (hooks 1992). Whiteness is the immovable mover, unmarked marker, and unspoken speaker.

Although it would be interesting to focus on race discussions within a homogeneous group, or same-race dialogues, the imagined situation we put forth is a mixed company because it projects the ideal of public integration and the educational challenges to it. Given that integration is the goal, many students of color who seek 'safe' race discussions in public rarely find them, having to settle for the reality that most pedagogical situations involving race are violent to them. They realize quite quickly that public race talk is not for them but for whites, or at least a white mindset. In other words, it caters to a white racial frame, a white imaginary (Leonardo 2009), which is a collective unconscious that tolerates race dialogue in small amounts. Often, as Fanon's (1967a) critique of Sartre (1948) indicates, whites turn racism into an intellectualist problem, rather than a lived one (132–5).[4] Following a Fanonian dialectic, at root racism is a material problem, which suggests displacing an idealist framework with a concrete one. Public race discussions are examples of white racial hegemony insofar as they represent whites' accommodation to demands of color as long as white common sense is observed and kept intact. As a result, most race discussions benefit whites and patronize people of color; they project a white audience, both real and imagined. In this interaction, the otherwise deep and intimate understanding that people of color have to offer is forsaken in exchange for an epiphenomenal, intellectualist interpretation of race.

There are genuine fears that must be confronted when educators publicly discuss race in the classroom. Both whites and people of color face certain dangers that prevent an authentic exchange. Not only do whites fear that they will be exposed as racist; they also fear being found out as racial beings. People of color already know that whites comprise a racial group, therefore white raciality would not represent a shocking discovery for them. However, whites' discovery of their own raciality is precisely what is at stake. Hiding behind the veil of color-blindness means that lifting it would force whites to confront their self-image, with people of color acting as the mirror. This act is not frightening for people of color but for whites. In the light of day, this fact of whiteness would have led Fanon to declare, 'Look a white person!' Although this pale façade is becoming more difficult to sustain, whites cultivate a color-blind mask that even Fanon would not have predicted. To be clear, color-blindness in a color-obsessed nation appears oxymoronic and whites would have to work hard to maintain the mask. In a race-saturated society, such as the United States, *color-blind racism is accurately described as a mode of feigning an oblivion to race.* In short, color-blind perspectives are attempts to observe – indeed to see – race in a way that maintains whites' equilibrium. It is not literally a form of blindness but its precise opposite: seeing race in a selective way that makes whites acceptable, not to people of color per se, but to themselves. *It would be a mistake to regard color-blindness as a non-racial move and more accurate to construct it as a particular deployment of race.*

Authentic race discussions are violent to whites for the very reason that such discussions would expose their investment in race, their full endorsement of, rather than, flippant regard for it. It speaks to the inauthentic education that whites experience. This does not suggest that their fear has no basis. In fact, it has a material basis for it represents one of the many walls that people of color have to scale as they attempt to convince whites that race matters in a manner different from whites' understanding of it. Some whites who are open minded enough, often feel enlightened and enlivened by discussions that confront racism, vowing their commitment to the cause. That established, whites often conceive of race talks as intellectually stimulating – as in a discovery or another topic in which they can excel – rather than a lived experience that students of color in good faith share with their white colleagues. Meanwhile, students of color walk away from the same discussions barely advancing their understanding of race and racism, sometimes satisfied departing with their legitimacy and mindset intact. After all, these confrontations were not for their benefit; they were not meant to advance people of color. A Fanon-inspired race dialogue is not anti-intellectual, but precisely anti-intellectualist. Said another way, it is materialist.

Minority fears are quite different from white apprehensions concerning public race talk. Despite the countless occasions where people of color expose their intimate thoughts and hurts about racism, then followed by white dismissal (not always overt), their desire for authentic race dialogue represents their hope not only in themselves but a hope projected onto whites. It is, on one hand, naïve and a sign of wishful thinking on the part of minorities to expect more out of whites than whites expect out of themselves. On the other hand, it is a humanizing desire and commitment to the other that prevents people of color from disengaging from whites. People of color may suspend their memory of white aggressions in order to start anew, of renewing their hope that *this time it will be different*. Then they are reminded of the pattern they know so well and their disappointment haunts them. They may even strike back against empire and voice their disapprobation at whites. Too often, whites interpret minority anger as a distancing move, or the confirmation of the 'angry' person of color archetype, rather than its opposite: an attempt to engage the other, to be vulnerable to the other, to be recognized by the other, to be the other for the other.

As Freire (1993) once remarked, protestation from the oppressed is an act of love insofar as it represents an act of engagement. When the oppressed open their wounds through communication, they express the violence in their dehumanization that they want the oppressor to recognize. People of color do not only fear overt violence from whites (although this would be enough) but rather their wantonness, their lack of recognition of people of color, a certain violence of the heart rather than the fist. This is what Fanon (2004) describes as 'violence rippling under the skin' (31). This secondary form of violence confirms a daily assault that often goes unnoticed. It is a double violence that fails to acknowledge the other on whom one imposes an unwelcome will. It may sound like a slave's maneuver to desire recognition from the master but such is the relationship of bondage within a colonial relationship. It would be enough to suggest that people of color fear overt white violence in the form of physical aggression. People of color have other fundamental fears in becoming invisible to whites, of becoming merely an idea to them.

Some minority students willingly participate in otherwise problematic race conversations because they refuse to surrender to absolute cynicism, where racism would have succeeded. They realize that participation maintains their sense of humanity and disengagement subverts the kind of person they want to cultivate, the kind of self or student they want to be. In other words, disengagement is one of the symptoms of structural racism, which succeeds at isolating us from one another, of subverting our ability to live through the other. Still some people of color give into despair, tired as they are of educating whites from ground zero … every time, again and again. Who can blame them? It is a survival mechanism that people of color have practiced over the years in order to prevent their anger and frustration from consuming them, of turning to self-destructive forms of violence in the form of rage. Or, it is a defense against white violence – in the form of microaggressions – which strikes at the academic legitimacy of scholars and students of color when they violate the color-blind codes of conduct that regulate the classroom. People of color sometimes overlook white violence *so they can get through their daily life*. Like a child who has been abused, people of color avoid white violence by strategically playing along, a practice that whites, whose racial development stunts their growth, underestimate when they mistake consensus as the absence of coercion. Like abused children who do not possess the ability to consent and defend themselves against the verbal and physical power of a parent, people of color have become masters at deflection. This is how they secure safety in violent circumstances.

It is apparent that both whites and people of color want to avoid violence from being enacted against them. They enter race dialogue from radically different locations – intellectual for the former, lived for the latter – and an unevenness that the critical race pedagogue must accept and becomes the constitutive condition of any progressive dialogue on race. It is the risk that comes with violence but one worth taking if educators plan to shift the standards of humanity. In an apparently common quest for mutual racial understanding, whites and people of color participate in a violence that becomes an integral part of the process and seeking a 'safe space' is itself a form of violence insofar as it fails to recognize the myth of such geography in interracial exchange. As it concerns people of color within the current regime, safe space in racial dialogue is a projection rather than a reality. This is the myth that majoritarian stories in education replay and retell in order to perpetuate an understanding of race that maintains white supremacy. Safe spaces are violent to people of color and only by enacting a different form of violence, of shifting the discourse, will race dialogue ultimately become a space of mutual recognition between whites and people of color.

If people of color observe the current call for safety, this process defaults to white understandings and comfort zones, which have a well-documented history of violence against people of color. It is a point of entry that is characterized by denials, evasions, and falsehoods (Frankenberg 1993; Mills 1997). Its shell is non-violent for in public most whites prize self-control. Race dialogue within a white framework is rational, if by that we mean a situation that preserves, as Angela Davis (1998) mentioned, peace and order. This procedural arrangement has much to recommend it if we want to avoid uprisings and outright violence. But its kernel is already violent to people of color because a certain irrational rationality is at work. Both parties leave the interaction relatively 'intact', which should not be equated with the absence of violence. Whites depart the situation with their worldview and value systems unchallenged and affirmed, and people of color remain fractured in theirs. Whites would need to experience violence if they expect to change. But this is different from a hegemonic understanding that violence is always a form of dehumanization. In our appropriation of Fanon's dialectics of violence, we find transformative possibilities in violence depending on the political project to which it is attached. Moreover, in this framework violence is not so much a description of this or that act qualifying as a form of violence, but a theoretical prescription of a different state of affairs, a response to oppression that equals its intensity. Thus, we do not describe what violence looks like, but assess its consequences.

A race education worth the name: shifting the ground of pedagogy

Given that education requires an overhaul if the ship of racism may be steered differently, then violence is warranted as a way to shift the standards. In this last section, we advance some ideas around the criteria for a more authentic dialogue around race in education. In so doing, we do not suggest that dialogue alone can turn the tide without addressing the structural changes that give racism its force. We do not harbor such illusions of grandeur. We offer the following thoughts on dialogue as a form of social practice: *dialogue as a method of violence and violence as dialogical.* A critical race education requires a pedagogy of violence that transcends fear without conveniently forgetting that it structures the learning moment. Our suggestion is not to escalate the pedagogy of fear that students and people of color experience by turning the proverbial table on whites. In saying this, we want to acknowledge that fear is already in the room, not as a form of cul-de-sac or pessimistic analysis but a realistic appraisal of an existing limit situation, an act of defiance in Bell's (1992) sense. But just as fear may be turned against itself in order to produce conditions for courage, so we suggest that fear is an emotion that does not necessarily paralyze the educator or scholar.

One, a race dialogue assumes already racialized participants. Therefore, safety is relational and asks the question, 'Who feels safe and toward what ends?' Working against the pretences of color-blindness, the race literate educator is not a post-race subject, if by that we mean achieving a position outside the universe of race. In race literacy, one works with race from within, not without (see Twine 2004; Guinier and Torres 2003). In this sense, race has no outside (Leonardo 2005). Even imagining a condition that hails 'after race' (which is possible), is an event within racialization for our imagination is itself racial. Fanon's was a racial analysis with post-racial implications. Therefore, race dialogues and the regulative ideals that educators establish as rational procedures that guide the discourse, are racialized ideals rather than race-neutral. As Omi and Winant (1994) have reminded us for a couple decades, procedures require a racial formation to give them meaning and significance. Discursive regulations are racial for they speak to the issue of power and who can say what to whom in the course of an exchange. They are part of a larger understanding of the self as belonging to a racial universe, not in the sense of an inherently limiting system (for all systems are limiting) but one that defines possible expressions within a given condition (see Goldberg 1993).

Two, a pedagogue may begin a course simply by having a meta-dialogue (dialogue about dialogue) about the assumptions of safety so pervasive in the academy when it comes to the topic of race. By redefining classroom space as a place of risk, educators encourage students to experiment with their self-understanding, and to promote the audacious notion that they may change their minds by the end of a term. We need to be clear that a place of risk does not promote hostility but growth. It does not promote discomfort for its own sake, as if learning only happens when one is uncomfortable. As we have noted, many students of color experience discomfort in public race forums, which hardly leads to new learning for them. Yes, something is learned, but discomfort is not the precondition to worthwhile learning. Against much of anti-racist writing, we do not suggest that a pedagogue's *goal* is to encourage white discomfort. Rather, whites must take ownership of feeling uncomfortable in critical race dialogue. Pedagogues can encourage them to take responsibility for their feelings of inadequacy and defensiveness. When paired with clarity in purpose and solidarity with the other, where judgment is practiced but one is never judged, discomfort can be liberating because it enables whites and people of color to remove the mask. They may end up knowing each other more fully as complex human beings rather than the shell of one: whites assumed to be more superior than they are, people of color more inferior than they are. After many years of experience in the university setting, we have learned that this apostasy – of creating risk as the antidote to safety – leads to more transformative learning opportunities. It humanizes students of color because it legitimates their voice and affirms whites' incompleteness, for it is guided by an ethic of concern for and not a desire to expose whites as simply racist. Not only does risk discourse encourage looking behind the dialogue (a hermeneutics of suspicion) but it also appreciates what it opens up in front (a hermeneutics of empathy). This lack of safety ironically produces a condition where whites are more able to empathize with people of color as both groups assume the consequences for risk, whereas people of color usually assume the burdens of a 'safe race dialogue'. A comfortable race dialogue belies the actual structures of race, which is full of tension. It is literally out of sync with its own topic.

Finally, violating the discourse on safety means aiming at rigor. It opens up deeper engagements on race, both in the intellectual and practical sense as a lived reality. In an educational system that prides itself on excellence, pedagogues paradoxically aim low when it comes to race dialogue, settling instead for mediocrity. They fail to take advantage of the deep competencies that students of color have to offer and instead rely on the shallowness of whiteness. It is a pedagogy guided by the least competent students in the room, a strategy that most educators would not endorse or tolerate in any other condition. It means helping the children most left behind (and who invest in being the last one in) when it comes to race literacy: mainly, white students. They are often racially illiterate and unable to decode the fundamental racial lessons of daily life. Using a Fanonian analytics of the oppressed to drive race dialogue does not mean that the oppressed are correct most of the time even if it means they are correct more of the time. It does not focus on their individual accuracy but on their collective experiences and the perspectives born from a life of risk. For their important decisions rely on race literacy as if their life depended on it. A humanizing violence would restore their education in the proper sense. This means increasing the violence in education, of disrupting its inhumane dimensions toward new standards of humanity that liberate rather than oppress.

Notes

1. We would like to take this moment to thank the anonymous reviewers for their excellent suggestions to improve the manuscript. Much appreciation goes to REE Chief Editor, David Gillborn, for giving our perspective space in the journal and working with us from beginning to end. It is a pleasure to publish in what has become the definitive venue for critical thought on race and education.
2. We recognize that Paulo Freire took up Fanon's project on the question of violence in *Pedagogy of the oppressed*. Furthermore, Freire theorized the nature of liberatory dialogue in the same text. Our project differs from Freire's to the extent that racial violence, and particularly its US iteration, figures more centrally in our analysis.
3. Homi K. Bhabha (2004) asserted that the glorification of violence that is attached to *The wretched of the earth* is the result of Jean-Paul Sartre's preface rather than Fanon's arguments (xxi).
4. One of the authors of this essay has seen this phenomenon play out during his own participation in a race-based discussion where, after the designation of safety, several African American and Latino students left the group after being accused of attacking white participants, leading one African American student to declare, 'Fuck safe space!' as she retreated from the group. Whites looked on in amazement.
5. Fanon (2004) writes, 'Antiracist racism and the determination to defend one's skin, which is characteristic of the colonized's response to colonial oppression, clearly represent sufficient reasons to join the struggle. But one does not sustain a war, one does not endure massive repression or witness the disappearance of one's entire family in order for hatred or racism to triumph. Racism, hatred, resentment, and "the legitimate desire for revenge" alone cannot nurture a war of liberation' (89).

4\. In *Black skin, white masks*, Fanon takes Sartre to task for reducing black experience to an idea rather than a brutal fact. Fanon writes, '*Orphée Noir* is a date in the intellectualization of the *experience* of being black. And Sartre's mistake was not only to seek the source of the source but in a certain sense to block that source' (134).

References

Alridge, D. 1999. Conceptualizing a Du Boisian philosophy of education: Toward a model for African American education. *Educational Theory* 49, no. 3: 359–79.

Alridge, D. 2008. *The educational thought of W.E.B. Du Bois.* New York: Teachers College Press.

Altbach, P., and G.P. Kelly, eds. 1978. *Education and colonialism.* New York: Longman.

Anderson, P. 1976. The antinomies of Antonio Gramsci. *New Left Review* I, no. 100: 5–65.

Appiah, K. 1990. Racisms. In *Anatomy of racism,* ed. D. Goldberg, 3–17. Minneapolis, Minnesota: University of Minnesota Press.

Bell, D. 1992. *Faces at the bottom of the well: The permanence of racism.* New York: Basic Books.

Bernal, D.D., and O. Villalpando. 2005. An apartheid of knowledge in academia: The struggle over the 'legitimate' knowledge of faculty of color. In *Critical pedagogy and race,* ed. Z. Leonardo, 185–204. Malden, Massachusetts: Blackwell.

Bhabha, H. 2004. Foreword: Framing Fanon. In *The wretched of the earth,* F. Fanon, vii–xli. New York: Grove Press.

Bobo, L., and R. Smith. 1998. From Jim Crow racism to laissez-faire racism: The transformation of racial attitudes. In *Beyond pluralism: The conception of groups and group identities in America,* ed. W. Katkin, N. Landsman, and A. Tyree, 182–220. Urbana: University of Illinois Press.

Bourdieu, P. 1977. *Outline of a theory of practice.* Trans. R. Nice. Cambridge: Cambridge University Press.

Bordieu, P., and J. Passeron. 1990. *Reproduction in education, society, and culture.* Thousand Oaks, California: Sage.

Brayboy, B. 2005. Toward a tribal critical race theory in education. *The Urban Review* 37, no. 5: 425–46.

Césaire, A. 2000. *Discourse on colonialism.* New York: Monthly Review Press, 1955.

Davis, A. 1998. Political prisoners, prisons, and black liberation. In *The Angela Y. Davis reader,* ed. J. James, 39–52. Malden, Massachusetts: Blackwell Publishing.

De Lissovoy, N. 2008. *Power, crisis, and education for liberation.* New York: Palgrave.

Derrida, J. 1985. Racism's last word. *Critical Inquiry* 12, no. 1: 290–9.

Dixson, A.D., and Rousseau, C.K. 2005. And we are still not saved: Critical race theory ten years later. *Race Ethnicity and Education* 8, no. 1: 7–27.

Du Bois, W.E.B. 1989. *The souls of black folk.* New York: Penguin Books, 1904.

Fanon, F. 1965. *A dying colonialism.* Trans. H. Chevalier. New York: Grove Press.

Fanon, F. 1967a. *Black skin, white masks.* Trans. C. Markmann. New York: Grove Press.

Fanon, F. 1967b. *Toward the African revolution.* Trans. H. Chevalier. New York: Grove Press.

Fanon, F. 2004. *The wretched of the earth.* Trans. R. Philcox. New York: Grove Press, 1963.

Foucault, M. 1980. *Power/knowledge.* Ed. C. Gordon. New York: Pantheon Books.

Foucault, M. 1990. *The history of sexuality,* vol. 1. Trans. R. Hurley. New York: Vintage Books, 1978.

Frankenberg, R. 1993. *White women, race matters: The social construction of whiteness.* Minneapolis, Minnesota: University of Minnesota Press.

Fraser, N. 1997. *Justice interruptus: Critical reflections on the 'postsocialist' condition.* New York: Routledge.

Freire, P. 1993. *Pedagogy of the oppressed.* Trans. M. Ramos. New York: Continuum.

Fuss, D. 1994. Interior colonies: Frantz Fanon and the politics of identification. *Diacritics* 24, nos. 2–3: 20–42.

Gillborn, D. 2008. *Racism and education: Coincidence or conspiracy?* New York: Routledge.

Goldberg, D.T. 1993. *Racist culture.* Malden, Massachusetts: Blackwell.

Gordon, L. 1995. *Fanon and the crisis of European man: An essay on philosophy and the human sciences.* New York: Routledge.

Gordon, L. 2008. Fanon dans la pensée politique africaine récente [Fanon in recent African political thought. Starting from Frantz Fanon]. Article in English. http://www.csprp.univ-paris-diderot.fr/gordon.html.

Gordon, L., T.D. Sharpley-Whiting, and R. White. 1996. Introduction. In *Fanon: A critical reader,* ed. L. Gordon, T.D. Sharpley-Whiting, and R. White, 1–8. Malden, Massachusetts: Blackwell.

Gramsci, A. 1971. *Selections from prison notebooks.* Trans. and ed. Q. Hoare and G. Smith. New York: International Publishers.

Grosfoguel, R. 2007. The epistemic decolonial turn: Beyond political-economy paradigms. *Cultural Studies* 21, no. 2: 211–23.

Guinier, L., and G. Torres. 2003. *The miner's canary.* Cambridge, Massachusetts: Harvard University Press.

Hall, S. 1996. Gramsci's relevance for the study of race and ethnicity. In *Stuart Hall: Critical dialogues in cultural studies,* ed. D. Morley and K. Chen, 411–40. London: Routledge.

Hegel, G.W.F 1977. *Phenomenology of spirit.* Trans. A.V. Miller. New York: Oxford University Press.

hooks, b. 1992. *Black looks: Race and representation.* Boston: South End Press.

King, M.L., Jr. 1996. Letter from a Birmingham jail. In *African intellectual heritage: A books of sources,* ed. M. Asante and A. Abarry, 740–50. Philadelphia, Pennsylvania: Temple University Press.

King, M.L., Jr. 1999. The power of nonviolent action. In *Social theory: The multicultural and classic readings,* ed. C. Lemert, 343–8. Boulder, Colorado: Westview Press.

Ladson-Billings, G. 1998. From Soweto to the South Bronx: African Americans and colonial education in the United States. In *Sociology of education: Emerging perspectives,* ed. C. Torres and T. Mitchell, 247–64. Albany, New York: State University of New York Press.

Ladson-Billings, G. 2004. Just what is critical race theory and what's it doing in a nice field like education. In *The Routledge Falmer reader in multicultural education,* ed. G. Ladson-Billings and D. Gillborn, 49–67. New York: Routledge Falmer.

Ladson-Billings, G., and W.F. Tate IV. 1995. Toward a critical race theory of education. *Teachers College Record* 97, no. 1: 47–68.

Leonardo, Z. 2002. The souls of white folk: Critical pedagogy, whiteness studies, and globalization discourse. *Race Ethnicity and Education* 5, no. 1: 29–50.

Leonardo, Z. 2003. Resisting capital: Simulationist and socialist strategies. *Critical Sociology* 29, no. 2: 211–36.

Leonardo, Z. 2005. Through the multicultural glass: Althusser, ideology, and race relations in post-civil rights America. *Policy Futures in Education* 3, no. 4: 400–12.

Leonardo, Z. 2009. *Race, whiteness, and education.* New York: Routledge.

Leonardo, Z. In press. After the glow: Race ambivalence and other educational prognoses. *Educational Philosophy and Theory.*

Lynn, M. 1999. Toward a critical race pedagogy: A research note. *Urban Education* 33, no. 5: 606–26.

Macedo, D. 2000. The colonialism of the English-only movement. *Educational Researcher* 29, no. 3: 15–24.

Maldonado-Torres, N. 2006. Césaire's gift and the decolonial turn. *Radical Philosophy* 9, no. 2: 111–38.

Maldonado-Torres, N. 2007. On the coloniality of being: Contributions to the development of a concept. *Cultural Studies* 21, no. 2–3: 240–70.

McLaren, P., Z. Leonardo, and R.L. Allen. 1999. The gift of si(gh)ted violence: Toward a discursive intervention into the organization of capitalism. *Discourse: Theoretical Studies in Media and Culture* 21, no. 2: 139–62.

Memmi, A. 1965. *The colonizer and the colonized.* Boston: Beacon Press.

Mills, C. 1997. *The racial contract.* Ithaca, New York: Cornell University Press.

Nayak, A. 2006. After race: Ethnography, race and post-race theory. *Ethnic and Racial Studies* 29, no. 3: 411–30.

Omi, M., and H. Winant. 1994. *Racial formation in the United States: From the 1960s to the 1990s.* 2nd ed. New York: Routledge.

Osamu, N. 2006. Anthropos and humanitas: Two Western concepts of 'human being'. In *Translation, biopolitics, colonial difference,* ed. N. Sakai and J. Solomon, 259–74. Hong Kong: Hong Kong University Press.

Parker, L., and D. Stovall. 2005. Actions following words: Critical race theory connects to critical pedagogy. In *Critical pedagogy and race,* ed. Z. Leonardo, 159–74. Malden, Massachusetts: Blackwell.

Provenzo, E. 2002. *Du Bois on education.* Lanham, Maryland: Alta Mira Press.

Quijano, A. 2000. Coloniality of power, Eurocentrism, and Latin America. *Nepantla* 1, no. 3: 533–80.

Sandoval, C. 2000. *Methodology of the oppressed.* Minneapolis, Minnesota: University of Minnesota Press.

Sartre, J.-P. 1948. Orphée Noir. In *Anthologie de la nouvelle poésie nègre et malgache,* ed. L. Senghor, ix–xliv. Paris: Presses Universitaires de France.

Sartre, J.-P. 2004. *Preface to* The wretched of the earth. New York: Grove Press, 1961.

Solorzano, D. 1998. Critical race theory, racial and gender microaggressions, and the experiences of Chicana and Chicano scholars. *International Journal of Qualitative Studies in Education* 11: 121–36.

Tate, W. 1997. Critical race theory and education: History, theory and implications. *Review of Research in Education* 22: 193–243.
Taylor, E. 1998. A primer on critical race theory: Who are the critical race theorists and what are they saying? *Journal of Blacks in Higher Education* 19: 122–124.
Thompson, A. 2003. Tifanny, friend of people of color: White investments in antiracism. *Qualitative Studies in Education* 16, no. 1: 7–29.
Twine, F.W. 2004. A white side of black Britain: The concept of racial literacy. *Ethnic and Racial Studies* 27, no. 6: 878–907.
Wallerstein, I. 2009. Reading Fanon in the 21st century. *New Left Review* 57, http://www.newleftreview.org/?view=2784.
Weber, M. 1978. The three pure types of authority. In *Economy and society,* ed. G. Roth and C. Wittich, vol. 1, 215–6. Berkeley: University of California Press.
Weedon, C. 1997. *Feminist practice & poststructuralist theory.* 2nd ed. Cambridge, Massachusetts: Blackwell.
Wynter, S. 1995. 1492: A new world view. In *Race, discourse, and the origin of the Americas: A new worldview,* ed. V.L. Hyatt and R. Nettleford, 5–50. Washington, DC: Smithsonian Institution.
Wynter, S. 2001. Towards the sociogenic principle: Fanon, identity, the puzzle of conscious experience, and what it is like to be 'black'. In *National identities and sociopolitical changes in Latin America,* ed. M.F Durán-Cogan and A. Gómez-Moriana, 30–66. New York: Routledge.
Yosso, T. 2006. *Critical race counterstories along the Chicana/Chicano educational pipeline.* New York: Routledge.
Zizek, S. 2008. *Violence.* New York: Picador.

Index

Note: Numbers in *italics* indicate a figure; those followed by 'n' indicate chapter note numbers

Abel, E. 145
academic achievement: achievement gap 85–91, 96–98, 99, 102, 103–104, 107–111, 177–186; African American students 21–22, 32, 50, 58, 60, 62–63, 67–68, 72, 74–75, 97, 103, 173–174; Asian American students 97; Black students 86–90, 97; Chicano/a students 83, 97, 123; data reporting 169; ethnic minority students in the UK 86–90; impact of competition on 163–164; Latino/a students 50, 83; in relation to school spending 23; Samoan students 97; students of color 172–186; White students 87, 88–90, 97, 177
academy schools 86–87, 91
activism 5, 6, 47, 80
admissions: color-blindness 29, 31, 32, 33; higher education 20, 29, 30–33; high school 50–52; selective enrollment 51–52, 168
affirmative action: abandonment of 19, 29; as benefitting Whites 14; conservative Right 44; constitutionalized 7; higher education admissions 29, 30–33; origins of 20
African Americans: communal bonds 124; cultural capital 126–127; effects of affirmative action on 14; effects of education reform on 165, 166, 167–168, 169; experiences of racial microaggressions 138, 139–140, 145–148, 152–153; narratives 33–34; person-as-property status 17–18; political representation 12; relations with Mexican-American community 51; resistant capital 126; social capital 125
African American students: academic achievement 21–22, 32, 50, 58, 60, 62–63, 67–68, 72, 74–75, 97, 103, 173–174; access to curriculum 20–21; assessment 21; effects of affirmative action on 29, 30–33; experiences in majority White schools 173–186; experiences of racial profiling 153; graduation rates 58, 61; high-achieving 173, 180; instruction 21; male athletes' experiences 57–75; as property 73–74; selective enrollment 51–52; in under-resourced schools 48, 50–52; *see also* Black students
Albach vs Odle 73
American Civil Rights Institute 44
American Indians 29, 117; *see also* First Nation; Indigenous students; Native Americans
Anderson, Perry 196
Ansley, Frances Lee 42
Anzaldúa, Gloria 114, 115, 122, 127
Appiah, K. 197, 198
Arizona 14, 34, 44, 83, 170, 196
Asian Americans 29, 30, 37n10, 117
AsianCrit 46, *116*, 117
Asian students 28, 86–90, 97, 178–186
aspirational capital 122–123
assessment 21–22, 87–90
athletics 5, 57–75

Bangladeshi students 88–90
Banks, James 24, 184
Barnes, R. 13
basketball 62, 68–69, 73, 181
Bell, Derrick: early work on CRT 12, 13, 116; *Faces at the bottom of the well* 13, 202; interest-convergence 5, 57–58, 69–71, 74, 81, 82, 166–167, 176; interest-divergence 82, 83; property rights 17; racial realism 155n5; storytelling 5, 23, 33
Benson, K. F. 72
bilingualism 123–124
Black narratives 33–34
Blackness 11, 126, 198
Black students: academic achievement 86–90, 97; access to curriculum 177; experiences in majority White schools 173–174; high-achieving 174; *see also* African American students

Black/White binary 46, 49, 117, 118
Bode, P. 175
Bonilla-Silva, E. 42–43, 46, 49, 175
Bourdieu, Pierre 4, 115, 121–122
Brown, John 13
Brown, K. 181–182
Brown, Michael 155
Brown vs. Board of Education 18, 19, 32, 57–58, 70–71, 74, 82, 144, 176

California 19, 29, 33, 35, 44, 47, 48, 125
Calmore, J. 47
Cameron, David 80, 85, 86
capitalism 5, 6, 17, 21, 43, 44–46, 48, 54, 81, 126, 129n8, 193
Carbado, D.W. 4, 6–7
Carter, D. J. 173–174
Carter, R. 147
Castagno, Angelina E. 5, 97
Caucus of Rank-and-File Educators (CORE) 169–170
Center for Constitutional Rights (CCR) 151
Center for Equal Opportunity 44
Center for Individual Rights 44
Césaire, Aimé 190
Chapman, Thandeka K. 5
charter schools 164, 167, 168–169, 176
Chicago Public Schools (CPS) 161–170
Chicago Teachers Union (CTU) 169–170
Chicanos/as: academic achievement 83, 97, 123; aspirations 123; Chicano/a Studies 118; cultural capital 121–122; effects of affirmative action on 29, 30, 32, 33; LatCrit 46, *116*, 117; *see also* Latinos/as
citizenship 16–19
civil rights 12–13, 42, 44
civil rights legislation: as focus of CRT research 41, 117; ineffectiveness of 17; school desegregation 19; Whites as primary beneficiaries of 14, 23
civil rights movement 49, 82, 194–196
civil unrest 80–81, 82, 90–91
class issues: CRT scholarship 3, 6, 12, 30, 44–46, 48, 50–51, 54, 65, 81, 119; deficit thinking 120; discrimination 45; hegemony 44–45; intersection with race 43, 45, 49, 54, 185; microaggressions based on class 138, 150
class society 44, 48
Clemson University 61
Clinton administration 12
Cohen, E. G. 24
Coleman, J. S. 23
collective identity 59, 103–105, 109, 126
Collegiate Commissioners Association (CCA) 66
Collins, Marva 21
colonialism 6, 43, 83, 190, 191–194, 198–199, 201
color-blindness: CRT research 36n6, 41, 64, 96, 118, 179; in education policy 48, 86, 178, 185; effect on curriculum 20, 175, 177, 181; experiences of students 35, 174, 183, 186; higher education admissions 29, 31, 32, 33; interest-convergence principle 70; post-racialism 172, 198; and race dialogue 189, 197, 200, 202–203; Supreme Court decisions on 154; White teachers 34–35, 178
communism 18, 70–71
community cultural wealth 114–129
community engagement 6, 42, 54, 151–152
community mobilization 50–54, 126, 165, 166, 169
conflict theory 61–62, 63
Connerly, Ward 44
Conservative/Liberal Democrat Coalition 85–87, 91
Conservative Party (UK) 85
conservativism 44, 45, 47
contract schools 164, 167, 168
Cooper, R. 174, 181
cooperative learning 24
counterstories and counternarratives: Bell's use of 5; in CRT methodology 5, 6, 41; definition 1; education reform 166, 168; social justice 50–51; *see also* storytelling
Creighton University 68–69
Crenshaw, Kimberlé: on the civil rights movement 13–14; on critical legal scholarship 12, 44; development of CRT 3–4, 116; intersectionality 1–2; on racial stereotypes 21
critical hope 162
Critical Legal Studies (CLS) 12–13, 44, 64, 116
Critical Race Praxis 42, 46, 49, 50–53, 169
Critical Race Theory (CRT): citizenship and 16–19; class analysis 3, 6, 12, 30, 44–46, 48, 50–51, 54, 65, 81, 119; common misinterpretations of 45–50; concepts and central tenets 1–4, 15, 29, 41, 46, 50, 53, 63–64, 96, 115–116, 118–119, 140–141, 174–175; critique of 2–3, 43–44; as framework for educational equity 24; future of 24, 35–36; genealogy of 5, 116, 118; gender and 6, 30, 64–65, 117, 119; origins 3–4, 9–10, 12–15, 63, 116–117
Critical Studies in Education Association (CRSEA) 6
cultural awareness 95, 97–98, 103, 109, 111
cultural capital 6, 115, 121–122, 126, 181
cultural difference 98–99, 104, 106, 108–109, 111, 120

cultural wealth 5, 114–127
curriculum: color-blindness and 30, 175; development 53, 120; effect of structural racism on 5; master scripting 20; as property 180–182, 186–187; race neutrality 20; restricted access to 20–21, 167, 174, 177; as tool for marginalization 177; tracking 180; White privilege and 177

Daley, Richard J. 162
Daley, Richard M. 163
Darder, A. 43–44, 45, 46, 50
Davis, Angela 193, 202
Davis, Timothy 69, 71–72
Deaf CRiT 6
decolonization 190–194, 198
deficit approach to minority education 21, 72, 120–121, 127
Delgado, Richard 12, 15, 33, 83
Delgado Bernal, Dolores 114, 126
Delpit, L. 16
democracy 11, 17, 24, 43, 71, 82, 85
desegregation 19, 23–24, 173, 174, 175, 179–180
Deyhle, D. 34
Diamond, J. B. 173, 174, 185
Disability Critical Race Theory (DisCrit) 2
discipline policies 182–183
discrimination: class 45; cumulative 32–33; employment 7, 29; racial 17, 31–35, 60, 70–71, 105, 109, 155; reverse 29–31, 37; school policies 30, 34
distributive justice 110–111
Di Toro, J. A. 33–34
diversity, in education 5, 29, 30–33, 35
Dixson, A. 42
Donnor, Jamel K. 5
Dred Scott vs Sandford 18, 74
DuBois, W. E. B. 115, 191, 192
Dudziak, Mary L. 71
Duke University 61
Dumas, M. 144
Duncan-Andrade, J. M. R 162, 169
Dyson, M. E. 72

economic capital 121–122
economic downturns 81, 83, 90
educational reform 86–91, 161–170, 184–185, 186
education policy 5, 47–48, 80–91, 161–170, 185–186
education: market-driven reforms 161–170; multicultural 24, 83, 97–98, 176, 184–185; public-private partnerships 161–170; relationship with colonialism 190–206; school desegregation 19, 23–24, 179–180; social justice in 40–54; *see also* higher education; schools
Edwards, Harry 58, 63
elites, White 2, 45, 81–82, 83
employment discrimination 7, 29
empowerment: community empowerment 6; in education 29; and race theory 29; relation to law 18
England 80–81
English Baccalaureate (E.Bacc.) 87–90, 91
English Defence League (EDL) 85
epistemology 30, 65, 102, 114–115
equal opportunity 19–20, 60, 118
Escalante, Jaime 21
ethnic studies programmes 83
ethnographic studies 96–98, 125, 126
Evers, Medgar 32

Fabricant, M. 162
Faces at the bottom of the well (Bell) 13, 202
faculty, hiring of 31, 33
family/familial capital 23, 43, 104, 115, 119, 121, 122, 124–125
Fanon, Frantz 189–202
Faulstich Orellana, Marjorie 121, 123, 124
Feagin, J. R. 32
FemCrit *116*, 117
feminism 29, 30, 44, 46, 48, 64, 97, 117, 118
Fine, M. 162
First Nation 97, 101, 107; *see also* American Indians; Indigenous students; Native Americans
Floyd et al v. City of New York 145, 147–153, 154, 155
Foley, Douglas 121
football 57–75, 181
foreign policy 70–71
Foster, M. 34
Foucault, Michel 4, 196
Fourteenth Amendment 70, 73
Franklin, V. P. 126
Freeman, Alan 12, 116
Freire, Paulo 120, 126, 154, 179, 199, 201, 204n2

Gándara, Patricia 123
Gandhi, Mohandas Karamchand 194, 195
García, Shernaz 120
Gay, Geneva 24
gender: and CRT 6, 30, 64–65, 117, 119; deficit thinking 120; intersection with race 6, 117, 138, 142, 166, 185; microaggressions based on 138, 147, 150, 156n10, 156n11; students of color 121
General Certificate of Secondary Education (GCSE) 87–90
Gillborn, David 4, 5

Gordon, Lewis 190, 195, 198
Goss vs Lopez 73
graduation rates 58, 61, 75n5, 76n7, 97
Gramsci, Antonio 12, 107, 193, 196
Grant, Carl 24, 184
Greene, Maxine 40–41
Guerra, Patricia 120
Guinier, Lani 12, 24, 82–83

Hacker, Andrew 17
Hall vs. University of Minnesota 73
Haney López, I. 10–11
harassment 35, 83
Harrell, Shelley 156n9
Harris, Cheryl 17, 21, 46, 95, 96, 101, 102, 105, 107, 110–111
Harris, O. 61
Harrison, C. K. 64
Harvard University 137
Hayes-Tilden compromise 74
Hayman, R. 46
Hegel, Georg Wilhelm Friedrich 198
hegemony: class 44–45; Gramscian notion of 12, 107, 193; racial 13, 15, 21, 43, 199; in schools 185
Henfield, M. S. 174
hierarchies 43, 83, 101, 115, 185
higher education: admissions 20, 29, 30–33; diversity claims 5; experiences of African American student athletes 57–75; graduation rates of African American students 58, 61; navigational capital 125; revenue generation 60–61; voice of teachers of color 16; *see also individual institutions*
high school: academic achievement 58, 172–186; admissions 50–52; experiences of students of color in majority White schools 172–186; race neutrality 35; racism in 5, 95–111, 183–184, 186; school funding 22–23, 47–48, 50–52, 109–110, 126, 177; teachers' attitudes to race 95–111
Hirsch, E. D. Jr. 127
homophobia 28, 35, 36
hooks, bell 189
Hoover Institute 44
Hopwood v. Texas 29, 30–33, 34–35
housing 162, 163, 164–165, 166, 167–168, 177
Huidor, O. 174, 181
hunger strikes 52–53

identity 48, 62, 69, 96, 121; *see also* racial identity
immigration status 29, 35, 83, 117, 118, 121, 138, 150
Indian students 88–89, 91n4
Indigenous students 17, 20, 25n4; *see also* American Indians; First Nation; Native Americans
individualism 44, 95, 98–109
Initiative 200 (Washington) 44
institutional racism: color-blindness and 174, 175; cumulative discrimination 32–33; limitations of legal scholarship 116; microaggressions as evidence of 138, 141–147, *149*, 152; qualitative research into 34; school funding as example of 22; teachers' awareness of 101, 105, 107; White privilege and 96; White supremacy as foundation for 141–142; *see also* racism; structural racism
instruction 19–24, 185
intelligence testing 21
interest-convergence 5, 14, 57–59, 69–75, 81–82, 90, 119, 166–167, 175, 176–177, 179, 180
interest-divergence 80, 82–85, 90–91
intersectionality 1–2, 6, 117–118, 140, 150, 185

Jencks, C. 23
Jervis, K. 36
Jim Crow era 31, 32, 36n7, 47, 145–147, 156n12, 175
Journal of African American History 126

Kang, E. 175
King, Martin Luther, Jr. 20, 194–195, 196; Martin Luther King Jr. Holiday 14
kinship 124
knowledge: cultural wealth 5, 114–127; experiential knowledge 1, 13, 15, 46–47, 49, 64, 118–119, 140, 166; 'Outsider' knowledge 115, 116
Kozol, Jonathan 20–21, 22

labor unions 169–170
Labour Party (UK) 86
Ladson-Billings, Gloria: on CRT in education 2, 29; CRT origins and central tenets 9–10, 12–15, 28, 41, 50, 53, 64–65, 128n2; curriculum as property 181–182; on knowledge 114; on obstacles to progress under Obama presidency 4
language: bilingualism 123–124; discrimination based on 138; linguistic capital 123–124; linguistic racism 190; of race 11, 43, 44; as racism 29
LatCrit 46, *116*, 117
Latinos/as: academic achievement 50, 83; cultural knowledge 121; effects of education reform on 165, 166, 167–168, 169; experiences in majority White

schools 178–186; experiences of racial microaggressions 147–148, 152–153; Raza Studies 83, 170; resistant capital 126; segregation 50; selective enrollment 51–52; under-resourced schools 48, 50–52; *see also* Chicanos/as
law enforcement 7, 47, 81, 145, 147–148, 151–153, 154, 155
Lawrence, C. 15, 107
LeCompte, M. D. 179
Lee, Sharon 10
legal literature 9–19, 46, 57–75
legal storytelling 15
Leonardo, Zeus 5, 54
liberalism 13–14, 41, 44, 69, 107, 193, 198
linguistic capital 123–124
Lipman, Pauline 35, 85, 162, 164
Lomotey, K. 23
Lopez, G. R. 186
Lopez, I. H. 176
Lorde, Audre 21
Lynn, M. 65

Mail on Sunday 90–91
Malia Lawrence, S. 64
malpractice 68–69
Marable, Manning 21, 117, 143
marginalization 1, 7, 15, 16, 20, 29, 30, 35, 41, 54, 63, 65, 114, 115, 119, 122, 146, 162, 167, 169
market-based education reform 161–170
Martinez, George 83–84
Martin Luther King High School (MLKHS) 99–100, 109
Marxism/Marxist theory 2, 4, 44, 48, 64
master scripting 20
Matsuda, Mari 15, 116
McIntosh, P. 18, 99
McLaren P. 184
media 90–91, 148
meritocracy 2, 13, 35, 44, 104, 118
mestiza knowledge 115, 122
Mexican Americans: in census data 10–11; community engagement 51–53; funds of knowledge 124; navigational capital 125; relations with African-American community 51; social capital 125
Mexico 196
microaggressions 6, 137–155, 201
Milliken v. Bradley 176
Mills, Charles 48, 81, 196–197
Missouri 155
Moore, J. L. 174
Moraga, Cherrie 118
Moreno, Melissa 126
Morris, Jerome 126–127
Morrison, Toni 11
multicultural education 24, 83, 97–98, 176, 184–185
multiculturalism 41, 84, 91, 99
Music Television Network (MTV) 137–138

NAACP *see* National Association for the Advancement of Colored People
naming one's own reality 15–16
narratives 33–34, 41, 48, 65, 106
National Association for the Advancement of Colored People (NAACP) 18, 70, 144
National Association of Colored Women's Clubs 125
National Basketball Association 14
National Collegiate Athletic Association (NCAA) 58, 62, 66, 73
National Football League (NFL) 14, 58
National Letter of Intent (NLI) 66
Native Americans 20, 34, 117, 178–186; *see also* American Indians; First Nation; Indigenous students
navigational capital 125
neoliberalism 69, 81, 161, 162–163, 165, 166, 169, 170
New York Police Department (NYPD) 145, 147–148, 151–153, 154
New York Times 148
Nieto, S. 175, 184–185
No Child Left Behind (NCLB) 47–48, 166, 177
North Carolina 145

Obama, Barak 4, 172
O'Connor, C. 173
Ohio State University 61
Oliver, Melvin 122
Omi, M. 11, 203
oppression: CRT as means to eliminate 64; forms of 1, 46, 117–119; racialized 1, 4–5, 13, 16, 21; state of nature theory 83–84; storytelling 13, 15, 16; structural 126
Osamu, Nishitani 199
'Other' 13, 25n2, 63, 64, 104, 198
'Outsider' knowledge 115, 116

Pacific Islanders 5, 103, 117
Pakistani students 88–89, 91n4
Palmer, D. 177
Parham, W. D. 62
Parker, Laurence 3, 5, 65
Parks, Rosa 20
patriarchy 29, 44, 48, 126
pedagogy 36n4, 118, 120, 127, 154, 175, 185, 189–190, 197, 198–204
Pedroni, T. 167
Pennsylvania State University 72
people of color: experiences of racial aggressions 137–155, 200–201;

marginalization of 7, 15, 16, 20, 29, 30, 41, 54, 63, 65, 83, 115, 119, 146, 162; voice 1, 15–16, 20, 22, 33–34, 41, 53, 115, 120, 170, 174, 203; *see also* students of color
Pérez Huber, Lindsay 5, 156n10
Pierce, Chester 138, 139–140, 141, 144, 150, 151, 153, 154, 155n4
Plan for Transformation (Chicago) 164, 165–166, 167, 168
Plessy v. Ferguson 18, 156n14
policing 7, 81, 145, 147–148, 151–153, 154, 155
political mobilization 82
political protest 80–81, 82, 90–91, 156n15
politics of desperation 161, 167–169
Porter, Ronald K. 5
post-racialism 172, 197–198, 202–203
poverty 119, 182
power: access to 121; misuse of by researchers 34; racial 4, 14, 49, 64, 69, 81, 99–103, 105–106, 108–111, 119, 189–190, 196, 198, 203; resistance as 196; structures 44, 45; White people 4, 81, 82, 84, 90–91
praxis 6, 40–43, 46, 49–54, 169–170, 185
privilege *see* White privilege
professional development 95–111
property: and citizenship 17; impact on school funding 22; intersection with race 73–74; student athletes as 73–74; *see also* Whiteness as property
Propositions: Proposition 187 (California) 35; Proposition 203 (Arizona) 44; Proposition 209 (California) 29, 33, 44
public policy 29, 44, 47; *see also* education policy

qualitative research methods 5, 33–35, 65, 179
Quebec 170

race: distinction between race and racism 43; diversity in higher education admissions 29, 30–33; as ideological concept 11; interaction with citizenship 16–19; intersection with class 43–49, 50–51, 54, 185; intersection with gender 6, 117, 138, 142, 166, 185; marginalization of 10, 11, 45; and neoliberal education policies 161–170; safety discourses 189–204; as social construct 3, 6, 10, 43–44, 64, 119
race inequity: CRT approach to 3–4, 64; in schools 86–91, 95–111; White power and 81–82
race neutrality: CRT research 41, 96, 118; curriculum 20; in higher education 29, 30–33, 34; instruction 21
racial bias 1, 31, 95, 97–100, 103–104, 137
racial classification 10–11
racial hegemony 13, 15
racial identity: in census data 10–11; color-blindness as disregarding 175; students of color in majority White schools 173–174, 184
racial inequality: in Bourdieu 121; constitutionalization of 7; counterstories as examples of 1; experiences of students of color in majority White schools 172–186
racial (in)justice 15, 39n4, 60, 70, 81, 82, 84, 126–127, 166
racialized social systems 42–43, 49, 54
racial profiling 145, 147–148, 152–153, 156n11
racial realism 3, 155n5, 176, 179
racism: categories of 46; critical theory of 43; CRT analysis of 2–3, 36–37, 41, 43, 45, 69, 96, 101, 118–119; in higher education admissions 31–32; impact on school funding policies 22; intellectualization of 198–202; judicial relief for 70; microaggressions as evidence of 137–155; narratives 15; normalized 13, 83; psychological and physiological effects of 146, 150–151; in schools 5, 95–111, 183–184, 186; social psychology of 5; state-sanctioned 5; systemic 22, 47, 54, 64, 96, 99, 101, 104–106, 138, 141–143, 146, 154; teachers' awareness of 95–111; towards Black student athletes 58; *see also* institutional racism; structural racism
Raible, J. 175
Raza Studies 83, 170
Regents of the University of Minnesota vs National Collegiate Athletic Association 73
Renaissance 2010 164, 165–167
resilience 122, 125
resistant capital 125–126
Rice University 61
Robeson, Paul 18–19
Roediger, D. 11
Ross vs Creighton University 68–69, 72
Rousseau, C. K. 42
ruling class 45–46, 54

safety, discourse on 189–204
Saltman, K. J. 162
Samoan students 97
Sartre, Jean-Paul 193, 199, 204n3
SAT (Scholastic Aptitude Test) 61, 97
Savage inequalities (Kozol) 22
scholarships 58, 66–69, 124
schools: desegregation 19, 23–24, 173, 174, 175, 179–180; discipline 182–183;

funding 22–23, 47–48, 50–52, 109–110, 126, 177; governance 109; inequity in 22–24, 95–111; performance 47–48, 168; policies 34, 182–183; racism in 5, 95–111, 183–184, 186; restructuring 35; urban areas 47–48, 50–54, 161–170, 176; White supremacy 5
segregation 31–32, 50, 57, 70–71, 82, 145–147, 178
selective enrollment 51–52, 168
self-awareness 107–110
self-determination 36
sexism 29, 35, 36, 119, 151
sexual orientation 30, 121, 138, 150, 156n10, 185
Shapiro, Thomas 122
Shelby County v. Holder 156n14
Shuette v. BAMN 154–155
Símon, Laura 35
Simpson, O. J. 13
slavery 31, 72, 74, 98–99, 125, 182, 190, 201
Sleeter, C. E. 184
Smith, W. 145, 153
social activism 42
social capital 121, 124–125, 181
social class *see* class issues
social hierarchy 43
social justice 11, 35, 40–54, 65, 118–119, 126–127, 141, 184–185
social mobility 121
social networks 121, 125
social psychology 5, 62–63
social reality 15, 63
social transformation 13–14
socioeconomic status 42, 63, 64, 180
Solorzano, Daniel G. 5, 6, 41, 118, 126, 128n3, 140, 156n10
South Africa 12, 196
sport 5, 57–75, 181
Stanfield, J. H. 34
Stanford University 61
stereotypes: internalization of 16; racial 21, 31, 32, 47, 58, 87–88, 99, 104, 173, 183–184
storytelling: aspirations 122; examples of 10, 27–28, 50–52; as linguistic capital 123–124; racially marginalized students 33; use in CRT scholarship 13, 15–16, 119; use of legal literature to substantiate 74; *see also* counterstories and counternarratives
Stovall, David 6
structural racism: as common framework for stories 15; definition 143; navigation through 125; professional development as means to address 95–111; race neutrality and 35; school funding as example of 22, 109–110; teachers' awareness of 99–105, 108–109; use of CRT in the study of 5; *see also* institutional racism; racism
structural transformation 108, 110–111
student advocacy 6
students of color: achievement gap 177–186; high-achieving 180; impact of racism on relations with teachers 5; in majority White suburban schools 172–186; safe spaces 197–199; *see also* African American students; Asian students; Black students
subordination 21, 29, 42, 44, 116, 117–119, 125, 126, 143
suburban schools 5, 22, 176–186
Sue, Derald Wing 141, 156n10
Supreme Court (US) 7, 82, 154; *see also specific cases*
Swartz, E. 20
Sweatt v. Painter 32

Tate, William 28, 64–65, 128n2
taxes 22, 29, 45, 164, 176, 177
Taylor vs. Wake Forest University 67–68, 72
teacher education 16, 95–111
teachers: attitudes to race 95–111; awareness of racism 95–111; color-blindness 34–35; cultural awareness 95, 97–98, 103; expectations of Black students 87; impact of racism on relations with students 5; racial bias 95, 97–100, 103–104; racialized responses to anti-racist training 95–111; strikes 169–170
Teranishi, R. T. 178
terrorism 7, 85
Torres, R. D. 43–44, 45, 46, 50
TribalCrit *116*, 117
Tribal Nation/Indigenous Studies 5
Trump administration 7

unemployment 84, 91
United Kingdom: Academy schools 86–87; criticism of CRT scholarship 2; education reform 80–91; effect of recession on racial and ethnic minorities 4, 80–91
United States: Black unemployment 84; class structure 12; community cultural wealth 114–129; education reform 161–170; majority White suburban schools 172–186; racial microaggressions 137–155; student athletes 57–75; structural racism 95–111; Supreme Court 7, 82, 154
universities *see* higher education
University of Alabama 32
University of Arizona-Tucson 61
University of California, Los Angeles (UCLA) 61
University of California-Berkeley 33
University of Colorado-Boulder 61

University of Florida-Gainesville 61
University of Michigan-Ann Arbor 61
University of Minnesota-Twin Cities 62, 73
University of Mississippi 32
University of Southern California 62
University of Texas-Austin 29, 30–33
urban schools 47–48, 50–54, 161–170, 176
Utah 34

vandalism 106
Vaught, Sabina E. 5, 96
Villenas, Sofia 126
violence 80, 190–204
voice of people of color 1, 15–16, 20, 22, 33–34, 41, 53, 115, 120, 170, 174, 203
voting rights 7, 156n14

Wake Forest University 67–68
Wallerstein, I. 191
Ware, L. 31
Warmington, P. 2–3, 4
Washington 44
Watkins, William 43
Weber, Max 196
West, Cornel 13
WhiteCrit *116*, 117
Whiteness: conceptual categories 11; CRT as framework for studying 35; deconstructing 11; Fanonian theory 198, 199; normative standards of 29; social value of 17, 83
Whiteness as property 17–18, 46, 95–96, 98, 101–108, 109, 110–111
White privilege 18, 36n4, 46, 48–49, 82, 95–96, 98–103, 105, 107–111, 117–119, 121, 175–176, 177, 179, 182, 190
Whites: as beneficiaries of affirmative action 14; as beneficiaries of color-blindness 70; effect of racial pedagogy on 189; middle and upper-class 60, 70, 115, 121–122, 127; as power-holders 4, 81, 82, 84, 90–91; as primary beneficiaries of civil rights legislation 14; working-class 21, 83, 85
White students: academic achievement 87, 88–90, 97, 177; curriculum as property 180–181, 185–186; selective enrollment 51
White supremacy: color-blindness as maintaining 175; counter-hegemonic challenge to 195; CRT analysis of 41, 44, 45, 49, 54, 81, 84; definition 42; as foundation for racial microaggressions 138–139, 141–142, 144, 145, 147, 153–154; impact on education 5, 48, 107, 110, 166; institutionalized 107, 138, 141; and interest-divergence 82; as structural phenomenon 42; in suburban schools 5; systemic 2, 7
Williams, Gregory 13
Williams, Patricia 14, 15, 18, 33–34
Winant, H. 11, 59, 203
women 14, 17, 25n2, 31, 33–34, 37n8, 48, 117, 125, 126, 168
Women's Studies 5, 116, 119
Wood, C. 174
workers' movement 49
World War II 18–19, 71
Wretched of the earth, The (Fanon) 190, 192, 197, 204n3
Wynter, S. 24

Yamamoto, Eric 40, 42, 50, 169
Yosso, Tara J. 5, 41

Žižek, S. 190